Family Theory Development in Nursing:
State of the Science and Art

Family Theory Development in Nursing:
State of the Science and Art

Ann L. Whall, PhD, FAAN
Professor
University of Michigan School of Nursing

Jacqueline Fawcett, PhD, FAAN
Professor
University of Pennsylvania School of Nursing

 F.A. DAVIS COMPANY • Philadelphia

PREFACE

Family scientists and clinicians of many disciplines have devoted much time and effort to develop a theoretical base which enhances understanding of that basic unit of society, the family. Nurses have always been interested in families and have continuously been on the cutting edge of family-centered practice. In recent years, nurse scholars extended the theoretical work done in other disciplines and developed conceptualizations of family phenomena consistent with nursing's disciplinary perspective.

The two goals of this book are to describe existing work done by family nurse scientists and to identify the potential of that work for development of formal middle-range family nursing theories. Family theory, as used throughout the book, refers to a set of relatively specific and concrete concepts and propositions that describe, explain, or predict something about the family. The focus is, therefore, on middle-range family theories, rather than more abstract formulations such as conceptual models and grand theories or even more concrete partial theories. The contributions of conceptual models of nursing to theory development are, however, explained.

In preparing the book, we worked from a relatively broad and contemporary view of the family. We regarded the family as a self-identified group of two or more individuals whose association is characterized by special terms, who may or may not be related by bloodlines or law, but who function in such a way that they consider themselves to be a family. Our ideas have been shaped by literature focusing on individuals within the context of their families, such as parents and children, as well as the literature reflecting a focus on the family as a single entity or unit of analysis.

The book is organized in two main sections. Part I includes five original chapters dealing with critical issues underlying development of family theory within the discipline of nursing, ranging from a historical analysis of nursing's interest in the family to empirical measurement of family phenomena in nursing research. Chapter 1 presents a review of the nursing literature dealing with the family from the birth of modern nursing in the mid-1800s to the present time. Chapter 2 offers an analysis of the concept family and provides a clear and precise definition of the family. Chapter 3 outlines various philosophies of science and their implications for family theory development in nursing. Chapter 4 is an extension of previously published work on the major conceptual and methodological issues surrounding research of families. Chapter 5 builds on the content of Chapter 4 by identifying the advantages and disadvantages of different approaches to the measurement of family phenomena.

Part II of the book contains reprints of publications by family nurse scholars that reflect various aspects of family nursing theory development. An effort was made to classify the papers so as to further describe the existing knowledge base in family nursing. We hope that the classification will lead to further work in each category as well as identification of new categories.

Each reprinted paper in Part II is accompanied by a brief commentary that focuses on contributions to middle-range family theory development and serves as a link between Part I and Part II of the book. Taken together, the contents of Parts I and II should facilitate the reader's understanding of the current state of family nursing science and the challenge of advancing the art of formal family theory development in nursing.

ACKNOWLEDGMENTS

We express our gratitude to the many nurse scholars whose original work made this book possible. We also are grateful to the publishers who gave permission to reprint important papers. We acknowledge the special and continuing contributions our students have made to our thinking about nursing theory development. We also acknowledge the encouragement we have always received from our families to go on with our work despite the disruptions and inconveniences created in their lives. And we acknowledge the support and patience of Senior Editor Robert G. Martone as well as the invaluable editorial assistance of Ruth De George, Executive Secretary of the F.A. Davis Company. Finally, we acknowledge the people who contributed to the production of this book.

CONTRIBUTORS

Nancy Trygar Artinian, PhD, RN
Assistant Professor
Wayne State University College of Nursing
Detroit, Michigan

Suzanne L. Feetham, PhD, FAAN
Special Expert
National Center for Nursing Research
National Institutes of Health
Bethesda, Maryland

and

Senior Fellow
University of Pennsylvania
School of Nursing
Philadelphia, Pennsylvania

Meryn E. Stuart, PhD, RN
Assistant Professor
School of Nursing

and

Adjunct Hannah Professor in the
History of Medicine and Health Care
Faculty of Health Sciences
University of Ottawa
Ottawa, Ontario
Canada

Jacqueline Sullivan, MSN, RN, CCRN, CNRN
Clinical Nurse Specialist and Clinical Assistant Professor
Thomas Jefferson University
Philadelphia, Pennsylvania

and

Doctoral Candidate
University of Pennsylvania
School of Nursing
Philadelphia, Pennsylvania

CONTENTS

PART

I

MAJOR ISSUES IN FAMILY NURSING THEORY DEVELOPMENT

INTRODUCTION

The phenomena of interest to any discipline are identified in the meta-paradigm concepts and propositions of that discipline. The phenomena of interest to the discipline of nursing are capsulized in the metapara-digm concepts person, environment, health, and nursing. These concepts are linked and given a distinctive nursing context in three propositions:

1. Nursing is concerned with the principles and laws that govern the life-process, well-being, and optimum function of human beings, sick or well
2. Nursing is concerned with the patterning of human behavior in interaction with the environment in normal life events and critical life situations
3. Nursing is concerned with the processes by which positive changes in health status are effected (Donaldson and Crowley, 1978; Gortner, 1980).

The "person" of nursing's metaparadigm, albeit implicit, is the individual. Thus, the family must be seen as either a group of separate individuals identified by position and relationship terms, such as parent and child, or as the environment for an individual (Friedemann, 1989; Murphy, 1986). The nursing literature reviewed in Chapter 1 revealed that individual family members have been a concern of nursing since Nightingale's time. But a growing body of literature, also reviewed in Chapter 1, reflects nursing's concern with the family as a whole, using terminology such as the *family unit* or the *family system* (Friedemann, 1989). This literature provides the rationale for modification of nursing's metaparadigm to account for family phenomena and to place family theory development within a nursing perspective. The concepts become family, family environment, family health, and nursing within the context of the family. The propositions then may be modified as follows:

1. Family is concerned with the principles and laws that govern family process, family well-being, and optimum function of families in various states of illness and wellness
2. Family is concerned with the patterning of family behavior in interaction with the environment in normal life events and critical life situations
3. Family is concerned with the processes by which positive

changes in family health status may be effected (Whall, 1984).

The modification of nursing's metaparadigm underscores the centrality of the family unit to nurses. Iveson-Iveson's (1982) comments highlight the importance of family theory development in nursing. She stated:

> Nurses are part of families, whether large or small. They work in a profession that has as its aim the common good of [human] kind, so to them understanding the meaning and value of kinship is essential (p. 19).

The modified metaparadigm of nursing articulates a perspective of the family different from that of other disciplines interested in family theory development, such as sociology and psychology. First, the focus on the family in nursing is distinguished from that of other disciplines by consideration of environmental influences on family health and the effect of actions taken by nurses on behalf of or in conjunction with the family. Second, the family focus in nursing is distinguished from that of other disciplines by a comprehensive biopsychosocial or holistic perspective of health. And third, there is considerable concern in nursing for family well-being rather than pathology, which frequently is the focus of other disciplines (Friedemann, 1989).

Metaparadigms provide direction for knowledge development by identifying phenomena of interest to each discipline and articulating the particular perspective from which the phenomena will be viewed. The knowledge of each discipline is then codified in its conceptual models and the theories that are derived from the more abstract models.

Conceptual models are abstract and general approaches to the study of the phenomena identified by the metaparadigm. Thus, the conceptual models of nursing present diverse approaches to the study of the person, environment, health, and nursing. In Chapter 1, an explanation is given of how several conceptual models of nursing have been extended to account for family phenomena.

Theories are statements that purport to account for or characterize some phenomenon (Stevens, 1984). According to Merton (1957), the most useful theories are of the middle range, which lie between partial theories made up of minor working hypotheses and all-inclusive grand or unifying theories. A middle-range theory, then, is a set of relatively specific and concrete concepts and propositions that describe, explain, or predict something about a phenomenon. For the purposes of this book, the phenomenon of interest is, of course, the family. References to family theory in Part I of this book are references to middle-range theories, rather than to more abstract grand theories or even more concrete partial theories.

Middle-range theories are characterized by explicit theoretical or constitutive definitions of concepts. Chapter 2 presents a clear definition of the concept family. This definition represents the critical starting point for development of middle-range theories about the family.

Middle-range theories are developed by means of empirical research, the components of which include instruments, procedures, and data analysis. Chapter 3 offers a review of different philosophies of science that undergird empirical research and their implications for development of middle-range family nursing theories. Chapter 4 extends previously published work on the conceptual and methodological issues underlying research designed to generate and to test family nursing theories. In this chapter, the terms *family-related research* and *family research* are introduced. This distinction in research of families does not imply a value judgment with regard to one category over another. Rather, the two categories are introduced as a means of clarifying the unit of analysis in research of families. Finally, Chapter 5 contributes a discussion of the advantages and disadvantages of different types of data about the family.

Throughout Part I, reference is made to formal theory development. A formal theory is an explicit set of concepts and propositions that is labeled with a particular name. The propositions of a formal theory may be presented concisely and precisely as equations or diagrams (Burr, Hill, Nye, and Reiss, 1979). For example, *quantum theory* is the label given to a set of concepts and propositions about the physical world. A well-known proposition of quantum theory is the relationship between the concepts energy (E), mass (m), and the speed of light (c). Written as an equation, the proposition is $E = mc^2$. Another example is *social support theory*, which is the label given to a set of concepts and propositions about the positive affect, affirmation, and aid available to people. A proposition of this theory states that support from others influences the relationship between life-change events and health status. This relationship may be diagramed as follows:

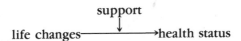

The contents of Part I reveal little evidence of formal family theory in nursing. The state of family theory development in nursing mirrors the state of all theory development in nursing and most other disciplines. Although the current state of theory development is of concern, the editors of this volume agree completely with Burr, Hill, Nye, and Reiss (1979) that "the process of theory construction is a long-term activity that is still in its early stages with respect to family phenomena, and they want to do what they can to motivate others to become involved in the process of further improving these theories" (p. 14). It is the editors' hope, then, that the five chapters of Part I of this book will help readers understand where nursing has been and where nurse scholars need to go to advance the specialty of family nursing through enhanced formal theory development.

REFERENCES

Burr, W. R., Hill, R., Nye, F. I., & Reiss, I. R. (Eds.). (1979). *Contemporary theories about the family* (Vol. 1). New York: The Free Press.

Donaldson, S. K., & Crowley, D. M. (1978). The discipline of nursing. *Nursing Outlook, 26,* 113–120.

Friedemann, M. L. (1989). The concept of family nursing. *Journal of Advanced Nursing, 14,* 211–216.

Gortner, S. R. (1980). Nursing science in transition. *Nursing Research, 29,* 80–183.

Iveson-Iveson, J. (1982). Time to celebrate the family. *Nursing Mirror,* 155(24), 18–19.

Merton, R. K. (1975). *Social theory and social structure* (rev. ed.). New York: The Free Press.

Murphy, S. (1986). Family study and nursing research. *Image: Journal of Nursing Scholarship, 18,* 170–174.

Stevens, B. J. (1984). *Nursing theory. Analysis, application, evaluation* (2nd ed.). Boston: Little, Brown.

Whall, A. L. (1984, November). *The relationship of theory to family research.* Paper presented at First Wingspread Conference: Advancing Family Research in Nursing, Racine, WI.

CHAPTER

1

The Family as a Focal Phenomenon in Nursing[1]

ANN L. WHALL, Ph.D., F.A.A.N.
JACQUELINE FAWCETT, Ph.D., F.A.A.N.

This chapter presents an analysis of the contributions to middle-range family theory development made by nurses since the beginning of modern nursing in the mid-1800s. The chapter begins with a historical overview of interest in the family reflected in the nursing literature, commencing with Nightingale's work, and continuing until the present time. Next, a review of the attention given in standards of nursing practice to family phenomena is presented. Then, the influence of conceptual models of nursing on family theory development is discussed. The chapter concludes with recommendations for future work that is directed toward formalization of existing knowledge about the family into explicit middle-range theories.

HISTORICAL OVERVIEW OF INTEREST IN FAMILY NURSING

A review of the nursing literature was undertaken to identify instances in which the family or family unit was discussed as a focus of nursing care. More specifically, published works were reviewed for references in ei-

---

[1]This chapter is an expanded version of Whall, A. L. (1986). The family as the unit of care in nursing: A historical review. *Public Health Nursing*, 3, 240–249.

ther title or text for the term *family* or *family unit*, as well as for position or relationship terms, such as *mother, father,* and *child.* The review started with the works of Nightingale and two of her early biographers. After the time of Nightingale, the nursing literature was grouped into 20-year time periods from 1890 to 1950 and then the 40-year period of 1950 to 1990. The literature search strategy involved hand searches of all volumes of the *Nursing Studies Index* and the *Cumulative Index to Nursing and Allied Health Literature.* Subject terms used were *family* and family relational terms, such as *mother, father,* and *child. Citations* with titles that appeared relevant were selected for review. In addition, the stacks of the historical nursing collection at the Wayne State University library were searched for relevant textbooks in various clinical specialties.

Nightingale and the Family

Florence Nightingale's (1863) concern with the family was underscored by her emphasis on the need to improve hospital accommodations for the sick wives and children of soldiers and for a separate delivery room. Her concern was further noted in a letter addressed to a friend to whom she referred a soldier's widow so that the widow might receive some dark clothing as a sign of her mourning (Nightingale, 1855). Moreover, she discussed the privacy and financial needs of families when they joined the soldiers at military camp (Nightingale, 1858). And she graphically depicted the treatment of the women and children in military camps and offered detailed directions to the army for improvement of these conditions (Nightingale, 1858).

Biographers of Nightingale also have noted her concern with the family. Tooley (1905) stated, "Miss Nightingale found the wives of soldiers, respectable women, without decent clothing, living in three or four rooms of the damp basement of a hospital. There by light of rush-light, measures were taken, the sick attended, and their babies born and nourished" (p. 153). Tooley explained that 22 babies were born to these women. In winter, due to a broken drain in the basement, a fever epidemic broke out. "Miss Nightingale procured a house, had it cleaned and furnished; she organized a plan to give employment to soldiers' wives . . . she started a school for the children and got a chaplain to visit them and help them" (Tooley, 1905, p. 153). Tooley noted that Nightingale later wrote that as improvements suggested by the Crimean War were made, care should be taken that the wives and children of soldiers not be forgotten.

Cook's (1913) biography points to Nightingale's interest in district nursing and its involvement with families. She claimed that Nightingale "was . . . possessed by the idea of the district nurse as a health missioner [who would] introduce to village mothers particular knowledge [such as] sanitation and skillful hands" (Cook, 1913, p. 383).

Analysis of Nightingale's original works, as well as those of her biographers, indicates that she recognized family members, including husbands, wives, and children. She explicitly mentioned needs of both mothers and infants and frequently used the family position or relationship terms *wife* and *child*. The family position terms *husband* and *father* were implicit as Nightingale wrote of soldiers and their family members. Furthermore, Cook (1925) suggested that Nightingale would have developed her ideas about family nursing more fully and explicitly had she had the opportunity to continue her work. Cook explained, "The movement for district nursing was always dear to Miss Nightingale's heart. [She regretted] that once district nursing came, it was too late [in her career] for her to help" develop the branch of nursing that at the time dealt primarily with families (p. 340).

It is clear, then, that family phenomena were of interest from the beginning of modern nursing. Although formal middle-range family theory development efforts were not undertaken by Nightingale, she sensitized nurses to the view that family members were an important focus for nursing care. Furthermore, although the "myriad empirical observations recounted in her writings never developed into a coherent [family] theory of nursing, . . . its potential still exists" (Donnelly, 1986, p. 2).

1890 to 1910

The literature of the period 1890 to 1910 reflected continued concern for the family. In *Trained Nurse*, Brooks (1890) pointed out that nurses who cared for the insane in their homes would relieve the families. Furthermore, Stewart (1908) told of a nurse who took care of three children with diphtheria and two who were not yet stricken. She noted that in one family the parents were so frightened by the children's illness that it took them almost two hours to decide what was best to do. After seeing the older boy successfully treated, the parents agreed that the nurse should treat the baby to prevent diphtheria.

Wald (1904) set forth general principles of home nursing, including advice about how to approach the family. She maintained that before removing "children lying upon the bed of the sick mother [and] washing their faces, [the nurse should first] establish herself" (p. 430). Wald recommended evaluation of whether a family could care for an invalid without becoming demoralized and discussed the relationship of the family with their neighbors and service agencies. She also presented several case studies in which the nurse assessed the ability of the family to care for the ill member and taught a family member to give care and/or put the family in touch with community agencies.

Analysis of the nursing literature of this period yielded no evidence of development of formal middle-range family theory. There was, however, a definite emphasis on the beneficial effects of nursing care provided to families in their own homes.

1910 to 1930

The literature of the period 1910 to 1930 continued the emphasis on nursing care of families in their own homes. Beard (1915), for example, noted that the ideal of bringing nursing to every home was "an idea that is little more than thirty years old" (p. 47). She had read a report of a home nursing visit conducted in 1890 in which the child had "double pneumonia" and the nurse gave instructions "to the mother about medication and nourishment" (p. 47). Beard quoted Nightingale (n.d.) as stating that success in nursing is "to keep whole families out of pauperism [by] nursing the breadwinner back to health."

By 1917, Beard had extended her discussion and stated that the public health nurse must have as "her conviction, that upon her observation and foresight depends the health of [the] whole family" (p. 247). She went on to claim that the family "as a unit more than any other individual member of it must be her thought . . . the correction of defects may be the pivot upon which family health turns" (p. 247). Beard included descriptions of several cases in which the family was approached as a unit by the public health nurse.

During this period, nursing care of families began to be recognized as a topic to be included in the nursing curriculum. This emphasis is evident in the 1917 *Standard Curriculum for Schools of Nursing*, which was prepared by the Committee on Education of the National League for Nursing Education (NLNE). In the outline of subject matter, the committee stated that students were to receive instruction in "Household Science," which pertained to "housekeeping problems of an industrial family." The overall objective of this course was to prepare "pupils who intend to go into families either as a public health or as a private duty nurse" (p. 62). The most satisfactory teaching method was to "have the pupil study individual families" (p. 62).

Laird (1923) was primarily concerned with the control of communicable disease when she maintained that "any plan of health education which does not include the whole family is not adequate" (p. 40). When a patient was hospitalized, she wondered, "What about the other members of the family? Even though the patient is adequately cared for . . . may not his progress be dependent on the condition and attitude of his family in the home?" (P. 40).

Faville's (1925) presentation of several case studies underscored the need to consider the family in terms of all relationships. "The public health nurse visiting homes has the priceless opportunity for seeing the family as a whole, for securing the solution of many of the social maladjustments at the root of illness" (p. 22).

As a result of major revisions, the NLNE's 1927 edition of *A Curricu-*

lum for Schools of Nursing excluded many previous references to preparation of nurses for work with families. The thrust of the 1927 guide was clearly different from that of the 1917 edition. For example, in the section "Practical Objects for Nursing Education," no explicit mention was made of families. In addition, the section "Household Science" was removed. A clue to these omissions is the introductory statement that there was no need to separate the preparation of "bedside" nurses from that of "public health nurses."

Analysis of the literature from 1910 to 1930 yielded still no evidence of formal middle-range family theory in nursing. There was, however, emphasis on preparation of the public health nurse for family nursing practice.

1930 to 1950

The literature of the period 1930 to 1950 emphasized preparation of nurses for care of families. Textbooks of this period, as well as a curriculum guide, included content about the family. Indeed, the exclusion of explicit family subject matter from the NLNE curriculum guide was short-lived, for the third edition, published in 1937, identified "The Modern Family" as a major unit of study, with 10 to 15 hours allocated. An emphasis in this edition was on the development of "the 'normal' family and the influence [that modern life] is tending to make in the functions and organization of the family" (p. 216).

On the subject "Nursing and Health Services in the Family," the authors of the curriculum guide declared, "The entire program outlined in this curriculum is based on the assumption that participation in health conservation and prevention of disease is inherent in the whole concept of nursing . . . also that the patient should not be considered as an individual only, but as a member of a group" (p. 510). In addition, courses that were directed toward family health care were not "specific preparation for public health nursing." The courses were, instead, intended to round out the nursing students' "experience, to meet more common situations found in family health" (p. 510). This theme continued in the statement that "the nurse must consider the family as a unit" (p. 513).

During this period, textbooks for various clinical areas began to include explicit content about the family. In her 1931 text on school nursing, Chayer stated, "The visiting nurse must be given the credit for pioneering work in the education of parents. . . . Before public schools went into the home, the visiting nurse was there" (p. 206). Chayer also commented that it had "taken 50 years for Florence Nightingale's vision of the Health Nurse going into homes in the community" to come about (p. 4).

In her 1935 medical-surgical nursing textbook, Harmer stated,

> Very often patients although pronounced cured, require further care. When this is the case, the nurse in charge of the social service

department will see that patients are properly cared for. As previously stated, the patient can never be rightly understood or adequately cared for considered apart from the family . . . in the homes of rich and poor alike, rural or army nursing includes all of this (p. 367).

Zabriskie (1934) addressed aspects of family care in her obstetrical nursing textbook. She maintained,

A thorough study of the cause and effect relationships entails not only a knowledge of the factors operating as determinants in the parent's attitude toward the child . . . but accepting the fact that the child reacts to given situations in the family. [Moreover,] in families where the parental adjustment to each other is inharmonious, the conflict problem for the child becomes markedly increased (p. 199).

The literature of this period increasingly emphasized the family unit. Bean and Brockett's (1937) article, "The family as a unit for nursing service," is an example. They noted that when going into a home, the public health nurse should not only give nursing care to individuals but also address the health needs of the entire family and work out a health plan for its members. The authors also identified ways to ascertain whether nurses were carrying out the commitment to care for the entire family. They described a one-year survey by the United States Public Health Service conducted at three county health departments. The purpose of the survey was presented as follows: "In view of the emphasis that has been placed on the principle of 'the family as a unit' for nursing service, it seemed appropriate to investigate the degree to which nurses in actual practice broadened their visits to include the entire family" (p. 1924). Bean and Brockett's review of over 3000 records revealed that in 62 percent of the cases, nurses addressed problems other than those for which they first came into the home. The authors concluded, however, that services tended to be confined to just a few family members on any one visit. This did not meet their criteria for total family service.

Analysis of the literature of this period revealed continued lack of formal middle-range family theory development. However, the family remained a focal phenomenon for nursing, with discussion of the needs of various family members included in textbooks directed toward diverse clinical areas. Furthermore, explicit content on the family was returned to the NLNE's curriculum guide. Moreover, the notion of the family as a unit began to appear in the literature.

1950 to 1990

Nursing literature dealing with the family has increased dramatically since 1950. Given the volume of books and articles, only a sample of these publications was reviewed. An attempt was made to select literature that reflected continuation of themes noted in previous eras as well as new thinking about and approaches to the family. Furthermore, given that no significant differences in emphasis were identified between the 1950-to-1970 and the 1970-to-1990 time periods, these two eras are considered together.

Beasley (1954) continued the discussion of the role of public health nurses in family nursing. In particular, she identified services that were available to families who had a mentally ill member. She explained, "It was this concept of supportive services to the families of the mentally ill that became the basis for an experimental program" (p. 482). The function of public health nurses in this regard was in part to help the family accept the patient's illness and understand the patient's need to be hospitalized, to help the patient be accepted back into the home, and to arrange for several families to meet together to discuss common problems. Beasley noted that the emphasis of service was placed purposefully on the family's needs, rather than on those of the individual patient.

Garside (1958) explained the role of school nurses in family nursing. She stated, "The home visit provides for a closer observation of intangibles such as family relationships and intergroup personality reactions" (p. 153). She also indicated that school nurses tended to address the needs of schoolage children and thereby unintentionally neglect family health. She stated further that the health of individual family members must be addressed "in order to protect the family as whole" (p. 155).

Maternity nursing texts of this period focused increasing attention on the impact of pregnancy and childbirth on the family. The 13th edition of *Maternity Nursing* (Reeder, Mastroianni, Martin, and Fitzpatrick, 1976), for example, included a chapter on the contemporary family and family theory, with an emphasis on role theory. The 15th edition of this book (Reeder, Mastroianni, and Martin, 1983) gave even more attention to the family, with whole chapters dealing with the philosophy of family-centered maternity care, the family in a changing world, and evolving family forms.

Pediatric textbooks of this period also noted the centrality of the family. Steele (1981), for example, viewed the family as a social subsystem.

Explicit emphasis on the family unit as the client was noted in many publications in the early years of this period, including articles by Kvarness (1959), Reinerston (1963), Hess (1966), Mereness (1968), and Smiley (1973). Furthermore, textbooks focusing entirely on the family, with the family unit or family system as the phenomenon of interest, began to appear. Relatively early entries in this category are Smoyak's *The Psychiatric Nurse as a Family Therapist*, published in 1975; Knafl and Grace's *Families across the Life Cycle: Studies for Nursing*, published in 1979; Miller and Janosik's *Family-Focused Care*, published in 1980; and

Jones's *Family Therapy: A Comparison of Approaches*, also published in 1980.

Later texts focusing entirely on the family include Friedman's *Family Nursing: Theory and Assessment*, the first edition of which was published in 1981 and the second edition in 1986; Miller and Winstead-Fry's *Family Systems Theory in Nursing Practice*, which appeared in 1982; Wright and Leahey's *Nurses and Families: A Guide to Family Assessment and Intervention*, published in 1984; and Bomar's edited volume, *Nurses and Family Health Promotion: Concepts, Assessment, and Interventions*, which appeared in 1989. These books are characterized by review of family theories from other disciplines and derivation of assessment tools and practice protocols for use in nursing practice. For example, Friedman (1981) used structural-functional theory to derive a family nursing assessment tool, and Wright and Leahey (1984) derived a model for family assessment from the structural, developmental, and functional theories of family analysis and therapy.

A different approach is apparent in Clements and Roberts's edited text, *Family Health: A Theoretical Approach to Nursing Care*, published in 1983. This book is distinguished by presentation of family nursing strategies derived directly from existing conceptual models of nursing. Several of these perspectives are descirbed in detail later in this chapter in the section on conceptual models and the family.

Still another approach was taken in Whall's (1986a) book, *Family Therapy Theory for Nursing*. This text continued the work begun by Fitzpatrick, Whall, Johnston, and Floyd (1982) on theory reformulation. This technique involves linkage of theories of other disciplines with conceptual models of nursing and reformulation of the theories to form logically congruent conceptual-theoretical systems of nursing knowledge. Examples from Whall's book are given in the section on conceptual models and the family later in this chapter.

Most publications of the 1970s and 1980s focused on the use of family theory for nursing practice. In her 1983 article, "The family as a unit of analysis: Strategies for the nurse researcher," Gilliss moved the focus to research and explained how various theoretical approaches influence the design of empirical studies of families. The reader is referred to Chapters 4 and 5 of this book for extensive discussion of nursing research of families.

A dual focus on research and practice is evident in Sherwen's (1987) *Psychosocial Dimensions of the Pregnant Family*. This text includes a discussion of family systems theory as well as reviews of theoretical and research literature dealing with psychosocial aspects of the pregnant family, such as body image, sexuality, and maternal role attainment. Most chapters include implications for nursing practice. The dual focus on research and practice also is evident in Gilliss, Highley, Roberts, and Martinson's (1989) edited volume, *Toward a Science of Family Nurs-*

ing. This book contains a chapter on major theories thought to undergird research and practice in nursing as well as in other disciplines including the interactionist, developmental, systems, and social exchange perspectives. Another chapter presents a critical review of family nursing research that was published in several scholarly nursing journals. Additional chapters present theoretically focused discussions of factors influencing family health, transitions in the family life cycle, and family health during chronic illness, as well as implications for nursing practice.

Although increasing emphasis was placed on the family as a unit or system in this latest period of modern nursing, attention also has been focused on individual family members within the context of their family environments. Four outstanding examples of this orientation are Hanson and Bozett's (1985) and Bozett and Hanson's (1990) edited volumes on fatherhood, and Rubin's (1984) and Mercer's (1986) book length presentations of their research programs dealing with motherhood.

In summary, review of the family nursing literature of 1950 to 1990 revealed emphasis on the practice and research implications of family theories from disciplines other than nursing. The family was further accepted as a client for nursing, and attention was given to caring for and studying the family as a unit. At the same time, nursing scholars devoted considerable time to studying individual family members. Despite the advances of the past 40 years, there remains virtually no evidence of formal middle-range family theory that is unique or distinctive to nursing.

STANDARDS OF NURSING PRACTICE AND THE FAMILY

A review of the standards for nursing practice for several clinical specialties revealed considerable interest in the family. The earliest *Standards of Community Health Nursing Practice* (American Nurses' Association, 1973a) included the term family approximately seven times. The opening statement for these standards declared, "Nursing practice is a direct service . . . to the individual, the family, and the community during health and illness" (p. 1). According to these standards, consumers of nursing care may be individuals and families. The standards went on to maintain that "active involvement of the individual, family, and community is necessary in attainment of positive health" (p. 3).

The term family was used more than 25 times in the earliest *Standards of Maternal-Child Health Nursing Practice* (American Nurses' Association, 1973b). One standard, for example, stated that maternal and child health nursing practice initiates changes to enhance family unity. Moreover, the idea of family solidarity was evident in several standards.

The earliest *Standards of Medical-Surgical Nursing Practice* (American Nurses' Association, 1974) included the term family approximately five times. These standards claimed that the nurse is to "ensure patient and family participation in health promotion" (p. 1), that "goals are formulated by the patient and his family" (p. 3), and that the nursing care plan "is communicated to the patient and family" (p. 3).

The family was mentioned more than 20 times in the *Standards of Pediatric Oncology Nursing Practice* (American Nurses' Association, 1978). These standards declared that "nursing care given to the pediatric oncology patient . . . incorporates the needs of the individual child and family" (p. 1). More specifically, the standards require systematic collection of data about the individual child and the family, as well as nursing actions that reflect consideration and appreciation of the integrity of the family unit.

The earliest *Standards of Psychiatric-Mental Health Nursing* (American Nurses' association, 1973c) mentioned the family. The 1982 edition of these standards was, however, more developed in terms of a family focus, with the term used or implied at least 10 times. Family therapy was described as interventions that focus on the family system and promote change toward adaptation in that system. Moreover, the standards require the nurse to utilize advanced clinical expertise in family psychotherapy.

In contrast, the earliest *Standards of Gerontological Nursing Practice* (American Nurses' Association, 1976) did not mention the term *family*. Instead, the term *significant other* was used to denote relationships. For example, the standards required plans for nursing care that were developed in conjunction with the older adult and/or significant others. The 1987 version of these standards, however, utilized the term family in an explicit manner.

In summary, the American Nurses' Association's standards of nursing practice include the family as a focal phenomenon and clearly link the family with nursing practice. Furthermore, as was found in the historical overview, the family is considered not only by the clinical specialties traditionally devoted to family-centered care, such as public health, maternity, and pediatric nursing, but also by the medical-surgical and gerontological nursing specialties. The standards do not, however, reflect a specific or explicit focus on formal middle-range family theory development.

CONCEPTUAL MODELS OF NURSING AND THE FAMILY

Several conceptual models of nursing models have been expanded by their authors to include a focus on the family. Furthermore, other scholars have derived family-focused works from the nursing models.

King's Perspective of the Family

King's (1981, 1987) work can be separated into an interacting systems conceptual framework and a middle-range theory of goal attainment. The conceptual framework encompasses the personal, interpersonal, and social systems as well as concepts that describe the central features of the three systems. The goal attainment theory proposes that when nurses and patients engage in mutual goal setting, there is a high probability of goal attainment.

King's 1981 text, *A Theory for Nursing: Systems, Concepts, Process* indexed the family extensively. She noted that most persons begin life as a part of a family and learn ways to meet basic needs in families, and that the family constitutes one of the groups in which one performs a certain role. King further noted that the family demonstrates the features of a social system, that is, structure, status, role, and social interaction.

King expanded her ideas about the family in a chapter published in Clements and Roberts's (1983) book. The family, according to King (1983), is "a social system that is seen as a group of interacting individuals" (p. 179). "As a social system," King went on to say, the family "influences individuals as they grow, develop, and move from dependence in childhood to interdependence in adulthood" (p. 180).

King (1983) also viewed the family as a small group or interpersonal system. When the family is viewed in this manner, the theory of goal attainment may be used by nurses "to assess and diagnose real and potential problems of individuals and families . . . [and to assist] family members to set goals, select means to achieve goals, and plan for resolution of problems or ways to cope with events" (p. 180).

The theory of goal attainment encompasses several concepts that are relevant to families, including perception, interaction, communication, transaction, space, time, growth and development, and stress. King (1983) claimed that *perception* "is a key concept in dealing with families and their health" (p. 181). The nurse's task is to assess and to verify the family's perception of a member's health state through *interactions* with the family. King explained,

> Within nurse-family interactions, each is perceiving the other and making some mental judgments about the other. The nurse, through direct observation of behavior and through purposeful *communication*, gathers information, interprets the information, and shares information with family members to identify real or potential problems and concerns. Family members reciprocate by sharing information with the nurse. In the course of their interactions, they arrive at mutual goals. . . . Values, wants, and needs of each person are communicated, and *transactions* are made. When transactions are made, goals are achieved (p. 181).

King went on to point out that interactions between nurses and family members are influenced by family movement through social space and physical space, as well as by the personal space requirements of each family member. Interactions also are influenced by each family member's concept of time. Still other influences on interactions are the growth and development profiles of family members and the stress in family environments.

Other work dealing with the extension of King's conceptual framework and theory of goal attainment has been done by Gonot (1986). She derived a theoretical model of family therapy that may be used with various family structures. Gonot explained,

> The interpersonal system of the family is the focal system of the [theoretical] model. The personal systems of family members are the subsystems, and the environmental social systems comprise the familial suprasystem. . . . During the therapeutic process, the nurse enters into an interpersonal system with the family client. Assessment focuses on the perceptions, communications, roles and developmental stages of members, as well as the stressors being experienced within the system. Through purposeful interaction, the nurse-therapist facilitates the process whereby family members establish shared goals and negotiate means to achieve them. As transactions occur, the health of the family system is promoted (p. 46).

King's definition of family and her theory of goal attainment provide direction for nurses as they develop middle-range theories for their work with families. King's theory of goal attainment needs to be tested with families, and other theories about interactions focused on mutual goal setting and goal attainment need to be generated and tested, because "achievement of goals related to family health is a measure of the effectiveness of nursing care" (King, 1983, p. 181).

Neuman's Perspective of the Family

Neuman's (1982, 1989b) Systems Model focuses on factors that influence the client system's response to stressors from the internal and external environment. The client system may be an individual, a family, or a community. The first edition of Neuman's (1982) book contains many references to the family. A chapter by Reed (1982) presented an explanation of how the model guides family psychosocial assessment and intervention. A chapter by Goldblum-Graff and Graff (1982) adapted Neuman's model to family therapy by linking its concepts and propositions to those of a theory of contextual family therapy. The second edition of Neuman's (1989b) book contained a chapter focused on the linkage between the Neuman Systems Model and family theory (Reed, 1989). In a separate publication, Buchanan (1987) presented a modification of Neuman's conceptual model that she claimed was appropriate for aggregates, families, and the community. Furthermore, Ross and Helmer (1988) identified the similarities and differences between individuals explain and predict the effects of nursing interventions that facilitate stability of the family system.

Orem's Perspective of the Family

Orem's (1985) work can be separated into a self-care conceptual framework and three middle-range theories: the theory of self-care, the theory of self-care deficit, and the theory of nursing systems. The conceptual framework and theories focus on determination of the relationship between the individual's therapeutic self-care demand—which is made up of universal, developmental, and health-deviation self-care requisites—and his or her self-care agency, or ability to care for self. When the demand exceeds agency, a self-care deficit exists. If the deficit cannot be met by a significant other through dependent-care agency, then nursing is required. Legitimate recipients of nursing care are, therefore, those individuals who have self-care or dependent-care deficits.

The first edition of Orem's text, *Nursing: Concepts of Practice*, published in 1971, did not index the term *family*. Orem did, however, indicate that the nurse "learns to work in cooperation with patients and their families" (p. 119), and that in terms of achieving goals, "one had to be aware of family implications" (p. 71). Orem also mentioned that parents are "child care agents" for their children (p. 29). In the second edition of Orem's book, which was published in 1980, the term *family* is cited several times. In this edition, Orem stated, "In search of valid ways to provide health care to families . . . it has been recognized that it may be essential to work with all members of the unit" (p. 200). Here Orem began to discuss the role of family members as dependent-care agents, that is, providers of care for other family members who are not capable of self-care agency. In the third edition of her book, which was published in 1985, Orem indicated that people receive nursing as individuals or as members of a multiperson unit. However, she maintained that "it should be recognized that only individuals have human needs that can be met through nursing" (p. 251). This feature of Orem's work has obvious implications for her view of nursing with regard to the family. Indeed, Orem views the family as only a backdrop for individuals. More specifically, family system elements compose just one category of basic conditioning factors, that is, factors that influence therapeutic self-care and self-care agency.

Orem's view of the family as a basic conditioning factor was introduced in her contribution to the Clements and Roberts (1983) text. She stated, "The system of family living, the physical and social environment of the family, and the family's culture [are] basic conditioning factors for all family members" (Orem, 1983b, p. 368). Another basic conditioning factor is "family roles and responsibilities" (Orem, 1983a, p. 386). Orem (1983b) also stated that "the system of family support should be

and families as client systems when using the Neuman Syst.
Moreover, Herrick and Goodykontz (1989) developed a fan
ment format based on Neuman's model. And Neuman (1989a)
trated the use of her nursing process format with a family. Alth
assessment focused on individual family members, family syst
ables were considered and interventions aimed at the family syste
described. Finally, Berkey and Hanson (1991) recently published
length treatment of the use of the Neuman Systems Model for t
assessment and intervention.

Neuman discussed her own ideas about the family in Clements
Roberts's 1983 book. A family, according to Neuman (1983), "is a grc
of two or more persons who create and maintain a common culture;
most central goal is one of continuance" (p. 241). The family system
Neuman claimed, "can be viewed as individual family members harmoni
ous in their relationship—a cluster of related meanings and values that
govern the family and keep it viable in a constantly changing environment" (p. 241). Individuals are viewed as subcomponents of family
systems in Neuman's perspective. The basic structure of the family system
consists of the composite of the relationships among the family members
and their patterns of interaction. Major categories of family system components are psychosocial relationship characteristics, physical status, developmental characteristics, and spiritual influence.

Neuman (1983) explained that the family system is exposed to
stressors that affect its stability, that is, its relative wellness state. The
integrity of the basic structure of the family system must be preserved to
maintain stability. If exposure to stressors leads to instability, an illness
state prevails. Stressors may be intrafamily, or those occurring within the
family unit, such as individual interactions among family members; inter-
family, or those occurring between the family and the immediate or
direct external environment, such as individual or family interactions
with other families, community groups, or agencies; and extrafamily
stressors, or those occurring between the family and the distal or indirect
external environment, such as influences from political and social issues.

Neuman's (1983) definition and description of family and her view
of the family as a client system exposed to environmental stressors provide direction for nurses as they develop theories for work with families.
Within the context of interventions as primary, secondary, and tertiary
prevention, the goal of nursing is to discern and to manipulate "environmental factors [that are] adversely affecting the family's ability to attain or
maintain itself in an optimal state of health or wellness" (p. 241). "The
role of the nurse," according to Neuman, "is to control vigorously factors
affecting the family with special goal-directed activities toward facilitating stability within the system" (p. 243). Research, then, should be
directed toward generation and testing of middle-range theories that
describe the factors that affect family system stability and those that

examined and adjusted as needed and then incorporated into the family system of living" (p. 368).

A somewhat different perspective of the family within the context of Orem's conceptual framework was provided by Tadych (1985), who linked selected concepts from Orem's framework with concepts from family theories. She explained,

> It appears that Orem intends that the nurse relate to both the responsible adult and the dependent person as individual units. A systems theory conceptualization of this type of nursing situation might be that of the nurse attending to the responsible adult and dependent person as a dyadic relationship and, therefore, the target focus and unit of service. If, as such, they were also members of the same family unit, the dyad could be viewed as a subsystem of that family. The family itself could be considered a primary focus and become the unit of nursing service if such a contract were established between the nurse and the family (p. 50).

Tadych went on to explain that although analysis of therapeutic self-care demand, self-care agency, and dependent-care agency occurs for each individual member of the family, the family unit as a whole is analyzed in terms of family structure, family functions, and family developmental stage.

Chin (1985) also endeavored to modify Orem's conceptual framework for use with families. Her approach involved redefining universal self-care requisites for the family. She stated, "Many noted authorities on families and family health have derived universal functions demanded of families. . . . We reasoned that these family functions were the universal self-care [requisites] of a family" (p. 57).

Orem's perspective provides direction for nurses as they develop middle-range theories about their work with members of families. Inasmuch as self-care and dependent-care agency are abilities only of individuals, nursing is directed toward enhancing the self-care and dependent-care agency of individuals who are family members. Thus, Orem's theories of self-care, self-care deficit, and nursing systems need to be tested with special attention to the basic conditioning factor of family system elements.

Rogers's Perspective of the Family

Rogers's (1990) conceptual system, which currently is referred to as the Science of Unitary Human Beings, focuses on the human being as a unitary multi-dimensional energy field engaged in continuous mutual process with the environment, which also is viewed as a multi-dimensional energy field. The human and environmental energy fields are continuously open, negentropic, and characterized by constantly changing pattern.

Roger's first major presentation of her conceptual system was published in her 1970 book and revised in later publications (Rogers, 1980, 1986, 1990). These publications did not include explicit references to the family. Fawcett (1975), however, based her conceptual framework of the family as a living open system on Rogers's early work. Fawcett (1989) then used that conceptual framework to develop and to test an explicit middle-range theory of wives' and husbands' pregnancy-related experiences in a series of studies. Furthermore, Whall (1981) constructed a logically congruent conceptual-theoretical system of nursing knowledge from Rogers's conceptual system, Fawcett's (1975) extension of Rogers's works to the family system, and theories of family functioning. She then developed a guide for assessment of families, organized according to individual subsystem considerations, interactional patterns, unique characteristics of the whole family system, and environmental interface synchrony. Moreover, Smith (1983) noted that the view of family used in her study of family development when a teenage mother and her infant are incorporated into the household was consistent with Rogers's work. And Johnston (1986) and Reed (1986) derived family therapy protocols from Rogers's work.

Johnston (1986) maintained, "In Rogers' view, the goal of family therapy is not analysis but rather synthesis" (p. 15). She then presented a modification of Whall's (1981) assessment guide, based on the thesis that

> the family is characterized by rhythmic developmental sequences which are in mutual process with the environmental field. Family field and environmental fields are four-dimensional energy fields in continuous interaction, integral with each other, and coextensive with the universe. Family field and environmental fields are essentially boundaryless, are unique (p. 28).

Reed (1986) reformulated the family developmental framework so that it was consistent with Rogers's conceptual system. In the new framework, the nurse therapist's role is

> to facilitate family development by promoting synchronization of the changes that occur across positional careers. Interventions include but are not limited to: education for good life-cycle management; anticipatory guidance on developmental tasks; assisting in decision making on timing of positional career changes; and facilitating repatterning of members' developmental strivings by improving new patterns out of dysynchronous family patterns (p. 89).

Friedemann (1989a, 1989b) also used Rogers's conceptual system as one base for her work. She presented a detailed description of a framework of systemic organization that can be used to guide nursing care of families and family members. She also described the influence of the systemic organization framework on derivation of a control-congruence model for mental health nursing practice with families.

Rogers presented her own expansion of her conceptual system to the family in her contribution to Clements and Roberts's (1983) book. Family, according to Rogers (1983), "refers to a range of configurations which may be variously labelled as nuclear family, extended family, one-parent family, blended family, single person family, homosexual family, and others" (p. 226). She went on to say that "family members may or may not live in the same household. They may or may not be related by blood or by law" (p. 226). Rogers views the family as she does the individual human being, that is, as "an irreducible, four-dimensional, negentropic . . . energy field" (p. 226). The family, then, is viewed as an irreducible whole that is not understood by knowledge of individual family members. Furthermore, "family fields and their respective environmental fields are in continuous mutual process" (p. 226). Family characteristics are manifestations of family and environmental field processes. The family field is characterized by "non-repeating rhythmicities of growing diversity . . . and continuous innovative change" (p. 226).

Rogers's extension of her conceptual system to the family provides direction for nurses interested in developing middle-range theories about their work with families. Theories must reflect the perception of the family as an irreducible whole that is a knowledgeable participant in changes that involve both the family field and the environmental field. Theories about nursing intervention should be directed toward explanations and probabilistic predictions dealing with therapeutic modalities and health measures that maintain and promote family well-being by means of creative processes "in which knowledgeable participation by the family is of central importance" (Rogers, 1983, p. 227).

Roy's Perspective of the Family

Roy's (1976, 1984) Adaptation Model focuses on environmental stimuli that influence the adaptive system's responses in four modes: physiological, self-concept, role function, and interdependence. Stimuli are focal, or that factor most immediately confronting the adaptive system; contextual, or those factors providing the context for responses; and residual, or those factors that may affect responses but whose effects are not measurable. The adaptive system may be an individual, a family or other group, a community, or society.

Roy (1976) addressed the family primarily as it related to the individual in the first edition of her book. The notion of the family as an adaptive system was expanded in the 1981 text by Roy and Roberts. This notion was continued in the second edition of Roy's book, published in 1984, as well as in the Andrews and Roy (1986) text.

Roy's (1983) contribution to the Clements and Roberts book indicated that she views the family as an adaptive system that, like the individual, has inputs, internal control and feedback processes, and output. "The inputs for the family as an adaptive system," Roy (1983) noted, "include the entire complex of stimuli that affect the family as a group, both internal to each person and those coming from the external environment" (p. 274). More specifically, inputs include needs of individual family members, as well as changes within members, among members, and in the environment. Internal processes relevant to the family are support, nurturance, and socialization. Feedback mechanisms include transactional patterns and member control. Output of the family as an adaptive system focuses on behavioral goals, including survival, continuity, and growth. Roy regarded the inputs to the family adaptive system as focal environmental stimuli and the internal processes of support, nurturance, and socialization as contextual and residual stimuli. Furthermore, she equated the feedback mechanism of transactional patterns with the interdependence mode of adaptation and the mechanism of member control with the physiological and role function modes. Moreover, she equated the output of survival with the physiological mode, the output of continuity with the role function mode, and the output of growth with the self-concept mode.

In addition to Roy's efforts to extend her conceptual model to the family, Whall (1986b) constructed a conceptual-theoretical system of knowledge by reformulating and linking the theory of strategic family therapy with Roy's model. Here, the nurse therapist is "participative with or joins the family in terms of mutual goal setting. [The therapist] assesses four modes and stimuli, [and] helps to manage the stimuli to bring them within the family's adaptive range" (Whall, 1986b, p. 67).

Roy's extension of her conceptual model to the family provides direction for middle-range family theory development. More specifically, theories of family adaptation and nursing practice theories of family need to be generated and tested. Theories of family adaptation should focus on identification of specific and concrete inputs, processes, and outputs of the family adaptive system. "Nursing practice theories about the family," Roy (1983) noted, "will relate to how nurses diagnose and intervene with the family system to promote system adaptation" (p. 275).

In summary, the analysis of conceptual models of nursing indicates that these abstract and general formulations provide considerable direction for generation and testing of middle-range family theories from a distinctively nursing perspective. The extensions to family made by King, Neuman, Rogers, and Roy deal with the family as a distinct and whole unit of analysis. In contrast, Orem's conceptual model deals with family only as a context or factor to consider when dealing with individuals.

CONCLUSION

The literature review presented in this chapter indicates that interest in the family as a unit of nursing care originated with Nightingale's concern for family members. Continued interest in the family is documented in books and journal articles since Nightingale's time as well as in the American Nurses' Association standards of nursing practice. Most of these publications point to the importance of the family in nursing but do little to advance formal middle-range family theory development.

The fact that so much as been written by nurses about the family but not formalized as explicit sets of concepts and propositions mirrors the current sate of nursing theory development as a whole. But the current status of theory development about the family can be improved. Authors of textbooks and journal articles can begin to include reviews of current knowledge about the family and restate that knowledge as formal middle-range theories. Each author whose work is focused on family nursing practice can identify the theory underlying the practice protocols. And every nurse researcher who studies the family can summarize findings as a formal middle-range theory.

An explicit impetus for formal family theory development is now evident in several conceptual models of nursing, especially in their authors' perspectives of the family. And movement toward explicit and formal middle-range family nursing theories is evident in the work of a few scholars who have either linked family theories from other disciplines with conceptual models of nursing or attempted to derive a middle-range family nursing theory from a nursing model.

The value of conceptual models to theory development was highlighted by Nye (1988). He pointed out that although broad formulations do not contain the "theoretical propositions from which research-level hypotheses can be deduced" (p. 313), they do represent the precursors to middle-range theories. He recommended, therefore, that more effort be concentrated on derivation of middle-range theories from general conceptual models. Thus, the authors of conceptual models of nursing and their colleagues should continue their work directed toward extension of existing conceptual models to encompass family phenomena. Furthermore, other nurse scholars can follow Friedemann's (1989a, 1989b) lead and develop new conceptual models of nursing and related middle-range theories focused exclusively on the family.

REFERENCES

American Nurses' Association (1973a). *Standards of community health nursing practice.* Kansas City, MO: Author.

American Nurses' Association (1973b). *Standards of maternal-child health nursing practice.* Kansas City, MO: Author.

American Nurses' Association (1973c). *Standards of psychiatric-mental health nursing practice.* Kansas City, MO: Author.

American Nurses' Association (1974). *Standards of medical-surgical nursing practice.* Kansas City, MO: Author.

American Nurses' Association (1976). *Standards of gerontological nursing practice.* Kansas City, MO: Author.

American Nurses' Association (1978). *Standards of pediatric-oncology nursing practice.* Kansas City, MO: Author.

American Nurses' Association (1982). *Standards of psychiatric and mental health nursing practice* (revised). Kansas City, MO: Author.

American Nurses' Association (1987). *Standards of gerontological nursing practice* (revised). Kansas City, MO: Author.

Andrews, H. A., & Roy, C. (1986). *Essentials of the Roy Adaptation Model.* Nowalk, CT: Appleton-Century-Crofts.

Bean, H., & Brockett, G. (1937). The family as a unit for nursing service. *Public Health Report, 52,* 1923–1931.

Beard, M. (1915). Home nursing. *Public Health Nursing Quarterly, 7,* 44–51.

Beard, M. (1917). The family as the unit of public health work. *Modern Hospital, October,* 247–251.

Beasley, F. (1954). Public health nursing services for families of the mentally ill. *Nursing Outlook, 2,* 482–484.

Berkey, K. M., & Hanson, S. M. H. (1991). *Nursing handbook: Family health assessment/intervention.* St. Louis: Mosby.

Bomar, P. (Ed.). (1989). *Nurses and family health promotion: Concepts, assessment, and intervention.*

Bozett, F. W., & Hanson, S. M. H. (1990). *Cultural variations in American fatherhood.* New York: Springer.

Brooks, J. (1890). Nursing the insane. *Trained Nurse, 4,* 10–12.

Buchanan, B. F. (1987). Human-environment interaction: A modification of the Neuman Systems Model for aggregates, families, and the community. *Public Health Nursing, 4,* 52–64.

Chayer, M. (1931). *School nursing.* New York: Teachers College Press.

Chin, S. (1985). Can self-care theory be applied to families? In Riehl-Sisca, J. P. *The science and art of self-care* (pp. 56–62). Norwalk. CT: Appleton-Century-Crofts.

Clements, I. W., & Roberts, F. B. (1983). *Family health. A theoretical approach to nursing care.* New York: Wiley.

Cook, E. (1913). *The life of Florence Nightingale* (Vol. 2). London: Macmillan.

Cook, E. (1925). *The life of Florence Nightingale* (rev. ed.). London: Macmillan.

Donnelly, G. F. (1986). Nursing theory: Evolution of a sacred cow. *Holistic Nursing Practice, 1*(1), 1–7.

Faville, K. (1925). The nurse as counselor in troubled homes. *Red Cross Courier, 4,* 14–15.

Fawcett, J. (1975). The family as a living open system: An emerging conceptual framework for nursing. *International Nursing Review, 22,* 113–116.

Fawcett, J. (1989). Spouses' experiences during pregnancy and the postpartum: A program of research and theory development. *Image. The Journal of Nursing Scholarship, 21,* 149–152.

Fitzpatrick, J. J., Whall, A. L., Johnston, R. L., & Floyd, J. A. (1982). *Nursing models and their psychiatric mental health applications.* Bowie, MD: Brady.

Friedemann, M-L. (1989a). Closing the gap between grand theory and mental health practice with families. Part 1: The framework of systemic organization for nursing of families and family members. *Archieves of Psychiatric Nursing, 3,* 10–19.

Friedemann, M-L. (1989b). Closing the gap between grand theory and mental health practice with families. Part 2: The control-congruence model for mental health nursing of families. *Archives of Psychiatric Nursing, 3,* 20–28.

Friedman, M. M. (1981). *Family nursing. Theory and assessment.* New York: Appleton-Century-Crofts.

Friedman, M. M. (1986). *Family nursing. Theory and assessment* (2nd ed.). Norwalk, CT: Appleton-Century-Crofts.

Garside, A. (1958). The school nurse as a family counselor. *Journal of School Health, 28,* 153–157.

Gilliss, C. L. (1983). The family as a unit of analysis: Strategies for the nurse researcher. *Advances in Nursing Science, 5*(3), 50–59.

Gilliss, C. L., Highley, B. L., Roberts, B. M., & Martinson, I. M. (1989). *Toward a science of family nursing.* Menlo Park, CA: Addison-Wesley.

Goldblum-Graff, D., & Graff, H. (1982). The Neuman model adapted to family therapy. In B. Neuman, *The Neuman Systems Model. Application to nursing education and practice* (pp. 217–222). Norwalk, CT: Appleton-Century-Crofts.

Gonot, P. W. (1986). Family therapy as derived from King's conceptual model. In A. L. Whall, *Family therapy theory for nursing. Four approaches* (pp. 33–48). Norwalk, CT: Appleton-Century-Crofts.

Hanson, S. M. H., & Bozett, F. W. (1985). *Dimensions of fatherhood.* Beverly Hills, CA: Sage.

Harmer, B. (1935). *Textbook of the principles and practice of nursing.* New York: Macmillan.

Herrick, C. A. & Goodykoontz, L. (1989). Neuman's systems model for nursing practice as a conceptual framework for a family assessment. *Journal of Child and Adolescent Psychiatric Mental Health Nursing, 2*(2), 61–67.

Hess, G. (1966). Family nursing experience. *Nursing Outlook, 14,* 51–53.

Johnston, R. L. (1986). Approaching family intervention through Rogers' conceptual model. In A. L. Whall, *Family therapy theory for nursing. Four approaches* (pp. 11–32). Norwalk, CT: Appleton-Century-Crofts.

Jones, S. L. (1980). *Family therapy: A comparison of approaches.* Bowie, MD: Brady.

King, I. M. (1981). *A theory for nursing. System, concepts, process.* New York: Wiley.

King, I. M. (1983). King's theory of nursing. In I. W. Clements & F. B. Roberts, *Family health. A theoretical approach to nursing care* (pp. 177–188). New York: Wiley.

King, I. M. (1987, May). *King's theory.* Paper presented at Nurse Theorist Conference, Pittsburgh, PA (Cassette recording)

Knafl, K., & Grace, H (Eds.) (1979). *Families across the life cycle: Studies for nursing.* Boston: Little, Brown.

Kvarness, M. (1959). The patient is the family. *Nursing Outlook, 7,* 142–146.

Laird, M. (1923). The value of follow-up work in the family. *American Journal of Nursing, 24,* 4043.

Mercer, R. T. (1986). *First-time motherhood. Experiences from teens to forties.* New York: Springer

Mereness, D. (1968). Family therapy: An evolving role for the psychiatric nurse. *Perspectives in Psychiatric Nursing, 6,* 259.

Miller, J., & Janosik, E. (1980). *Family-focused care.* New York: McGraw-Hill.

Miller, S. R., & Winstead-Fry, P. (1982). *Family systems theory in nursing practice.* Reston, VA: Reston.

National League for Nursing Education. (1917). *Standard curriculum for schools of nursing.* Baltimore: Waverly Press.

National League for Nursing Education. (1927). *A curriculum for schools of nursing.* New York: Author.

National League for Nursing Education. (1937). *A curriculum guide for schools of nursing.* New York: Author.

Neuman, B. (1982). *The Neuman Systems Model. Application to nursing education and practice.* Norwalk, CT: Appleton-Century-Crofts.

Neuman, B. (1983). Family intervention using the Betty Neuman health-care systems model. In I. W. Clements & F. B. Roberts, *Family health. A theoretical approach to nursing care* (pp. 239–254). New York: Wiley.

Neuman, B. (1989a). The Neuman nursing process format: Family. In J. P. Riehl-Sisca, *Conceptual models for nursing practice* (3rd ed., pp. 49–62). Norwalk, CT: Appleton and Lange.

Neuman, B. (1989b). *The Neuman Systems Model. Application to nursing education and practice* (2nd ed.). Norwalk, CT: Appleton and Lange.

Nightingale, F. (1855, August 6). Letter to Lady Alicia Blackwood. Written at Scutari.

Nightingale, F. (1858). *Notes on matters affecting the health, efficiency, and hospital administration of the British army.* London: Harrison & Sons.

Nightingale, F. (1863). *Notes on hospitals.* London: Longman, Green.

Nye, F. I. (1988). Fifty years of family research, 1937–1987. *Journal of Marriage and the Family, 50,* 305–316.

Orem, D. E. (1971). *Nursing: Concepts of practice.* New York: McGraw-Hill.

Orem, D. E. (1980). *Nursing: Concepts of practice* (2nd ed.). New York: McGraw-Hill.

Orem, D. E. (1983a). The family coping with a medical illness. Analysis and application of Orem's theory. In I. W. Clements & F. B. Roberts, *Family health. A theoretical approach to nursing care* (pp. 385–386). New York: Wiley.

Orem, D. E. (1983b). The family experiencing emotional crisis. Analysis and application of Orem's self-care deficit theory. In I. W. Clements & F. B. Roberts, *Family health. A theoretical approach to nursing care* (pp. 367–368). New York: Wiley.

Orem, D. E. (1985). *Nursing: Concepts of practice* (3rd ed.). New York: McGraw-Hill.

Reed, K. (1982). The Neuman Systems Model: A basis for family psychosocial assessment and intervention. In B. Neuman, *The Neuman Systems Model. Application to nursing education and practice* (pp. 188–195). Norwalk, CT: Appleton-Century-Crofts.

Reed, K. S. (1989). Family theory related to the Neuman Systems Model. In B. Neuman, *The Neuman Systems Model. Application to nursing education and practice* (2nd ed., pp. 385–395). Norwalk, CT: Appleton and Lange.

Reed, P. G. (1986). The developmental conceptual framework: Nursing reformulations and applications for family therapy. In A. L. Whall, *Family therapy theory for nursing. Four approaches* (pp. 69–91). Norwalk, CT: Appleton-Century-Crofts.

Reeder, S. R., Mastroianni, L., Martin, L. L., & Fitzpatrick, E. (1976). *Maternity nursing* (13th ed.). Philadelphia: Lippincott.

Reeder, S. R., Mastroianni, L., & Martin, L. L. (1983). *Maternity nursing* (15th ed.). Philadelphia: Lippincott.

Reinerston, B. (1963). The patient is part of a family. *American Journal of Nursing, 63,* 106–107.

Rogers, M. E. (1970). *Introduction to the theoretical basis of nursing.* Philadelphia: F. A. Davis.

Rogers, M. E. (1980). Nursing: A science of unitary man. In J. P. Riehl & C. Roy, *Conceptual models for nursing practice* (2nd ed., pp. 329–337). New York: Appleton-Century-Crofts.

Rogers, M. E. (1983). Science of unitary human beings: A paradigm for nursing. In I. W. Clements & F. G. Roberts, *Family health. A theoretical approach to nursing care* (pp. 219–228). New York: Wiley.

Rogers, M. E. (1986). Science of unitary human beings. In V. M. Malinski (Ed.), *Explorations on Martha Rogers' science of unitary human beings* (pp. 3–8).

Rogers, M. E. (1990). Nursing: Science of unitary, irreducible, human beings: Update, 1990. In E. A. M. Barrett, *Visions of Rogers' science-based nursing* (pp. 5–11). New York: National League for Nursing.

Ross, M. M., & Helmer, H. (1988). A comparative analysis of Neuman's model using the individual and family as the units of care. *Public Health Nursing, 5,* 30–36.

Roy, C. (1976). *Introduction to nursing. An adaptation model.* Englewood Cliffs, NJ: Prentice-Hall.

Roy, C. (1983). Roy adaptation model. In I. W. Clements & F. B. Roberts, *Family health. A theoretical approach to nursing care* (pp. 255–278). New York: Wiley.

Roy, C. (1984). *Introduction to nursing. An adaptation model* (2nd ed.). Englewood Cliffs, NJ: Prentice-Hall.

Roy, C., & Roberts, S. L. (1981). Theory construction in nursing. An adaptation model. Englewood Cliffs, NJ: Prentice-Hall.

Rubin, R. (1984). *Maternal identity and the maternal experience.* New York: Springer.

Sherwen, L. N. (1987). *Psychosocial dimensions of the pregnant family.* New York: Springer.

Smiley, O. (1973). The family-centered approach—challenge to public health nurses. *International Nursing Review, 20,* 49–50.

Smith, L. (1983). A conceptual model of families incorporating an adolescent mother and child into the household. *Advances in Nursing Science 6,* (1), 45–60.

Smoyak, S. (1975). *The psychiatric nurse as a family therapist.* New York: Wiley.

Steele, S. (1981). *Child health and the family. Nursing concepts and management.* New York: Masson Publishing USA.

Stewart, H. (1908). In quarantine with diphtheria. *Trained Nurse, 41,* 92–94.

Tadych, R. (1985). Nursing in multiperson units. The family. In Riehl-Sisca, J. P., *The science and art of self-care* (pp. 49–55). Norwalk, CT: Appleton-Century-Crofts.

Tooley, S. (1905). *The Life of Florence Nightingale* (2nd ed.). London: Macmillan.

Wald, L. (1904). The treatment of families in which there is sickness. *American Journal of Nursing, 4,* 427–428, 515–519, 602–606.

Whall, A. L. (1981). Nursing theory and the assessment of families. *Journal of Psychiatric Nursing and Mental Health Services, 19*(1), 30–36.

Whall, A. L. (1986a). *Family therapy theory for nursing. Four approaches.* Norwalk, CT: Appleton-Century-Crofts.

Whall, A. L. (1986b). Strategic family therapy: Nursing reformulations and applications. In A. L. Whall, *Family therapy theory for nursing. Four approaches* (pp. 51–67). Norwalk, CT: Appleton-Century-Crofts.

Wright, L. M., & Leahey, M. (1984). *Nurses and families. A guide to family assessment and intervention.* Philadelphia: F. A. Davis.

Zabriskie, L. (1934). *Nurses' handbook of obstetrics.* Philadelphia: Lippincott.

CHAPTER

2

An Analysis of the Concept of Family[1]

MERYN E. STUART, Ph.D., R.N.

This chapter presents a systematic analysis of the concept family. The analysis follows the guidelines for concept analysis proposed by Walker and Avant (1988). "Concept analysis," according to Walker and Avant, "is a strategy that allows us to examine the attributes or characteristics of a concept" (p. 35). The concept analysis presented in this chapter encompasses the following eight steps:

1. Select a concept.
2. Determine the aim or purpose of the analysis.
3. Identify all uses of the concept that you can discover.
4. Determine the defining attributes.
5. Construct a model case.
6. Construct borderline, related, contrary, invented, and illegitimate cases.
7. Identify antecedents and consequences.
8. Define empirical referents
   (Wilson, cited by Walker and Avant, 1988, p. 37).

[1]An earlier version of this chapter was completed during doctoral study at the University of Pennsylvania, for which the Ontario Ministry of Health generously provided the funds in the form of a fellowship.

SELECTION OF A CONCEPT

Family is the most basic concept of interest in any nursing theory about the family. Family was, therefore, selected for analysis over family phenomena such as family health or family nursing. Moreover, given the current early stage of family theory development in nursing, clarification of the basic underlying concept is necessary.

AIM OF THE ANALYSIS

The aim of this concept analysis is to develop a comprehensive theoretical definition of family and, therefore, to clarify the meaning of family. The theoretical definition developed through the analysis then can be used to formulate an operational definition that identifies one or more instruments that empirically measure the concept.

Family is a highly politicized concept that has been presumed to be "natural" and universal in its traditional form. A multiplicity of different issues and social alarms, such as relations between the sexes and child abuse, has been projected onto the family, depending on the historical and social context within which the concept is analyzed. A precise definition will enable scholars to reflect the theoretical basis of the concept accurately.

USES OF THE CONCEPT FAMILY

Uses of the concept family were gleaned from several sources, including dictionaries, thesaurusi, colleagues of the author, and recognized experts in the field of family study. In addition, a 15-year (1974–1989) review of the family literature in nursing, medicine, sociology, and psychology was conducted.

It is important to point out that the concept of family often is not explicitly defined in reports of family nursing research (Feetham, 1984), nor is it clearly defined in many theoretical and clinical discussions of the family. The definition may, however, be induced from the individuals who are the focus of attention, such as a mother and her child. It may be that the omission of an explicit definition is due to a common belief in our society that "we all know a family when we see one" (Walters, 1982, p. 841). Unfortunately, this omission has created difficulties in identifying all literature dealing with families.

ATTRIBUTES OF THE CONCEPT FAMILY

The dictionary (*Webster's Third*, 1971, p. 821) definition of the noun family alludes to a variety of meanings, including (a) a group of persons of common ancestry (clan); (b) a group of persons living under one roof;

(c) a group of things having common features or properties; and (d) the basic biosocial unit in society having as its nucleus two or more adults living together and cooperating in the care and rearing of their own or adopted children. Family has been used to denote one's children, as in "the young mother was seen shepherding her family down the street." Family also is used as an adjective in many colloquial ways, for example, "family farm," "family style," "family man," "family affair," and "in a family way." This chapter focuses on human families because human beings constitute nursing's distinctive perspective.

An analysis of the literature revealed the following attributes of the concept of family:

1. A social system or unit that is self-defined by its members and is not a constant, that is, change and development are inherent.
2. The members may or may not be related by birth, adoption, or marriage and may or may not live under one roof.
3. The unit may or may not contain dependent children.
4. There must be commitment and attachment among members that develop over time and have some notion of future obligation.
5. The unit carries out the relevant functions of caregiving, that is, protection, nourishment, and socialization of its members, including providing the primary source for children to learn cultural values.

The following section of this chapter will explicate and describe the basic attributes of the family's varying structure as a system that functions as caregiver. The unique family characteristic is a commitment to a future obligation to the integrity of its members, as well as to the unit as a whole.

The Family as a System

The view of the family as a system has received considerable attention in the past 20 years as general system theory has become one of the predominant perspectives in nursing and other disciplines (Murphy, 1986). Family system theorists conceptualize the family as an open system that functions in relation to its broader sociocultural life cycle (Walsh, 1982) and historical context (Whall, 1986). As interactional systems, families operate according to rules and principles that apply to all systems, including interdependence, interrelatedness, nonsummativity, circular causality, equifinality, and homeostasis. Major family theorists claim that family systems theory has provided a general theoretical orientation for many marital and family therapists (Olson, Russell, and Sprenkle, 1980; Walsh, 1982). Conversely, others claim that general system theory has been misused and misapplied in family situations, and that family specialists are unable to define the family as a system or even as a group (Galligan, 1982).

A review of family nursing literature revealed evidence that families are regarded as systems (Friedemann, 1989; Lewandowski and Jones, 1988; Whall, 1981; Wright and Leahey, 1984). Fawcett (1975) noted the utility of a systems approach, explaining that "the systems approach fosters a conception of the family as a complex system and provides an opportunity for incorporation of other theoretical models" (p. 113). She cautioned, however, that general system theory "cannot be fully and uncritically adopted for use by nursing" (p. 113). And Mercer (1989) pointed out that "many of the systems concepts or theories are difficult to operationalize" (p. 23).

More recently, major nursing theorists (King, 1983; Neuman, 1983; Rogers, 1983; Roy, 1983) have used the notion of the family as a system as a starting point for their particular perspectives of the family. Their conceptualizations of the family are discussed in Chapter 1 of this book.

The Structure of the Family Unit

Miller (1974) noted that "the definition of the family varies in different societies and for different purposes" (p. 480). For statistical purposes, the family frequently is defined as a household of those who live together and who are related by blood, marriage, or adoption. This definition, however, fails to include extended family members, cohabiting and gay or lesbian couples, "blended" (stepparent) families, groups of single people living together, and other variations. Even pets can be seen as family members. Indeed, Sussman (1979) and Macklin (1980) maintained that the traditional way of viewing the family as one man (the primary provider) and one woman with children in a legal, lifelong, sexually exclusive marriage is no longer tenable. In fact, the majority of households in the Unites States no longer represent traditional nuclear families (Macklin, 1980).

In nursing, almost all research dealing with the family focuses on the marital dyad or nuclear families with children (Gilliss, 1989). Very little has been published on nontraditional family forms, although recently a few nurses have begun to look at single-parent families (Duffy, 1984; Norbeck and Sheiner, 1982), stepfather families (Stern, 1982), and extended families (Bunting, 1989; Phillips and Rempusheski, 1986; Uphold and Harper, 1986; Robinson, 1988).

Commitment and Attachment

Most literature dealing with the family includes some mention of an attachment and a commitment that bind family members together and obligate them to a future. These characteristics are thought to differentiate families from ad hoc groups. Walters (1982) explained:

> The qualities of commitment and attachment may so affect family processes as to produce a quality in family groups that is not duplicated in other groups. . . . Apparently, attachment can hold a family together even when the structure of the family is dysfunctional for some members and when relationships are hurtful (p. 847).

Walters acknowledged the complexity of commitment and attachment and noted the lack of knowledge about exactly what processes link family members together.

Mauksch (1974) maintained that the family unit consists of "two major components: the unit members and the 'linking processes'" (p. 522). Although the nature and meaning of the linking processes are virtually unexplored, Mauksch characterized them as "emissions and infusions which occur among the unit members [including] modes of relating and the emergence of meaning in verbal and other forms of communication" (p. 523).

In the nursing literature, emotional bonding and/or complementarity frequently are included in definitions of the family (Gilliss, Roberts, Highley, and Martinson, 1989; Leavitt, 1982; Logan, 1978; Murray and Huelskoetter, 1983; Sedgwick, 1981). Knafl and Grace (1978), however, decried the lack of knowledge about common family processes and experiences.

Family Functions

Most definitions of the family seem to be wedded, either implicitly or explicitly, to the functions of the family (Ericksen and Leonard, 1983; Forrest, 1981; Gantman, 1980; Gilliss, 1989; Pratt, 1976). Within nursing, many authors have discussed the importance of the family in the transference of values related to health and other behaviors (Forrest, 1981; Oseasohn, 1981; Warner, 1981). Moreover, a variety of nursing assessment tools (Edison, 1979; Ericksen and Leonard, 1983; Wright and Leahey, 1984) and research instruments (Roberts and Feetham, 1983) refer to the assessment of functioning as if this were a core attribute.

Caregiving, within the context of both health and illness, is central to the discussion of functioning. In what is commonly called "functional" or "healthy" families, the family provides the protection, nourishment, stimulation for growth, and socialization, among other things, that are necessary for an individual's health.

Family functioning in terms of coping processes, especially in situations involving chronic illness or disability, has been a topic of much recent nursing research (Blank, Clark, Longman, and Atwood, 1989; Bunting, 1989; Lewandowski and Jones, 1988; Phillips and Rempusheski, 1986; Robinson, 1988; Woods, Yates, and Primono, 1989). When a family member is ill, the unit must somehow find the resources to care for that individual and still maintain homeostatic functioning. Frequently, people look to the community for the resources, yet "community care for the elderly or disabled is, to a very large extent, family care" (Goodman, 1986, p. 705).

A MODEL CASE OF THE CONCEPT FAMILY

The next step of the concept analysis is to develop a model case. Walker and Avant (1988) explained that "a model case is a 'real life' example of the use of the concept that includes *all* the critical attributes and *no* attributes of any other concept. That is, the model case should be a pure case of the concept, a paradigmatic example" (p. 40).

The model case, which contains all of the attributes of the concept of family, may be stated as follows:

> A father, mother, and two children, aged 10 and 12 years, are seated around a dinner table discussing how the family will integrate their grandmother, who is coming to live with them permanently in a few days. They want to be sure that they make her feel welcome and wanted when she arrives. Each member of the family takes a turn at discussing how he or she might make grandmother feel "at home" and loved because the family members believe it is important for everyone to feel this way. The children discuss with each other and their parents how they will help each other adjust to sharing a bedroom, because grandmother will need one of their rooms. The parents praise the children for their caring attitude.

This is a paradigmatic example of the concept of family because it depicts parents and children, who are related by marriage and birth, interrelating and coping with the change required by incorporating another family member into the household. The system must use feedback, readjust itself, and find innovative ways to deal with the change. There is a clear commitment to the future together which will involve new challenges and may result in different patterns of dependence and relationship. There also is a clear regard for the emotional and social needs of the children, as they are being asked for their input into the process. They are being nourished with praise and a respect for their points of view. The children also are being socialized according to the family values of sharing information and resources, in this case physical space within the home.

OTHER CASES OF THE CONCEPT FAMILY

The next step of the concept analysis is to construct borderline, related, contrary, invented, and illegitimate cases.

A Borderline Case

"Borderline cases," according to Walker and Avant (1988), "are those examples or instances that contain some of the critical attributes of the concept being examined but not all of them. . . . These cases are inconsistent in some way and as such they help us see why the true or model case is not [inconsistent]" (pp. 40–41). Borderline cases are especially helpful in clarifying the critical attributes of the concept.

The following borderline case contains all of the attributes of the concept of family except carrying out the functions of providing necessary nourishment and protection for one of its members. This member has been the victim of physical and sexual abuse by the father, and yet the family remains together, committed to a future attachment and coping in some way with system change. The family may be characterized as "dysfunctional" because one member is scapegoated and abused.

> A father, mother, and two children ages 10 and 12 are sitting around the dinner table. The father looks very angry, the mother and younger daughter seem nervous and anxious, and the elder daughter looks angry and defiant as she argues with her father about going out with her boyfriend and other friends. The father insists that his daughter is "grounded" and cannot go out with her friends because she was late for supper and did not do all of her chores. The daughter, not wanting to be grounded on a Saturday night, continues to argue and threatens that she will go out anyway. In a violent rage, the father jumps out of his chair, pulls the daughter so roughly from the table that her feet fly up in the air and land in the food and hot gravy on the table. The father then takes her into her room and beats her. The mother, shaking with fear, instructs the younger daughter to be quiet and eat her supper. The younger daughter, crying, screams her anger at her father's outburst, then finishes her meal.

A Related Case

Walker and Avant (1988) noted that related cases "demonstrate ideas that are very similar to the main concept but . . . differ from them when examined closely" (p. 41). In other words, related cases are similar to the concept of interest and are connected to the concept in some way, but they do not contain the critical attributes. A concept that could be developed into a related case is "social support network." There is a sense that this concept is related to the concept of family, but the relationship is not clear.

More specifically, social support is a concept referring to "interpersonally supportive behaviors and relationships" (Tilden, 1985, p. 199). Meister (1984) pointed out that much of what the family contributes to members can be called social support, and that when a member is in need, social support may be seen as "the provision of direct aid, expression of affect and/or the affirmation of agreement or valuation of thoughts, feelings or actions" (p. 61). In contrast, family social support also has been conceptualized as "a process of relationships between the family [unit] and its social environment" (Kane, 1988, p. 24).

The following example illustrates a social support network that functions for the benefit of both the individual and the family unit.

> A 40-year-old man with advanced multiple sclerosis finds that neither he nor his wife is able to care for him and he must be institutionalized. He has no relatives other than his wife, who is an active young professional. Friends and colleagues develop a social support network, and each makes a commitment to visit him at the hospital, take him out for recreational evenings, and handle his legal affairs. The network of friends is committed to support the man and his wife so that both can continue to get the most out of the remaining time of his life. The aims are to provide an atmosphere of caring and affirmation, assisting him to maintain a sense of belonging to an extended family that will meet his needs.

A Contrary Case

"Contrary cases," according to Walker and Avant (1988), "are those that are clear examples of 'not the concept'" (p. 41). It is clear that they contain none of the critical attributes of the concept of interest. An example of a contrary case would be a group of adults who are waiting in line for theater tickets. They may interact on a superficial level, but they will be together for only a short period of time. Furthermore, although they share the common goal of buying tickets, they will not commit themselves to any future interaction or attachment. They serve no caregiving function for one another, and they cannot be viewed as a system in the same sense as the family system.

Invented and Illegitimate Cases

Walker and Avant (1988) explained that "invented cases are cases that are constructed using ideas outside our own experience. They often read like science fiction" (Walker and Avant, 1988, p. 42). Taking the concept out of its ordinary context and putting it into an invented one facilitates understanding of the critical attributes of the concept of interest. Invented cases, then, may contain all the attributes of the model case, as is evident in the following example.

> Suppose that a group of large and small humanlike beings, of indeterminate gender, set up housekeeping on earth and appeared to look after one another, although they did not have the same emotional and physical requirements as earth people. Suppose also that the humanlike beings stayed together for years but did not appear to interact with earth people.

An illegitimate case is an example of the concept used in an improper manner. The meaning given the concept is completely different from all others (Walker and Avant, 1988). In this case, the meaning of "family" when used by a biologist to refer to the subdivision above a genus in the classification of plants and animals is entirely different from the meaning of the term as used in this chapter.

ANTECEDENTS AND CONSEQUENCES OF THE CONCEPT FAMILY

The next step in concept analysis is to identify antecedents and consequences of the concept. Walker and Avant (1988) explained that "antecedents are those events or incidents that must occur *prior to* the occurrence of the concept. . . . Consequences, on the other hand, are those events or incidents that occur as a *result* of the occurrence of the concept" (p. 43).

Identification of antecedents helps further clarify the attributes of the concept, because the two cannot overlap or be the same. One antecedent of the concept of family is the existence of a community of human beings, which is required as a source of potential family members. The community of human beings, in turn, implies a culture and a society or a social context for the family. Other antecedents can be marriage, moving in together, motivation for commitment and attachment, and need for care and protection.

Specification of consequences often facilitates identification of neglected ideas, variables, and relationships that require study. Consequences of the concept of family include status in society by virtue of being a member of a particular family, identity, illness, health, stress, joy, gratification of members' needs for protection and nourishment, as well as violence and abuse of members as a result of conflict and scapegoating. Articulation of the consequences of the concept family serves to remind us that not all families are healthy or happy environments for their members.

EMPIRICAL REFERENTS OF THE CONCEPT FAMILY

The final step in concept analysis is the identification of empirical referents. Empirical referents are actual phenomena that demonstrate the occurrence of the concept in the observable world. Critical attributes and empirical referents are essentially identical when the concept of interest is concrete, such as height or weight. In contrast, when the concept is abstract, its critical attributes usually are abstract as well, so that identification of the means by which the concept may be observed becomes important (Walker and Avant, 1988). In the case of the concept family, which is relatively abstract, one would have to look for observable evidence of the critical attributes, such as responses to instruments designed to measure self-definition as a family, commitment, attachment, and interdependence, as well as caregiving functions.

CONCLUSION

An analysis of the concept of family has been presented in this chapter. The analysis led to identification of five critical attributes:

1. The family is a system or unit.
2. Its members may or may not be related and may or may not live together.
3. The unit may or may not contain children.
4. There is commitment and attachment among unit members that includes future obligation.
5. The unit caregiving functions consist of protection, nourishment, and socialization of its members.

In concluding, it is important to point out that the analysis failed to clarify differences that might exist between the family and an ad hoc small group or a social support network. Neither of these entities may define itself as a family, but either one could exhibit the attributes of a family, depending on the definition of commitment and attachment used and the level of caregiving function. Future work should be directed toward a clear, unambiguous definition of family, especially as the concept is used within the discipline of nursing. Such a definition would serve as a starting point for development of instruments to measure the concept and for systematic middle-range family theory development in nursing.

REFERENCES

Blank, J. J., Clark, L., Longman, A. J., & Atwood, J. R. (1989). Perceived home needs of cancer patients and their caregivers. *Cancer Nursing, 12*, 78–84.

Bunting, S. M. (1989). Stress on caregivers of the elderly. *Advances in Nursing Science, 11*(2), 63–73.

Duffy, M. (1984). Transcending options: Creating a milieu for practicing high-level wellness. *Health Care for Women International, 5*, 145–161.

Edison, C. E. (1979). Family assessment guidelines. In D. P. Hymovich & M. N. Barnard (Eds.), *Family health care. Vol. 1. General perspectives* (2nd ed., pp. 264–279). New York: McGraw-Hill.

Ericksen, J., & Leonard, L. G. (1983). A framework for family nursing. *Nursing Papers, 15*(1), 34–50.

Fawcett, J. (1975). The family as a living open system: An emerging conceptual framework for nursing. *International Nursing Review, 22,* 113–116.

Feetham, S. (1984). Family research: Issues and directions for nursing. In H. H. Werley & J. J. Fitzpatrick (Eds.), *Annual Review of Nursing Research* (Vol. 2, pp. 3–25). New York: Springer.

Forrest, J. (1981). The family: The focus for health behavior generation. *Health Values: Achieving High-Level Wellness, 5,* 138–144.

Friedemann, M-L. (1989). The concept of family nursing. *Journal of Advanced Nursing, 14,* 211–216.

Galligan, R. J. (1982). Innovative techniques: Siren or rose. *Journal of Marriage and the Family, 44,* 875–886.

Gantman, C. A. (1980). A closer look at families that work well. *International Journal of Family Therapy, 2,* 106–119.

Gilliss, C. L. (1989). Family research in nursing. In C. L. Gilliss, B. L. Highley, B. M. Roberts, & I. M. Martinson (Eds.), *Toward a science of family nursing* (pp. 37–62). New York: Addison-Wesley.

Gillis, C. L., Roberts, B. M., Highley, B. L., & Martinson, I. M. (1989). What is family nursing? In C. L. Gilliss, B. L. Highley, B. M. Roberts, & I. M. Martinson (Eds.), *Toward a science of family nursing* (pp. 64–73). New York: Addison-Wesley.

Goodman, C. (1986). Research on the informal career: A selected literature review. *Journal of Advanced Nursing, 11,* 705–712.

Kane, C. F. (1988). Family social support: Toward a conceptual model. *Advances in Nursing Science, 10*(2), 18–25.

King, I. M. (1983). King's theory of nursing. In I. W. Clements & F. C. Roberts, *Family health. A theoretical approach to nursing care* (pp. 177–188). New York: Wiley.

Knafl, K. A., & Grace, H. K. (Eds.). (1978). *Families across the life cycle. Studies for nursing.* Boston: Little, Brown.

Leavitt, M. B. (1982). *Families at risk. Primary prevention in nursing practice.* Boston: Little, Brown.

Lewandowski, W., & Jones, S. L. (1988). The family with cancer. Nursing interventions throughout the course of living with cancer. *Cancer Nursing, 11,* 313–321.

Logan, B. (1978). The nurse and the family: Dominant theories and perspectives in the literature. In K. A. Knafl & H. K. Grace (Eds.), *Families across the life cycle. Studies for nursing* (pp. 3–14). Boston: Little, Brown.

Macklin, E. D. (1980). Nontraditional family forms: A decade of research. *Journal of Marriage and the Family, 42,* 905–922.

Mauksch, H. O. (1974). A social science basis for conceptualizing family health. *Social Science and Medicine, 8,* 521–528.

Meister, S. (1984). Family well-being. In J. Campbell & J. Humphreys (Eds.). *Nursing care of victims of family violence* (pp. 53–73). Reston, VA: Reston.

Mercer, R. (1989). Theoretical perspectives on the family. In C. L. Gilliss, B. L. Highley, B. M. Roberts, & I. M. Martinson (Eds), *Toward a science of family nursing* (pp. 9–36). New York: Addison-Wesley.

Miller, F. J. W. (1974). The epidemiological approach to the family as a unit in health statistics and the measurement of community health. *Social Science and Medicine, 8,* 479–482.

Murphy, S. (1986). Family study and nursing research. *Image: The Journal of Nursing Scholarship, 18,* 170–174.

Murray, R. B., & Huelskoetter, M. M. (1983). *Psychiatric/mental health nursing. Giving emotional care.* Englewood Cliffs, NJ: Prentice-Hall.

Neuman, B. (1983). Family intervention using the Betty Neuman health-care systems model. In I. W. Clements & F. C. Roberts, *Family health. A theoretical approach to nursing care* (pp. 239–254). New York: Wiley.

Norbeck, J. S., & Sheiner, M. (1982). Sources of social support related to single parent functioning. *Research in Nursing and Health, 5,* 3–12.

Olson, D. H., Russell, C. S., & Sprenkle, D. H. (1980). Marital and family therapy: A decade review. *Journal of Marriage and the Family, 42,* 973–993.

Oseasohn, C. (1981). Introduction to basic curriculum work. *Nursing Papers, 13*(1), 38–39.

Phillips, L. R., & Rempusheski, V. F. (1986). Caring for the frail elderly at home: Toward a theoretical explanation of the dynamics of poor quality family caregiving. *Advances in Nursing Science, 8*(4), 62–84.

Pratt, L. (1976). *Family structure and effective health behavior: The energized family.* Boston: Houghton Mifflin.

Roberts, C. S., & Feetham, S. L. (1983). Assessing family functioning across three areas of relationships. *Nursing Research, 31,* 231–235.

Robinson, K. M. (1988). A social skills training program for adult caregivers. *Advances in Nursing Science, 10*(2), 59–72.

Rogers, M. E. (1983). Science of unitary human beings: A paradigm for nursing. In I. W. Clements & F. C. Roberts, *Family health. A theoretical approach to nursing care* (pp. 219–228). New York: Wiley.

Roy, C. (1983). Roy adaptation model. In I. W. Clements & F. C. Roberts, *Family health. A theoretical approach to nursing care* (pp. 255–278). New York: Wiley.

Sedgwick, R. (1981). *Family mental health. Theory and practice.* St. Louis: Mosby.

Stern, P. N. (1982). Affiliating in stepfather families: Teachable strategies leading to step-father-child friendship. *Western Journal of Nursing Research, 4,* 76–89.

Sussman, M. B. (1979). Actions and services for the new family. In D. Reiss & H. Hoffman (Eds.), *The American family. Dying or developing.* New York: Plenum Press.

Tilden, V. P. (1985). Issues of conceptualization and measurement of social support in the construction of nursing theory. *Research in Nursing and Health, 8,* 199–206.

Uphold, C. R., & Harper, D. C. (1986). Methodological issues in intergenerational family nursing research. *Advances in Nursing Science, 8*(3), 38–49.

Walker, L. O., & Avant, K. C. (1988). *Strategies for theory construction in nursing* (2nd ed.). Norwalk, CT: Appleton and Lange.

Walsh, F. (1982). Conceptualizations of normal family functioning. In F. Walsh (Ed.), *Normal family processes* (pp. 3–44). New York: Guilford Press.

Walters, L. H. (1982). Are families different from other groups? *Journal of Marriage and the Family, 44,* 841–850.

Warner, M. (1981). Health and nursing: Evolving one concept by involving the other. *Nursing Papers, 13*(1), 10–17.

Webster's Third New International Dictionary (1971). Springfield, MA: Merriam.

Whall, A. L. (1981). Nursing theory and the assessment of families. *Journal of Psychiatric Nursing and Mental Health Services, 19*(1), 30–36.

Whall, A. L. (1986). The family as the unit of care in nursing: A historical review. *Public Health Nursing, 3,* 240–249.

Woods, N. F., Yates, B. C., & Primono, J. (1989). Supporting families during chronic illness. *Image: The Journal of Nursing Scholarship, 21,* 46–50.

Wright, L., & Leahey, M. (1984). *Nurses and families. A guide to family assessment and intervention.* Philadelphia: F. A. Davis.

CHAPTER

3

Philosophy of Science and Family Nursing Theory Development

NANCY TRYGAR ARTINIAN, Ph.D., R.N.

The scientific present and future of family nursing theory can benefit from philosophy of science. This chapter presents a discussion of the implications of the philosophy of science for progress in development of nursing knowledge about the family. The first section of the chapter provides a historical overview of philosophy of science. The second section presents different philosophical views of goals of knowledge development and scientific progress. The third section examines the implications of philosophy of science for middle-range family theory development and research in nursing.

PHILOSOPHY OF SCIENCE

Philosophy of science is generally regarded as a field of inquiry concerned with philosophical problems raised by science, such as the meaning of scientific concepts, laws, and theories; the structure of science; and the methodology by which science attains its results (Wallace, 1979). Philosophers of science are primarily concerned with three kinds of questions (Brody, 1970):

1. implications of new scientific findings for traditional philosophical issues

2. analysis of fundamental concepts of the scientific discipline
3. the nature of the goals of the scientific disciplines and the methods scientists employ to attain those goals

History of Philosophy of Science

During the past 60 years the philosophy of science has moved through five developmental stages (Polkinghorne, 1983). The first phase consisted of the received view or logical positivism developed by the Vienna Circle in the 1920s and 1930s. Members of the Vienna Circle included Schlick, Neurath, Feigl, Carnap, and Godel. The received view believed that knowledge was contained only in statements that were descriptions of direct observation. Phenomena needed to be observable or required a set of directly observable characteristics the presence or absence of which could be intersubjectively ascertained by direct observation. For example, verbal descriptions of pain, moaning, crying, pacing, withdrawal from social contact, and guarding the affected area could be a set of directly observable characteristics for the phenomenon of pain.

In addition, logical positivists believed that the goal of science was a network of knowledge statements linked together by deductive logic. The only kinds of statements assuring *certainty* or absolute truth were those grounded in observation and belonging to a deductive network system. Modus tollens is an example of deductive logic:

> If H is true, then so is I
> *But I is not true*
> H is not true (Hempel, 1966, p. 7).

Adherents to logical positivism were not interested in examining the activity of science — they wanted to see the results. Logical positivists were concerned with how theories were justified rather than on how they were discovered. Philosophers allied to this belief system were Hempel, Reichenbach, and Ayer (Polkinghorne, 1983).

The second developmental phase of the philosophy of science was a period of refinements and improvements by the proponents of the received view. The second phase of the development of the received view was expanded to include purely theoretical terms. Also, the aim of science broadened not only to include a description of events or phenomena but also to explain and to understand why events occur as they do.

> The expansion allowed for a form of explanation which answers the question of why an event has happened by describing the law under which the event has occurred. These laws were explained by being subsumed under more general laws, and finally all events were explained from a network of deductive relationships stemming from a few basic axioms (Polkinghorne, 1983, p. 71).

Explanations by deductive subsumption under general laws were called deductive-nomological explanations. The following is an example of this type of explanation:

> The probability for persons exposed to measles to catch the disease is high. (general law)
> *Jim was exposed to the measles.*
> Jim caught the measles (Hempel, 1966, p. 59).

All events could be explained from a network of deductive relationships stemming from a few basic axioms. Hempel continued to be a prominent philosopher during this phase.

The third phase took place in the 1960s and was a period of criticism of the received view which proposed to show that the received view was untenable and should be abandoned in favor of an alternative approach. One criticism generated about the received view was that it is impossible to distinguish between direct observation and theoretical terms; in other words, theory-independent observations do not exist. Achinstein and Quine were two philosophers during this phase who suggested that concepts are theory dependent. Achinstein argued that terms used by scientists are such, and that to understand the concepts they use, one must have at least some knowledge of the theory in which they appear. For example,

> To understand the expression "straight flush" one must know at least the rudiments of poker, whereas this is not so with the expression "queen of hearts" which is common to all card games and carries with it none of the "special language" of any of them (Achinstein, 1968, p. 182).

Another criticism about the received view was that theories cannot be viewed as entirely axiomatizable or formalizable; rather, the formalization involved in systematizing theories should be semantic, not syntactical. Suppe (1977) proposed that the importance of theory rested in its meaning rather than in its linguistic formations. For example, the statements "Chronic illness within a family alters family roles and responsibilities" and "Family roles and responsibilities are affected by chronic illness within the family" express the same meaning but are syntactically different (Polkinghorne, 1983).

The final criticism about the received view was that linking of the theory to the world must allow for time sequences (causal analysis) and experimental correlations (Polkinghorne, 1983). Inductive arguments or empirical generalizations as an alternative description of the nature of science was put forth. It was believed that research did not have to be a test of hypotheses derived from a theoretical network but may be a study of a circumscribed set of variables that produce statements of regularity in a set of observations. Empirical generalizations stand on their own, independent of theoretical deductions, and thus need to be judged by the degree of confirmation rather than by the criterion used for deductive arguments, which is that the truth of the conclusions is guaranteed (Polkinghorne, 1983).

During the 1960s and 1970s alternate descriptions of the nature of science were offered. The fourth developmental stage was a period referred to as Weltanschauungen, or world outlook analysis. During this period it was believed that knowledge was relative to one's perspective, that is, neither pure sense data nor formal logic could provide an absolute foundation for knowledge. The character of one's knowledge, the categories according to which experience is formed, were functions of one's Weltanschauung.

During the fourth phase truth was not based on absolute certainty; rather, truth was a function of one's world picture. Wittgenstein, a prominent philosopher of this phase, maintained that logic and grammar were historical products. "Logic does not lie outside one's world picture" (Polkinghorne, 1983, p. 108). The task of science became a task of discovering what was held to be true within a given community. The world view of scientists conceptually shaped the way in which the world was experienced and was closely associated with the language system one used to speak of understanding the world. One's conceptual apparatus determined what one experienced as fact. Purely objective fact could not exist independent of human nature. For example, to understand the concept family health, the concept would be examined from the perceptions of a particular family in the context of their environment and reality.

Prominent philosophers of the fourth period were Polanyi, Hanson, Feyerbend, and Kuhn. Philosophers of the fourth phase contended that all perspectives were equal in their attempts to approach knowledge. However, critics of this phase stated that the Weltanschauungen view destroyed the objectivity of scientific knowledge, making knowledge subjective and irrational and reducing knowledge to sociocultural group prejudice (Suppe, 1977, p. 700).

The fifth and current developmental stage of the philosophy of science, labeled historical realism by Suppe (1977), accepts the insight of the Weltanschauung position that science is a human activity that takes place in various historical contexts rather than a process of formal logic attaining timeless truths (Polkinghorne, 1983, p. 116). However, philosophers of this phase do not agree that being historical necessarily implies that various scientific statements are true only for their contexts. This phase is characterized by a renewed belief that science does work and that it provides reliable information about the world. Science does far more than make knowledge claims that are coherent only within a certain system; it seeks to say something that corresponds to how things really are (Polkinghorne, 1983, p. 117). It also became apparent during this phase that science should be concerned with the process of discovery as well as with the process of justification.

Philosophers of the fifth phase emphasize the use of various patterns of reason rather than simply logic to build knowledge. It is through the processes of reasoning that hypotheses are suggested and developed, and it is through the processes of reasoning that knowledge claims are evaluated. The patterns of reasoning yield conclusions that go beyond the logic entailments of deductive logic. These patterns are different systems of rules of science, and deductive logic is merely one pattern of rationality (Polkinghorne, 1983, p. 117).

Although the fifth phase has its roots in the 1960s, it is still in its beginning stages today. Some philosophers of this phase are Shapere, Radnitzky, Laudan, and Toulmin. The hope of the philosophers of the fifth phase is that a re-examination of science will reveal those essential features which allow it to produce knowledge. "Historical realism does not place science into a deductive-sensation position, but opens up knowing to the whole human repertoire of judgement and action" (Polkinghorne, 1983, p. 133).

An overview of the history of philosophy of science provides direction for the future of family nursing theory development. Empiricist approaches of the logical positivists, historicist approaches from the Weltanschauungen period, and the recognition of the need for various methodologies from the historical realist period supply fruit for family nurse theorists to harvest.

GOALS OF KNOWLEDGE DEVELOPMENT AND SCIENTIFIC PROGRESS

Knowledge development involves the idea of a process occurring through time. The progress of knowledge development is always relative to some set of aims (Laudan, 1984). Determination of progress must be relativized to a certain set of ends, but there is no one appropriate set of ends. "There is no single 'right' goal for inquiry because it is evidently legitimate to engage in inquiry for a wide variety of reasons and with a wide variety of purposes" (Laudan, 1984, p. 64).

There are several philosophical views about the goals of science. Truth as the object of science represents the realist philosophical position. The realist maintains that the goal of science is to find ever truer theories about the world (Castell and Borchert, 1983). A theory is approximately true if it is explanatorily successful (Castell and Borchert, 1983). In other words, it is an aim of science to come to knowledge of how the world really is; the correspondence between theories and reality is a central aim of science (Suppe, 1977, p. 649). In sum, realists seek true theories.

Critics of the realist position state that it is impossible to achieve truth. There is no way to recognize when we have achieved these aims, and there is no way to tell whether we are moving closer to the truth. For any two theories it is impossible to tell which is closer to the truth (Laudan, 1984).

Polkinghorne (1983) avoided the truth claim when he referred to assertoric knowledge as being a goal of science:

> In assertoric knowledge, some knowledge claims are better than others, but none is beyond doubt. This is a more common-sense understanding of knowledge, for it means one can have more confidence in some knowledge claims than in others and need not make a final choice between truth and falsity (Polkinghorne, 1983, p. 279).

This position is distinct from the logical positivism position that the aim of science was to produce absolutely certain knowledge, that is, apodictic knowledge (Polkinghorne, 1983). According to Polkinghorne (1983), the goal of science becomes the creative search to understand better, and it uses whatever approaches are responsive to the particular questions and subject matters addressed.

Laudan is a prominent critic of the realist philosophical position and represents the philosophy of pragmatism. According to Laudan (1977), the single most general aim of science is problem solving. "The maximization of the empirical problems we can explain and the minimization of the anomalous and conceptual problems we generate in the process are the raison d'être of science" (Laudan, 1977, p. 124).

Laudan (1977) viewed problems as the focal point of scientific thought and theories as its end results. There are two types of problems to be solved: empirical problems and conceptual problems. "Empirical problems are substantive questions about the objects which constitute the domain of any given science" (Laudan, 1977, p. 15). "Conceptual problems are characteristics of theories and have no existence independent of the theories which exhibit them" (Laudan, 1977, p. 48). Internal conceptual problems may mean that a theory is logically inconsistent or that there is conceptual ambiguity or circularity within a theory. External conceptual problems may include one theory that is logically inconsistent with another accepted theory, two theories that are inconsistent with another accepted theory, two theories that are logically compatible but jointly implausible, or one theory that ought to reinforce another theory but fails to do so and is merely compatible with it (Laudan, 1977).

In addition to scientific aims, several authors have addressed other criteria of scientific progress. Meleis (1985) stated that progress of a discipline is measured by the scope and quality of its theories and the extent to which the community of scholars is engaged in theory development. Isolated research projects make a limited contribution to scientific progress.

At the 1987 Boston Theory Conference, Meleis discussed the need for four factors in order to progress and to build nursing knowledge. Those four factors were

1. a clear vision of a clear mission

2. identification of the nature of what it is we want to know
3. maintenance of an atmosphere of openness and skepticism
4. persistence toward developing the whole

Meleis also suggested we must know something about the people who are developing knowledge. It is not enough to evaluate the number of answered questions.

Polkinghorne (1983) offers other criteria by which to evaluate scientific progress. He states that critique of scientific progress is based on the significance of the questions asked and the fruitfulness of the answers given, as well as on the persuasiveness of the evidence and the arguments.

Kuhn, Lakatos, and Laudan have offered models of scientific progress. Kuhn's (1970) model of scientific progress is based on the paradigm that defines the problems and methods of a research field. Once a paradigm is accepted by the scientific community, the community works to solve the problems of the paradigm. This period is known as normal science. The paradigm remains until anomalies accumulate. An accumulation of anomalies signals a period of crisis during which scientists consider alternate paradigms.

Many philosophers have cited criticisms of Kuhn's model of scientific progress, for example, obscurity of the concept of paradigm, historical incorrectness, and no continuity in content from one paradigm to the next (Suppe, 1977; Gholson and Barker, 1985). In addition, Laudan (1977) cites Kuhn's failure to see the role of conceptual problems in the role of scientific debate as well as Kuhn's inability to resolve the question between a paradigm and its constituent theories.

According to Lakatos (1970), greater empirical content makes one theory more progressive than another. Lakatos's model of scientific progress is based on research programs that consist of methodological rules and produce a series of theories. A scientific research program is better than a rival if the sequence of theories produced under it shows a greater increase in content than the sequence of theories produced under the rival program. A research program is better than a competitor and contributes to progress if it has increased empirical content, that is, it has produced successful predictions and has heuristic power (Radnitzky and Anderson, 1978).

Progress according to Laudan, is judged relative to research traditions.

> A research tradition is a set of general assumptions about the entities and processes in a domain of study, and about the appropriate methods to be used for investigating the problems and constructing the theories in that domain (Laudan, 1977, p. 81).

A research tradition is a set of ontological and methodological do's and don't's (Laudan, 1977). Every research tradition is associated with a series of specific theories, each of which is designed to particularize the ontology of the research tradition.

A successful research tradition is one that leads, via its component theories, to the adequate solution of an increasing range of empirical and conceptual problems. Research traditions have a higher rate of progress if over the course of time the problem-solving effectiveness of its components has increased. Laudan (1977) has identified three characteristics of progressiveness:

1. The research tradition solved the problems which it set for itself.
2. Few if any empirical anomalies or conceptual problems were generated in the problem-solving process.
3. Over the course of time the research tradition expanded the domain of explained problems and minimized the number and importance of its remaining conceptual problems and anomalies.

It is important to note that Laudan (1977) includes increase in conceptual clarity of a theory and specifications of meaning as an important way in which a science progresses.

Family nursing or even nursing as a whole does not have the exact equivalent of paradigms, research programs, or research traditions as originally set forth by the respective authors. Within nursing, global conceptual frameworks defining broad perspectives for ways of looking at nursing phenomena exist to guide development of middle-range theories (Walker and Avant, 1988). However, conceptual frameworks such as those developed by Roy, King, or Rogers have been used rarely to generate middle-range family nursing theories.

In summary, it is apparent that there is more than one philosophical position about the appropriate aims of science. However, aims must be determined in order to evaluate the progression of knowledge development. Other criteria put forth by philosophy of science to judge scientific progress are significance of research questions asked and fruitfulness of answers given, clarity of theoretical concepts, and empirical support for theories generated from a research program or amount of problem-solving ability of theories evolving from a research tradition.

IMPLICATIONS FOR FAMILY NURSING THEORY DEVELOPMENT

There are several implications from philosophy of science for family nursing theory development. First, philosophy of science suggests a philosopher of family nursing science would conduct the following activities:

1. Analyze concepts central to family nursing theories.

2. Analyze the structure of family nursing science and its component theories.
3. Evaluate the nature of the goals in family nursing science.
4. Assess the methods to attain those goals.

Philosophy of science suggests that all science does not follow the same reasoning patterns or follow the same methodology. Patterns of reasoning may be conditioned by the content of science (Suppe, 1977). Family nursing science can benefit from using multiple methodologies. Each methodology detects and describes some aspect of a phenomenon, but each of them also misses parts of the full experience. Various knowledge claims about the same topic, each in the context of a particular methodology, can be brought together and utilized to increase the fullness of our understanding of a family phenomenon (Polkinghorne, 1983).

No one method is correct for constructing family nursing theory or conducting family nursing research. The method or pattern of reasoning must be appropriate for answering the questions being addressed. For example, certain family research questions may focus on explaining variance, exploring the strength of variable relationships, or predicting family events in the future and therefore may dictate the need for empiricist methods such as deductive reasoning, objectivity, statistical techniques, and control. Other family research questions may focus on family pattern discovery, exploring family activities holistically, or describing family values, and therefore may call for historicist approaches such as inductive reasoning or subjectivity.

Philosophy of science suggests several guidelines that can be used to evaluate the progress of family nursing theory development. The following questions may be used as an assessment framework:

1. Who in the family nursing community is involved in theory development?
2. What are the cognitive aims or goals of family nursing theory development?
3. Do family theorists have a clear vision of the discipline's scientific goals?
4. What problems are of central importance to family nursing?
5. What is the significance of the questions being asked?
6. What is the scope and quality of family nursing theories?
7. Do we have conceptual clarity?
8. Are problems being solved or questions being answered? (a pragmatic perspective) Are we converging on the truth or an understanding of how reality really is? (a realist perspective)
9. Is there empirical support for theories?
10. Is the evidence provided for theories persuasive?
11. What research methods are being used?

Clearly some of the above questions have begun to be answered. There is a recognized cadre of family nursing scholars as evidenced by the recent text *Toward a Science of Family Nursing* (Gilliss, Highley, Roberts, and Martinson, 1989), the successful International Family Nursing Conference (See Bell, Wright, Leahey, Watson, and Chenger, 1988) and the National Conference on Family Nursing (See Krentz, 1989), and the planned Second International Family Nursing Conference in May of 1991.

Family nursing theorists do have a vision of developing theoretical explanations of family behavior in health and illness. The vision is not totally clear, as manifested by continued controversy related to the family member versus family unit as appropriate units of analysis (Gilliss, 1989). Literature reviews (Artinian, 1990; Gilliss, 1989) revealed several problems of concern to family nurses: family health promotion and health behavior, family responses to actual or potential health problems, factors influencing family responses in health and illness, and nurse-family interactions. Questions being asked relative to the preceding list of problems are significant because they are generating descriptive and correlational data that can be used as a basis for deriving and testing family nursing interventions.

Family nursing scholars need a means of tracking family nursing theories and determining the scope and quality of those theories. They need to examine the relevance of existing conceptual nursing theories for generating middle-range family nursing theories. Depending on the goals of family nursing theory development, more effort needs to be made at conceptualizing family nursing research within one of the current conceptual frameworks or others that may be designed specifically for family nursing.

Programs of research have been used and should continue within family nursing to enhance scientific progress. Although slightly different from the research programs described by Lakatos, programs of research within nursing consist of a series of investigations conducted by one researcher or a group of researchers that focus on a particular problem. The investigations are logically interrelated and have a goal or outcome that is clearly articulated. For example, Campbell's program of research began with a study of homicide of women which indicated the potential lethal outcomes of battering of female partners. The work has continued in three major directions:

1. midrange theory development to explain women's responses to battering as a major health problem
2. predication of homicide in battering situations
3. explorations of related phenomenon such as battering during pregnancy and sexual abuse in intimate relationships

The long-term goal is designing and testing nursing interventions for secondary prevention of battering. The program of research combines

qualitative and quantitative methods, feminist assumptions, and advocacy components (Campbell, 1981; Campbell, 1986a; Campbell, 1986b; Campbell, 1989a; Campbell, 1989b).

Finally, family nursing theorists need to continue to stride toward achieving conceptual clarity. The debate about what is family nursing must be settled so that energies can be devoted to clarifying other family concepts.

CONCLUSION

The development of explicit family nursing theory is just beginning. Various philosophies of science provide insights and guidelines to assist in the continued growth and development of middle-range family nursing theories.

REFERENCES

Achinstein, P. (1968). *Concepts of science: A philosophical analysis.* Baltimore: The Johns Hopkins Press.

Artinian, N. T. (1990). *Adult families and illness: A literature review.* Unpublished manuscript.

Bell, J. M., Wright, L. M., Leahey, M., Watson, W. L., & Chenger, P. L. (1988). *Proceedings of the International Family Nursing Conference.* Calgary, Alberta, Canada: Faculty of Nursing, The University of Calgary.

Brody, B. A. (1970). *Readings in the philosophy of science.* Englewood Cliffs, NJ: Prentice-Hall.

Campbell, J. C. (1981). Misogyny and homicide of women. *Advances in Nursing Science, 3,* 67–85.

Campbell, J. C. (1986a). A support group for battered women. *Advances in Nursing Science, 8*(2), 13–20.

Campbell, J. C. (1986b). Nursing assessment for risk for homicide with battered women. *Advances in Nursing Science, 8*(4), 36–51.

Campbell, J. C. (1989a). An exploration of two explanatory models of women's responses to battering. *Nursing Research, 38,* 18–24.

Campbell, J. C. (1989b). Women's responses to sexual abuse in intimate relationships. *Women's Health Care International, 8,* 335–347.

Gholson, B., & Barker, P. (1985). Kuhn, Lakatos, and Laudan: Applications in the history of physics and psychology. *American Psychologist, 40*(7), 755–769.

Gilliss, C. L. (1989a). Family nursing research, theory and practice: Our challenges. In L. Krentz (Ed.), *Proceedings of the National Conference on Family Nursing* (pp. 15–24). Portland, OR: Department of Family Nursing, Oregon Health Sciences University.

Gilliss, C. L. (1989b). Family research in nursing. In C. L. Gilliss, B. L. Highley, B. M. Roberts, & I. M. Martinson (Eds.), *Toward a science of family nursing* (pp. 37–73). Menlo Park, CA: Addison-Wesley.

Gilliss, C. L., Highley, B. L., Roberts, B. M., & Martinson, I. M. (1989). *Toward a science of family nursing.* Menlo Park, CA: Addison-Wesley.

Hempel, C. G. (1966). *Philosophy of natural science.* Englewood Cliffs, N. J.: Prentice-Hall.

Krentz, L. G. (1989). *Proceedings of the National Conference on Family Nursing*. Portland, OR: Department of Family Nursing, Oregon Health Sciences University.

Kuhn, T. S. (1970). *The structure of scientific revolutions* (2nd ed.). Chicago: University of Chicago Press.

Lakatos, I. (1970). Falsification and the methodology of scientific research programs. In I. Lakatos & A. Musgrave (Eds.), *Criticism and the growth of knowledge* (pp. 91 – 196). New York: Cambridge University Press.

Laudan, L. (1977). *Progress and its problems: Towards a theory of scientific growth*. Berkeley: University of California Press.

Laudan, L. (1984). *Science and values. The aims of science and their role in scientific debate*. Berkeley: University of California Press.

Meleis, A. I. (1985). *Theoretical nursing: Development and progress*. Philadelphia: J. B. Lippincott.

Meleis, A. I. (1987). Epistemilogy: The nature of knowledge. In C. Bridges & N. Wells (Eds.), *Proceedings of the fourth nursing science colloquium: Strategies for theory development in nursing — IV* (pp. 5 – 17). Boston: Boston University.

Polkinghorne, D. (1983). *Methodology for the human sciences: Systems of inquiry*. Albany, NY: State University of New York Press.

Radnitzky, G., & Anderson, G. (1978). Objective criteria of scientific progress? Inductivism, falsificationism, and relativism. In G. Radnitzky & G. Anderson (Eds.), *Progress and rationality in science* (pp. 3 – 19). Boston: D. Reidel Publishing.

Suppe, F. (1977). *The structure of scientific theories* (2nd ed.). Chicago: University of Illinois Press.

Walker, L. O., & Avant, K. C. (1988). *Strategies for theory construction in nursing* (2nd ed.). Norwalk, CT: Appleton and Lange.

Wallace, W. A. (1979). *From a realist point of view: Essays on the philosophy of science*. Washington, D. C.: University Press of America.

Conceptual and Methodological Issues in Research of Families

SUZANNE L. FEETHAM, Ph.D., F.A.A.N.

This chapter presents a discussion of the conceptual and methodological issues surrounding nursing research of families. Inasmuch as the function of research is to generate and to test theory, the issues explicated in this chapter have profound effects on the types and content of middle-range theories about family phenomena. Although emphasis in this chapter is placed on issues of particular importance to nursing research, some attention is given to issues that must be considered by all investigators of family phenomena, regardless of discipline.

CONCEPTUAL ISSUES

Conceptual issues encompass the distinctions between family-related research and family research, explication of the specific purposes of nursing research of families, and identification of criteria appropriate for evaluation of research of families.

Family-Related and Family Research

Family-related and family research together constitute research of families. Family-related research refers to research that focuses on relationships between family members, using data derived from individuals.

Family research, in contrast, refers to research that focuses on the family unit as a whole. Individual family members are not considered explicitly. Rather, family unit behavior is taken into account (Fisher, 1982). In family research, relationships are not considered linear; thus, A plus B plus C does *not* equal X. This is because A, B, and C are not independent units but, rather, comprise a D that transacts with X, rather then adding up to X. The hypotheses in family research may, therefore, need to be stated as sequences of actions or configurations of behaviors (Fisher, 1982). For example, in family research, a hypothesis may state that there will be an increased occurrence of the pattern of X family behavior in families experiencing high anxiety prior to a member's surgery. Stated another way, the hypothesis is that families experiencing preoperative anxiety will respond in a certain sequence of behaviors or pattern of family behaviors. The sequence or pattern of behaviors is examined in family research, rather than the presence or absence of a given behavior. The nonlinear complexity of family research is consistent with the thesis that the family is not greater than the sum of its parts but, rather, is a re-creation due to the interactions of the individual family members (Ranson, 1984).

Family-related research and family research are of equal importance, and both can contribute knowledge about families. Moreover, both types of research can be conducted within a single program of research. It is crucial, however, that the researcher clearly delineates which type of research is being conducted.

Purposes of Nursing Research of Families

Nursing research of families, like nursing research in general, is directed toward developing middle-range theories that will describe, explain, and predict human responses to actual and potential health problems. More specifically, one purpose of nursing research of families is to examine the responses of families and family members to various states of health. The second purpose is to examine responses of families and family members to expected and unexpected life transitions. The third purpose of nursing research of families is to test theories of the effects of nursing on family members and families. And the fourth purpose is to formulate theories of predictors of family outcomes. This last purpose is especially important to consider, for in a health care environment of declining economic and personnel resources, the ability to identify factors most predictive of successful family outcomes is critical.

Criteria for Evaluating Research of Families

Evaluation of the merit and contributions of research of families should be based not only on general criteria for all research, such as theoretical clarity and methodological rigor, but also on criteria that directly address the special conceptual issues of research involving families.

The criteria identified here reflect the concerns identified by Wakefield, Allen, and Washchuck (1979) regarding research of families. They reported that a review of funded research of families revealed few studies that had explicit conceptual or theoretical bases. Furthermore, most of the research was family-related, rather than family research, as those terms have been defined in this chapter.

The criteria presented in this chapter represent an expansion of Feetham's (1984a) earlier work. An attempt has been made here to clearly distinguish between family-related and family research.

Criteria appropriate for both family-related and family research are
- There is a conceptual or theoretical framework for the research.
- There is an explicit conceptualization of the family.
- There is a definition of the family that is consistent with the conceptualization.
- The research adds to the knowledge of family functioning and family structure.
- The research is relevant to nursing practice.

A criterion specific to family-related research is
- The research examines the responses of individual family members and/or examines concepts related to families or family members.
- Criteria specific to family research are
- The conceptualization, measurement, and analysis aspects of the research all reflect the family as a unit or system.
- The research adds to knowledge of the family system.

Taken together, the criteria serve as a standard or guideline for the development and review of research of families. The following section of this chapter presents a discussion of the current status of research of families with regard to each criterion and implications for future family-related and family research.

The first criterion for research of families states that a conceptual or theoretical framework should guide the research. This criterion has been met with increasing frequency in recent years by nurse researchers interested in the family. Indeed, 13 of the 15 articles dealing with family-related or family research published in refereed nursing journals from 1982 to 1987 included explicit conceptual or theoretical frameworks (Germino and Feetham, 1987). This finding contrasts sharply with a previously reported analysis of the literature from the 1920s to 1983 that revealed little use of an explicit conceptual or theoretical framework (Feetham, 1984b).

Despite the increased use of explicit frameworks for research of families, there is little evidence of nursing research derived from existing family theories in the family sciences. More specifically, theories most common to the family sciences, such as choice, exchange, symbolic interaction, and general system theory have not been frequently tested in the context of family and health. Rather, the frameworks were derived from crisis and stress and coping theories of psychology, from family therapy theory, and from sick role theory of sociology.

Furthermore, there was little evidence of clear linkages between the conceptual or theoretical framework and the empirical aspects of the research, including design, instrumentation, and data analysis (Germino and Feetham, 1987). In particular, few studies reported in the nursing literature and the literature of other disciplines used instruments that actually operationalized or measured the concept purported to be of interest.

Assessment of the first criterion for research of families supports the recommendation that nursing researchers of families present a clear and explicit conceptual or theoretical framework derived from existing family perspectives and actually use that framework to direct all other aspects of the study. Only when the complete and logical linkage of the framework to the empirical aspects has been achieved consistently can the first criterion be said to have been met.

The second criterion for research of families requires an explicit conceptualization of the family. A corollary of this criterion requires the conceptualization of the family to be congruent with the conceptual or theoretical framework for the research and to be reflected in the empirical aspects of the study. Review of relevant research indicates that this criterion is seldom met (Feetham, 1984a; Germino and Feetham, 1987).

Researchers interested in clarifying their ideas about the family and, therefore, meeting the second criterion have several alternative conceptualizations of the family from which to choose. One conceptualization views the family as a system. Particular attention was given to the family as a system by Broderick (1971), Fawcett (1975), Holman and Burr (1980), and Kantor and Lehr (1975). Family scientists from the field of human ecology have further refined the conceptualization of the family as a system by viewing the family as an energy transformation system within the ecosystem (Andrews, Bubolz, and Paolucci, 1980; Bubolz and Whiren, 1984; Thompson and Bubolz, 1986). An assumption of the human ecological framework is that the family system and individual members are interdependent with the environment. This assumption is particularly important in nursing research of families because the health care system is one component of the family's environment.

Viewing the family as a system requires examination of the notion that the family is greater than the sum of its individual members (Ranson, 1984; Rogers, 1983; White, 1984). Thus, the family system perceives and responds differently from any individual member. A summation of individual perceptions does not give a measure of the family system. Ranson (1984), however, has challenged this notion. He stated that it is not that a family is more than the sum of its individuals but, rather, that the individuals themselves are redefined and recreated in the process of their interactions. The recreation, in turn, restructures the family, which creates new conditions resulting in further recursive cycles. For Ranson, then, parts and wholes have equal status as hierarchical relations. Ranson's view of the family is consistent with the issues of family research raised by Gilliss (1983), Schumm and colleagues (1985), and Doherty and Campbell (1988) and reinforces the need for nonlinear designs and analyses when examining the family as a system.

Another conceptualization of the family is that the family is the environment for the individual family members. A review of nursing research of families revealed that few researchers have used this conceptualization (Feetham, 1984a). An extension of this conceptualization is the recognition that the family is a mediator between the individual family members and the environment. This conceptualization is evident in family therapy research, in which the family may be seen as adversarial. The cohesion and adaptation model of family (Olson, 1986) and the family environment model (Moos, 1974; Moos and Moos, 1976) incorporate this conceptualization of the family, as does the research focused on children with health problems in which cases the family is viewed as a mediator or a buffer (Drotar, 1981; Greg, Genel, and Tamborlane, 1980).

Recognizing the family as the environment reinforces the assumption of family systems theory dealing with the interdependence of individual family members with the family, and the interdependence of the individual and family with the environment. This is an especially salient conceptualization for nursing research of families because the primary environment for the individual family member with a health problem may be his or her family, and a primary environment for the family may be the health care system.

Another conceptualization identifies the family as the etiology of health and/or illness (Doherty and McCubbin, 1985; Lasky and colleagues, 1985; Litman, 1974; Speer and associates, 1985). Family research or family-related research often is designed so that families described as pathological are examined rather than normal families. In this type of research, the focus is on the ill family member as the independent variable, thereby implying direct causality between the presence of the ill family member and family outcomes. In contrast, investigators examining families regarded as healthy tend to use a measure of the healthy family as the independent variable, and outcomes related to the individual family members as the dependent variables.

The criterion of an explicit conceptualization of the family rarely has been met, despite the fact that several conceptualizations have been available in the literature for many years. It seems likely that most researchers do have a conceptualization of family in mind, yet they fail to make this explicit. It is, therefore, recommended that investigators strive to identify explicitly the conceptualization of family guiding their studies, as well as to explain how the selected conceptualization derives from the conceptual or theoretical framework and how it influences the empirical aspects of the study.

The third criterion for research of families is inclusion of an explicit definition of the family. A single definition of family for all research of families is not the issue. Rather, each investigator needs to define family within the context of his or her research. The definition of family may be in its more generic sense, such as the nuclear, biological, and/or legal group. Or the family could be defined by the study subjects as they identify their families through functional relationships. Howard's (1978) notion of the given family (biological members) and chosen family (individuals with functional relationships), which is an extension of the approach of study subjects providing their own definition of family, also could be used.

The criterion of an explicit definition of the family has not been met in most reports of research of families. The importance of meeting this criterion in every report should be underscored. Researchers have many definitions from which to choose, or they can provide their own definitions. It is, therefore, recommended that each study include a clear and explicit definition of family.

The fourth criterion requires the research to add to knowledge of family functioning and family structure. Structure and function are basic concepts within theories and research of families. Research of families that meets the first three criteria should, by virtue of the conceptualization of family employed and the methods used, add to knowledge of family structure and function as the roles and functions of individual family members and/or the family system are examined. Yet Feetham (1984a) reported that most nursing research titled *family research* did not examine family structure or functions in an explicit manner. It is, therefore, recommended that the concepts of family function and structure be addressed explicitly.

The fifth criterion states that research of families is relevant to nursing practice. Nursing is a practice discipline; it is, therefore, expected that much of the research conducted by nurses would be relevant to nursing practice. Research relevant to nursing practice also should advance knowledge in other disciplines. Indeed, it is important that nurses participate actively in the basic theory development work of the family sciences. It is, therefore, recommended that nurse researchers explain not only how their studies of families are related to nursing practice but also how their research findings advance family theory development in a general manner.

The preceding five criteria are appropriate for both family research and family-related nursing research. The next criterion is specific to family-related research. This criterion states that the focus of family-related research is on concepts related to individual family members rather than concepts of the family system as a whole. Most research of families meets this criterion (Feetham, 1984a; Wakefield and others, 1979). This important area of research contributes to knowledge of individual family members, such as their responses to illness in their mates.

The final two criteria are specific to family research. One criterion requires all aspects of the research clearly to reflect a focus on the family as a unit or system. The other criterion requires the research to add to knowledge of the family as a whole. Few studies meet these two criteria. The primary reason for this is relatively new understanding of what family research factually entails. Other reasons include the lack of valid and reliable measures of the family system as well as the lack of the techniques needed for analysis of nonlinear family concepts. It is anticipated that as researchers design studies that clearly take into account the criteria for family research, progress will be made in this important area of research of families.

METHODOLOGICAL ISSUES

Several methodological issues regarding nursing research of families are linked to the criteria for research of families and to the differences between family-related research and family research. The methodological issues encompass the source and level of family data, instrumentation, sampling, and data analysis.

Source and Type of Family Data

Increasing attention in the research of families has been given to the source of data. A shift from obtaining data from just one family member to collecting data from two or more family members is evident in recently reported research.

An issue related to the source of the data is what information is provided from individual family members versus multiple family members. Some family scientists maintain that data from the individual family member may provide a perception of another individual, a relationship between individuals, or the family unit. Data from two or more individuals about family relationships or functioning may represent shared meaning. Data collected from the family as a group may provide an average measure of the individuals' perceptions or may be the individuals' perceptions as allowed by the family group interaction (Oliveri and Reiss, 1984; Thomas, 1987).

Fisher and colleagues (Fisher, 1982; Fisher and associates, 1985) provide another perspective about information from different sources of data. They link the source of the data to three levels of data: individual, relational, and transactional. Individual data are from a single family member and make no reference to the perceptions or actions of other family members.

Relational data are individual level data collected from two or more family members and combined in some way. The relational dimensions of these data are determined by the researcher. The scores for relational data are calculated from the individuals' data. Analysis of these data results in descriptive statements about the family and may refer to a quality of family members' perceptions of family events, history, attitudes, and/or attributes. Relational data are obtained from family-related research designs.

Transactional data are measures of the family. These data are not indicators of contributions from individual family members but, rather, are derived from the functioning of the entire family unit and are different from the sum of the parts of the family. These data are obtained from family research designs.

There also are varying perspectives on what methods are appropriate to collect family data. Bavelas (1984) and Fisher and colleagues (1985) agreed that family level or transactional data may be obtained only from naturalistic observation and contingent, structured interaction. In contrast, other family scientists maintain that family level measures can be obtained from individual family members by means of both questionnaires and observations.

Agreement does exist with regard to the effect of context on family data. It is recognized that responses may differ when the same questions are asked of the same person alone or when in the presence of other family members.

Uphold and Strickland (1989) provided a cogent analysis of these issues and suggest that the underlying theory and the research questions determine the source of data. Thompson and Walker (1982) gave examples of data on the relational properties between family members using individual informants. Clearly, careful consideration should be given to the sources of data, and data from individual family members should not be totally negated in an attempt to follow research trends that seem to direct the investigator away from individual family members as important sources of family data.

Instrumentation

A conspicuous flaw in much of the research of families has been the lack of congruence between conceptual or theoretical framework and instruments. In fact, there is little evidence of a logical linkage between what the investigator stated was measured and the concepts the instruments were purported to measure. For example, Oliveri and Reiss (1984) reported that there were 12 known descriptions of family functioning under the heading of *family cohesion*. Although Oliveri and Reiss found a relatively common base in the theoretical description of family cohesion, a comparison of various instruments purported to measure family cohesion revealed little empirical evidence of associations between the instruments.

The results reported by Oliveri and Reiss raise questions about the interpretation of correlations between instruments purported to measure the same concept. A high correlation between the scores from two instruments would indicate that the instruments measure the same concept. A modest correlation would indicate that two instruments measure related but not identical family properties, or that they measure different aspects of the same family property. A low correlation would indicate that the family concepts measured are uniquely tied to specific instruments.

Investigators have, for example, reported low correlations between the Family Environment Scale (FES) (Moos, 1974; Moos and Moos, 1976) and the Card Sort Procedure (CSP) but also reported that both instruments distinguished families with known pathologies from families perceived to be normal (Oliveri and Reiss, 1984; Sigafoos and colleagues, 1985). Close examination of the instruments revealed that the FES measures each family member's perception of the family's internal relationships, and the CSP measures the family interaction with external relationships. This suggests that the two instruments measure different family properties.

There are, of course, other explanations for low correlations between scores obtained from different instruments. One explanation is the differential effect of other variables, such as family structure and socioeconomic status. For example, the FES is highly correlated with socioeconomic status, whereas the CSP is independent of socioeconomic status (Oliveri and Reiss, 1984). Thus, the differential effect of socioeconomic status may account for the low correlation between the FES and the CSP.

Another explanation is the measurement problems inherent in different methods used to obtain data. Self-report questionnaires tend to inform the respondent of the researcher's intent or objectives and, therefore, are subject to socially desirable responses. Furthermore, self-report instruments are administered to individual family members who determine what and how they will respond. Thus, it may be difficult to measure the family as a group or its intrinsic qualities versus each individual's perceptions. In contrast, the research purpose often is less obvious to family members when direct observation is employed. Moreover, the family may be observed as a group rather than as individual family members (Oliveri and Reiss, 1984; Olson, 1986; Sigafoos and colleagues, 1985). Thus, scores from self-reports and observations may not be highly correlated because of the quality of the data obtained from these two methods.

Still another explanation for low correlations between instruments is the variance of the scores obtained in a particular sample. When the variance is low, correlations tend to be low.

The magnitude of a correlation, then, should not be taken at face value. Rather, all possible explanations should be taken into account when inspecting the correlations between scores from instruments thought to measure the same concept.

A special problem of instrumentation in research of families is sensitization. More specifically, the instruments used for research of families can sensitize both families and researchers and, therefore, confound the interpretation of responses. Through questionnaires and interviews, family members are asked to process information about their families in a systematic, structured way. The sequencing and content of the questions may increase awareness of family issues and priorities, and the increased awareness may in turn alter responses of individual family members. Similarly, what scientists learn about families may influence their perceptions and observations as well as their responses to their own and other families. Furthermore, participation in the research can serve as an intervention for family members, which in turn can influence their responses to questionnaires and their subsequent behavior. These challenges to measurement can be controlled in the conceptualization of the research, design, instrumentation, and analysis. Selection of reliable and valid instruments that are true indicators of the conceptualization of the family being employed, training of data collectors, and debriefing families following data collection all can control for the sensitizing effects of instruments.

Sampling

There are two critical issues related to sampling in research of families. These are determining whether the sample is representative and identifying comparative samples. In the research of families and health, many factors influence the ability to obtain representative samples. The decision process for care, such as who is transferred to a tertiary center and who receives new or experimental care techniques, affects representativeness. Other factors include the variability of health resources among states, and in some situations the physician-controlled access to study subjects (Thomas, 1987). These factors should not deter the investigator from studying the health of families, but these factors must be addressed in the study's conceptualization, design, and analysis. Obviously the researcher should report whether it was possible to obtain a representative sample or how the sample differed from the population of interest.

Determining family membership is another sampling issue. For example, comparative studies of families with school-age children and one or two younger siblings must take several family variables into account. The parents may or may not be biological parents, there may be a gender difference in the index child and siblings, or there may be differences in involvement with health professionals. Moreover, parental age and the developmental level of the family may be major confounding variables inasmuch as the developmental age of the family may not be related to parental age, particularly in the situation of divorce and remarriage.

Data Analysis

Analysis of data obtained from studies of families poses both theoretical and statistical problems. When, for example, relational data are used, the technique used to combine scores from two family members may yield a score that lacks theoretical meaning. Furthermore, combined scores may result in reduction of the amount of information provided by the original scores, which in turn may lead to distortion in the interpretation of the data (Fisher and associates, 1985; Walters, Pittman, and Norrell, 1984). A more detailed discussion of the problems associated with relational data is given in Chapter 5.

Several data analytic techniques yield theoretically and statistically meaningful results for research of families. Schumm and colleagues (1985) presented one appropriate technique for family data analysis. They recommended determining the existence of a common family base or shared variance. For example, asking the same question of three family members results in three variables for one concept and provides three sources of variance. When there are high levels of family variance, it is appropriate to use statistical approaches for correlated data.

Exploratory analysis, as described for application to nursing research by Ferketich and Verran (1986) and Verran and Ferketich (1987), is another technique. This technique involves identification of patterns of distribution of scores across family members, which facilitates detection of outliers and should guide future analyses, such as the appropriateness of summated or mean scores (Appelbaum and McCall, 1983).

Other techniques for analysis of family data include path analysis (Alwin and Hauser, 1975; Godwin, 1985, 1986) and canonical correlation (Godwin, 1985, 1986; McLaughlin and Otto, 1981). Simultaneous equation methods also may be used. The latter methods are extensions of multiple linear regression and allow the researcher to analyze complex relationships with several dependent or endogenous variables in a system of linear equations (Godwin, 1985; Lehrer, 1986). Furthermore, simultaneous equation methods estimate relationships in a system of two or more equations in which there are conceptually or mathematically interdependent relationships between the dependent variables. A criterion for using this analytic technique is that the relationship between the dependent variables is not unidirectional. The relationship also must be prespecified. An advantage of this approach is that it allows the researcher to recognize the simultaneous influences involved in intrafamily behavior.

Different analytic techniques may be used with the same data. If several techniques provide the same results, the particular technique probably is not significant. The selection of a data analysis technique should not, however, be arbitrary. Rather, technique(s) must be linked conceptually to the study and must be appropriate for the data.

As scientists test theories derived from various conceptual frameworks, different analytic techniques may be tied to different frameworks. For example, one assumption of family systems theory is the interdependence of the individual family member, the family, and the environment. Inherent in this assumption is the view that the relationships are complex and multidirectional. Data analytic techniques that test simple linear relationships are, therefore, not consistent with family systems theory.

CONCLUSION

Several conceptual and methodological issues in the research of families have been discussed in this chapter. The distinction between family research and family-related research has been made. The criteria for research of families have been identified, and progress made by nurse scientists toward meeting each criterion has been discussed.

Instrumentation and data analysis are central to the resolution of the methodological issues in research of families. In this chapter, various interpretations of correlations between instruments were discussed, as were several different methods of analysis of data from studies of families. It is clear that multiple techniques for data analysis are needed in the research of families. It is also clear that continued efforts are needed to assure consistency of the conceptual framework, the design, the instrumentation, the data analysis, and the interpretation of findings. These complex methodological issues cannot be reduced to a few rules or guidelines. Nurse scientists and family scientists, while building from the existing work, also need to challenge and to test theories, methods, and analytic techniques. It is only through such tests and challenges that empirically valid theories of the family will be developed.

The criteria for the research of families, with particular attention to differentiation between family research and family-related research, should serve as a guide to structure the interpretation of the research findings. The interpretation must, of course, be consistent with the conceptual framework, the design, the instrumentation, and the data analytic techniques.

In conclusion, nursing research of families has the potential to affect practice and health policy for families (Meister, 1989). Continued and more diligent attention to the conceptual and methodological issues, building on the previous work in nursing and other disciplines, will strengthen this potential.

REFERENCES

Alwin, D. F., & Hauser, R. M. (1975). The decomposition of effects in path analysis. *American Sociological Review, 40,* 37–47.

Andrews, M., Bubolz, M., & Paolucci, B. (1980). Ecological approach to study of the family. *Marriage and Family Review 32,* 29–49.

Appelbaum, M., & McCall, B. (1983). Design and analysis in developmental psychology in B. Mussen (Ed.), *Handbook of child psychology* (4th ed., pp. 415–476). New York: Wiley.

Bavelas, J. B. (1984). On "Naturalistic" family research. *Family Process, 23,* 337–341.

Broderick, C. B. (1971). Beyond the five conceptual frameworks: A decade of development in family theory. *Journal of Marriage and the Family, 33,* 139–159.

Bubolz, M. M., & Whiren, A. P. (1984). The family of the handicapped: An ecological model for policy and practice. *Family Relations, 33,* 5–12.

Doherty, W. J., & Campbell, T. L. (1988). *Families and health.* Newbury Park, CA: Sage.

Doherty, W. J., & McCubbin, H. (1985). Families and health care: An emerging arena of theory, research, and clinical intervention. *Family Relations, 34,* 5–11.

Drotar, D. (1981). Psychological perspectives in chronic childhood illness. *Journal of Pediatric Psychology, 6,* 211–228.

Fawcett, J. (1975). The family as a living open system: An emerging conceptual framework for nursing. *International Nursing Review, 22,* 113–116.

Feetham, S.L. (1984a). Family research: Issues and directions for nursing. In H. Werley & J. J. Fitzpatrick (Eds.), *Annual review of nursing research* (Vol. 2, pp. 3–25). New York: Springer.

Feetham, S. L. (1984b, November). *Conceptualization of family for nursing research.* Keynote address presented at First Wingspread Conference: Advancing Family Research in Nursing, Racine, WI.

Ferketich, S., & Verran, J. (1986) Exploratory data analysis: Introduction. *Western Journal of Nursing Research 8,* 464–466.

Fisher, L. (1982). Transactional theories but individual assessment: A frequent discrepancy in family research. *Family Process, 21,* 313–320.

Fisher, L., Kokes, R. F., Ransom, D. C., Phillips, S. L., & Rudd, P. (1985). Alternative strategies for creating "relational" family data. *Family Process, 24,* 213–224.

Germino, B. B., & Feetham, S. (1987, October). *Measurement in family nursing research: Survey of nurse investigators.* Paper presented at Council of Nurse Researchers International Research Conference, Arlington, VA.

Gilliss, C. L. (1983). the family as a unit of analysis: Strategies for the nurse researcher. *Advances in Nursing Science, 5(3),* 50–59.

Godwin, D. G. (1985). Simultaneous equations methods in family research. *Journal of Marriage and the Family, 47,* 9–22.

Godwin, D. G. (1986). Simultaneous equation techniques revisited: A reply to Lehrer. *Family Process, 25,* 883–885.

Greg, M. J., Genel, M., & Tamborlane, W. V. (1980). Psychosocial adjustment of latency-aged diabetics: Determinant and relationship to control. *Pediatrics, 65,* 69–73.

Holman, T. B., & Burr, W. R. (1980). Beyond the beyond: The growth of family theories in the 1970s. *Journal of Marriage and the Family, 42,* 729–741.

Howard, J. (1978). *Families.* New York: Simon and Schuster.

Kantor, D., & Lehr, W. (1975). *Inside the family.* San Francisco: Jossey Bass.

Lasky, P., Buckwalter, K. C., Whall, A. L., Lederman, R., Speer, J., McLane, A., King, J. M., & White, M. A. (1985). Developing an instrument for the assessment of family dynamics. *Western Journal of Nursing Research, 7,* 40–52.

Lehrer, E. L. (1986). Simultaneous equations methods in family research: A comment. *Family Process, 25,* 881–882.

Litman, T. J. (1974). The family as a basic unit in health and medical care: A social-behavioral overview. *Social Science and Medicine, 8,* 495–519.

McLaughlin, S. D., & Otto, L. B. (1981). Canonical correlation analysis in family research. *Journal of Marriage and the Family, 43,* 716.

Meister, S. B. (1989). Health care financing, policy, and family nursing practice: New opportunities. In C. L. Gilliss, B. L. Highley, B. M. Roberts, & I. M. Martinson (Eds.), *Toward a science of family nursing* (pp. 146–155). New York: Addison-Wesley.

Moos, R. H. (1974). *Family environment scale.* Palo Alto: Consulting Psychologists Press.

Moos, R. H., & Moos, B. S. (1976). A typology of family social environments. *Family Process, 15,* 357–371.

Oliveri, M. E., & Reiss, D. (1984). Family concepts and their measurement: Things are seldom what they seem. *Family Process, 23,* 33–48.

Olson, D. H. (1986). Circumplex model VII: Validation studies and FACES III. *Family Process, 25,* 337–351.

Ranson, D. (1984). Random notes. The patient is not a dirty window. *Family Systems Medicine, 3,* 230–233.

Rogers, R. H. (1983). An introduction to the family development schema. In R. Rogers, *Family interaction and transaction. The developmental approach* (pp. 9–21). Englewood Cliffs, NJ: Prentice-Hall.

Schumm, W. R., Barnes, H. L., Bollman, S. R., Jurich, A. P., & Milliken, G. A. (1985). Approaches to the statistical analysis of family data. *Home Economics Research Journal, 14*(1), 112–122.

Sigafoos, A., Reiss, D., Rich, J., & Douglas, E. (1985). Pragmatics in the measurement of family functioning: An interpretive framework for methodology. *Family Process, 24,* 189–203.

Speer, J., McLane, A., White, M. A., King, J. M., Buckwalter, K. C., Lasky, P., & Lederman, R. (1985). Collaboration and the research process. *Western Journal of Nursing Research, 7,* 32–39.

Thomas, R. B. (1987). Methodological problems in family health care research. *Journal of Marriage and the Family, 49,* 65–70.

Thompson, J., & Bubolz, M. (1986, October). *Energy in the family system: Meaning usage and assumptions.* Paper presented at the Research and Theory Workshop, National Council of Family Relations Annual Meeting, Dearborn, MI.

Thompson, L., & Walker, A. (1982). The dyad as the unit of analysis: Conceptual and methodological issues. *Journal of Marriage and the Family, 44,* 889–900.

Uphold, C. R., & Strickland, O. L. (1989). Issues related to the unit of analysis in family nursing research. *Western Journal of Nursing Research, 11,* 405–417.

Verran, J. A., & Ferketich, S. L. (1987). Exploratory data analysis: Comparison of groups and variables. *Western Journal of Nursing Research, 9,* 617–625.

Wakefield, R. A., Allen, C., & Washchuck, G. (Eds.). (1979). *Family research: A source book, analysis and guide to federal funding* (Vol. 1). Westport, CT: Greenwood Press.

White, J. M. (1984). Not the sum of its parts. *Journal of Family Issues, 5,* 515–518.

CHAPTER

5

The Measurement of Family Phenomena

JACQUELINE SULLIVAN, M.S.N., R.N.
JACQUELINE FAWCETT, Ph.D., F.A.A.N.

This chapter focuses on the measurement of family phenomena. Here, the discussion about types of family data begun in Chapter 4 is extended. More specifically, descriptions of individual, relational, and transactional data as those types of data were defined by Fisher and colleagues (1985) are given. Throughout the chapter, empirical methods used to generate each type of data are explained and the advantages and disadvantages of these methods are discussed.

TYPES OF DATA ABOUT FAMILIES

During the last decade, increasing concern with the family in nursing practice, research, and theory development has been evident as the impact of the family on its members' health becomes clearer (Feetham, 1984; Uphold and Harper, 1986; Whall, 1986). Recently, questions have been raised about the validity of measures of family phenomena, especially when an attempt is being made to view the family as a whole, rather than as a collection of individual members. Fisher and his associates (1985) maintained that "a major problem facing family clinicians and researchers is creating data that will reflect the family as a unit" (p. 213). They claimed that this problem could be solved by using a framework for measurement of family phenomena that is based on three measurement strategies: individual, relational, and transactional.

Individual Level Data

Individual measurement strategies involve data collection from a single family member. This strategy has been used in much of the research on families, in which an individual with a particular family role is the study subject. Feetham (1984) noted that the mother is frequently the primary source of data in such studies. Children also have been used as subjects in many studies, as evidenced by the many instruments dealing with family phenomena that are designed for administration to children (Johnson, 1976; Straus and Brown, 1978). Fathers, grandparents, and other relatives are rarely used as subjects in family research, although a trend toward including fathers in nursing research of childbearing families appears to be growing (for example, Bozett and Hanson, 1990; Brown, 1988; Clinton, 1987; Fawcett, 1978; Fawcett and York, 1987; Ferketich and Mercer, 1989; Glazer, 1989; Strickland, 1987).

GENERATING INDIVIDUAL LEVEL DATA

Typically, individual level data are responses to self-report scales; answers to interview questions; or observations of individual, noncontingent behaviors occurring as individual family members perform investigator-directed tasks. Individual level data frequently are the individual family member's perceptions of his or her own behavior, but they may encompass that individual's perceptions of other family members' views, perceptions, or actions. Individual level data also may consist of one family member's report of family structure and function.

Sources of individual level data are the hundreds of questionnaires and rating scales now available (Grotevant and Carlson, 1989; Johnson, 1976; McCubbin and Thompson, 1987; Straus and Brown, 1978; Touliatos, Perlmutter, and Strauss, 1990). Grotevant and Carlson's book contains descriptions and critiques of 49 self-report questionnaires dealing with family functioning, family stress and coping, or parent-child relationships. McCubbin and Thompson's volume includes detailed descriptions of 17 self-report inventories used in a major research project designed to measure family stress, coping, and health. Abstracts of 813 instruments, the descriptions of which appeared in the psychological and sociological literature between the years 1935 and 1974, are presented in Straus and Brown's book. Almost 1000 abstracts of instruments are included in Touliatos and associates' book; more than 500 of these abstracts deal with instruments cited in the literature since 1975. Johnson's book includes at least 40 other instruments that generate data of interest to family researchers. The Feetham Family Functioning Survey (Roberts and Feetham, 1982), the Family Adaptability and Cohesion Evaluation Scales (Olson, Portner, and Lavee, 1985), and the Family Dynamics Measure (Lasky and associates, 1985) are examples of instruments the scores of which can be used as individual level data. These three instruments are discussed in detail below in the section on relational data.

ADVANTAGES AND DISADVANTAGES OF INDIVIDUAL LEVEL DATA

The primary advantages of individual level data are the relative ease with which this type of data is obtained and the relatively low cost of duplicating and administering instruments to individuals rather than to several family members. Another advantage is the availability of appropriate instruments, inasmuch as virtually all self-report questionnaires used to measure family phenomena are designed for administration to individuals. Other advantages are the relative ease of scoring instruments administered to one person and the relative simplicity of data analysis (Uphold and Strickland, 1989). These advantages of individual level data will become more obvious later in this chapter when relational and transactional data are discussed. Still another advantage is that individual level scores are useful in that they have intrinsic value and may predict outcomes with a high degree of precision (Fisher and colleagues, 1985). Yet another advantage is that an individual may express thoughts and emotions more freely if alone, rather than with other family members (Thomas, 1987).

The major disadvantage of individual level data is that they do not reflect the family as an entity in itself. Indeed, scholars especially interested in the family as a unit of analysis have pointed out that individual level data are not data generated by the family unit and, therefore, cannot be considered whole family data. Some scholars go so far as to claim that in the strictest sense, individual level data should not be considered family data (Fisher and associates, 1985). This claim is based on the view that measures obtained from individuals represent only that particular person's view or behavior and do not represent a quality or characteristic of the family unit or family system (Fisher and others, 1985).

Another disadvantage is that individual level data are measures of a single family member that are out of the context of the family unit. The data, then, do not reflect family interactions.

Individual level data may, however, yield information about family relationships. Thompson and Walker (1982) noted that data about dyadic family relationships may be obtained from a single member of a family. Their claim is based on the premise that the research meets the following criteria:

1. The research question is framed at the level of the relationship.
2. The sample reflects involvement in relationships.
3. Measurement encompasses some property of relationships, such as complementarity, congruence of perceptions, reciprocity, or interdependence.
4. The analysis provides information about relationships.
5. Interpretations of the data refer to a relationship.

Furthermore, Grotevant and Carlson (1989) claimed that self-report questionnaires can be used to obtain at least one family member's view of dyadic, nuclear, or extended family relationships. They also noted that some instruments "capture qualities of the family system" (p. 66).

The theoretical perspective of family is, of course, the most important factor to consider when discussing the advantages and disadvantages of individual level data. Certain approaches to the study of the family, such as symbolic interactionism, attribution theory, and crisis theory are based on assumptions of the primacy of the individual's perceptions and the influence of individual perceptions on values, beliefs, and behavior (Uphold and Strickland, 1989). It follows, then, that when the individual's perception is of theoretical import, instruments yielding individual level data are the most appropriate ones to use.

Relational Data

Relational measurement strategies use data generated from various family members but combine the data into a single score. Although most instruments designed to measure phenomena of interest to family scholars are administered to individuals, mathematical calculations can convert the individual level data to relational data, that is, data about the family. More specifically, relational data "are derived from the contributions of [individual] family members combined or contrasted in some way to indicate a characteristic of the [family] unit. Such data yield descriptive statements *about* the family" (Fisher and colleagues, 1985, p. 215).

Relational data, then, are obtained from two or more family members and related to each other by the researcher to yield a new single score that represents an attribute or characteristic of the family as a whole. Fisher and associates (1985) explained that

> this derived score is no longer a reflection of a single family member, as in individual level data, but instead is descriptive of the *combined products* of individual family members. Statements made from these data refer to characteristics or views of the contributing members. They are statements *about* the family in so far as they refer to a quality of family members' perceptions of some event or to aspects of their history, attitudes, or attributes. (pp. 214–215)

GENERATING RELATIONAL DATA

Relational data may be generated by a variety of techniques (Ball, McKenry, and Price-Bonham, 1983; Fisher and others, 1985; Glass and Polisar, 1987). Some techniques involve calculating an arithmetic mean of individual scores, summing individual scores, selecting the most deviant or extreme of two or more individuals' scores, computing differences to obtain a discrepancy or congruence score, or combining the magnitude of each individual's score with the difference between two individuals' scores. Other techniques use multivariate procedures, such as multiple regression, scatterplot regression, cluster or factor analysis, and structural modeling, that can account for score level, differences between scores, and order of magnitude of scores. Additionally, repeated-measures analysis of variance and multivariate analysis of variance procedures can be used to calculate difference scores for family members. Still other techniques require computation of correlation coefficients, percentages of agreement, and other measures of association to obtain similarity scores.

Relational data typically are single scores obtained from independent data provided by two or more family members who are paired by the researcher into sets of dyads. Dyads include mother-father, parent-child, or child-child. In one sense, then, these data represent dyadic relationships rather than more complex nets of relationships among several family members. It is, however, possible to calculate single scores from data provided by several family members. For example, a family mean score can be computed from the separate scores of any number of individuals in a family.

The need for data from at least two family members for generation of relational data must be emphasized. Computations made on data obtained from just one family member, such as discrepancies between responses to questions about actual versus ideal situations, remain individual level data and represent only that family member's perception.

Relational data generated in nursing research of families are exemplified by various scores used to test hypotheses about the relationship between wives' and husbands' strength of identification and similarities in their pregnancy-related experiences. One series of studies tested the hypothesis that spouses' strength of identification would be positively related to similarities in their body image changes during pregnancy and the postpartum (Drake, Verhulst, Fawcett, and Barger, 1988; Fawcett, 1978; Fawcett and associates, 1986). Other studies tested the hypothesis that spouses' strength of identification would be positively related to their reports of physical and psychological symptoms during pregnancy and the postpartum (Drake, Verhulst, and Fawcett, 1988; Fawcett and York, 1987).

In all studies, the strength of identification score was calculated from wives' and husbands' independent responses to the Identification

Scale (Lazowick, 1955). The Identification Scale is a semantic differential containing 10 concepts that are differentiated on nine 7-point bipolar adjective scales. Relational data are generated from this instrument by means of a variation of difference scores. Computation involves taking the square root of the sum of the squared differences between the wife's and the husband's separate scores for each scale item.

In the body image studies, the similarity score was computed from longitudinal data obtained independently from wives and husbands. Separate scores from instruments measuring body image were obtained at five data collection points during pregnancy and the postpartum. These scores were used to calculate a Pearson product moment correlation coefficient for each couple that was used as the single body image similarity score.

In the symptoms studies, the similarity score was computed from cross-sectional data obtained independently from each spouse. Separate scores from a Symptoms Checklist developed by the investigators were obtained from each wife and each husband comprising the sample. These scores were used to calculate a coefficient of agreement for each couple that represented the percentage of agreement of each wife-husband dyad for their affirmative responses to the checklist items. The coefficient of agreement was used as the single symptoms similarity score. The same computation technique was used in the Fawcett and York (1987) symptoms study to calculate a similarity score from data obtained from each spouse's response to each Beck Depression Inventory item (Beck and associates, 1961).

These examples illustrate the generation of relational data from instruments that were not originally developed to measure family phenomena. Similar computation techniques may be applied to instruments that were specifically designed to measure family-oriented concepts. Three examples of such instruments are given below.

The Feetham Family Functioning Survey (FFFS) was developed by Roberts and Feetham (1982) to assess family functioning across three areas of relationships, including the family and broader social units, such as the community and the economy; the family and subsystems, such as division of housework and other family-related labor; and the family and each family member, such as reciprocal relationships between spouses and between parents and children. This instrument was derived from the family ecological framework (Andrews, Bubolz, and Paolucci, 1980; Paolucci, Hall, and Axinn, 1977).

The FFFS consists of 21 family function items. The items are constructed in the Porter format, which measures magnitude, importance, and degree of satisfaction. Each item requires responses to three questions:

1. How much is there now?
2. How much should there be?
3. How important is this to me?

Each question is rated on a 7-point scale ranging from 1 (little) to 7 (much). Direct measures of magnitude for questions 1 and 2 are calculated by summing the scores across items. A direct measure of importance is obtained by summing the scores for question 3 across items. An indirect measure of satisfaction with family functioning is obtained when a discrepancy score is calculated by determining the absolute difference between how much there is and much there should be for each family function item, that is, by obtaining the absolute difference between the scores for question 1 and those for question 2. The higher the score, the greater the discrepancy between how much there is and how much there should be and, therefore, the greater the likelihood that the respondent is not satisfied with family functioning. As absolute numbers, discrepancy scores do not indicate the direction of differences. According to Roberts and Feetham, however, when the discrepancy score (question 1 minus question 2) is used with the importance score (question 3), both direction and degree of satisfaction with family functioning can be determined.

The FFFS yields individual level data from each family member. If both parents complete the FFFS, two separate individual level data sets are obtained. Relational data may be generated from the FFFS if scores from both parents are available and are combined in some manner. For example, a correlation could be calculated for the parents' individual discrepancy scores. Roberts and Feetham alluded to the notion of relational data when they noted a pattern of increasing differences between mothers' and fathers' scores at each data collection point in a longitudinal study. Actual relational data could be generated if discrepancy scores consisting of the differences between each mother's and father's response to each item were calculated.

The Family Adaptability and Cohesion Evaluation Scales version 3 (FACES III) was developed by Olson, Portner, and Lavee (1985) to measure the family adaptability and family cohesion dimensions of the Circumplex model of marital and family systems (Olson, Russell, and Sprenkle, 1983; Olson, Sprenkle, and Russell, 1979). Family adaptability refers to the family's ability to shift its power structure, roles, and rules of relationships in response to unfamiliar or stressful conditions. Family cohesion is defined as emotional, intellectual, and physical oneness that family members feel toward one another.

The FACES III contains 20 items requiring responses on a 4-point continuum ranging from rigid (low) to chaotic (high) adaptability and from disengaged (low) to enmeshed (high) cohesion. The resulting matrix provides 16 possible positions for describing types of family systems ranging from rigidly disengaged to chaotically enmeshed. A moderate balancing of adaptability and cohesion is viewed as necessary for optimal family functioning.

The FACES III can be used to measure the respondent's perceived and ideal descriptions of the family system. Separate administrations of the questionnaire are required to obtain both descriptions. The two descriptions then can be used to determine the perceived-ideal discrepancy, which is an indirect, inverse measure of family satisfaction. The greater the perceived-ideal discrepancy, the less the family satisfaction.

The FACES III can be used to generate both individual level and relational data. Individual level data are obtained when a single family member's responses to both the perceived and the ideal versions of the questionnaire are scored to classify that person on the continua of adaptability and cohesion as well as to determine the discrepancy between perceived and ideal. Relational data are obtained when the FACES III is administered to two or more family members and a family composite score is calculated by summing the scores of all family members. Relational level discrepancy scores are calculated by comparing responses of various family members to both the perceived and ideal versions of the FACES III (Forman and Hagan, 1984). Relational data also may be obtained by use of combined scaling (Fisher and colleagues, 1985). When applied to the FACES III, this method involves reduction of continuous data to categories. Thus, each family member's perceived and ideal FACES III scores are categorized as one of the 16 family system types. Family members then may be compared according to the discrepancies in each one's perceived and ideal family system types.

The Family Dynamics Measure (FDM) was developed by Lasky and her colleagues (1985) to assess family dynamics during health and illness. The FDM was based on assumptions that reflect nursing's traditional concern for holism and the holistic nature of the family.

The initial version of the FDM contains 112 items that are rated on a Likert-type response scale. The FDM items reflect six categories of family relationships identified by Barnhill (1979). Stated as bipolar dimensions, the categories are individuation versus enmeshment, mutuality versus isolation, flexibility versus rigidity, stability versus disorganization, clear communication versus unclear or distorted communication, and role compatibility versus role conflict.

The FDM yields individual level data that measure the perceptions of individual family members. The investigators indicated that individuals' responses are to be used to generate family profiles (Lasky and associates, 1985). Family profiles constructed from combining scores of two or more family members would, of course, represent relational data.

ADVANTAGES AND DISADVANTAGES OF RELATIONAL DATA

An advantage of relational data generated from the individual family member's responses is the lack of need for new instruments. Little or no revision in several existing instruments is required to generate relational data. Furthermore, although some calculations are tedious, such as those required for the strength of identification score, computation statements can easily be written within the framework of existing computer software. For example, calculation of the Identification Scale score was done by means of a "compute" statement in SPSS-X.

A disadvantage of relational data is the fact that there are theoretical and methodological problems associated with the techniques used to generate this type of family data. The computation technique may not yield a score that is theoretically meaningful. For example, Fisher and colleagues (1985) pointed out that relational data composed of arithmetic means or sums of scores do not take into account family members' characteristics that may be theoretically important, such as age; developmental state; family role (for example, parent or child); or status, influence, and power within the family. Furthermore, a sum of family members' scores frequently yields a score that exceeds the range of possible scores for the instrument, making interpretation of the relational data score difficult. Moreover, means and sums of scores may represent aggregates rather than relationships or patterns between family members (Thompson and Walker, 1982). Sums of scores also pose problems when comparisons are to be made of families of unequal sizes (Uphold and Strickland, 1989). This problem can, of course, be overcome if mean scores are used.

The use of similarity scores also poses theoretical problems. In particular, the use of similarity scores to generate relational data requires the researcher to decide what constitutes a similarity. In the pregnancy-related symptoms studies discussed earlier, a decision was made to calculate the percentage of agreement only for wives' and husbands' affirmative responses (that is, the yes-yes responses) to the symptoms listed. But the analysis also could have included the percentage of agreement on the nonaffirmative responses (that is, the no-no responses). A theoretical question in this instance is whether data regarding extent of similarity in the couples' responses, regardless of the direction, would have enhanced understanding of wives' and husbands' responses to pregnancy. Another theoretical question is whether the study hypotheses would have been more fully or accurately tested had both affirmative and nonaffirmative similarities been used in the data analysis.

Several methodological problems must be considered when generating relational data. Coding and other measurement errors may be compounded by combining individuals' scores (Thomson and Williams, 1984). Furthermore, use of arithmetic means and sums of scores do not reflect individual differences in the contributing scores, nor do these techniques reflect the order of score magnitude for various family members. These problems could arise when, for example, relational data are calculated from responses to the FACES III. Discrepancy scores reflect a difference between two individuals' scores, but they may not reflect the direction of the difference or each individual's score level. The latter problem has already been noted for the FFFS, in which absolute numbers are used for discrepancy scores.

The calculations involved in generating relational data also may fail to take into account statistical problems, such as regression to the mean and reduction of score variance which can result from derivation of a single score. For example, reduction in variance has been a continuing problem with the Identification Scale, inasmuch as samples of married couples exhibit less variance in strength of identification than randomly matched married women and men (Lazowick, 1955). The lack of variance in a relational data score has further ramifications, inasmuch as low variance is associated with low correlation coefficients. Thus, the depressed variance that results from creating a single score may obscure a relationship between variables. Another statistical problem dealing with variance occurs when correlations are used to compute similarity scores. For example, if similarity over time is of interest, as it was in the body image studies discussed above, changes must occur in both family members' scores for computation of correlation coefficients. If there is no change in one person's scores, the correlation is indeterminate; that is, it cannot be calculated due to lack of variance.

Multivariate techniques overcome at least some of the problems encountered when individuals' scores are combined. The utility of multivariate techniques was cited by Fisher and colleagues (1985), who noted that "by working with configurations of scores or score patterns rather than the scores themselves and by stepping to a higher level of abstraction, one creates a potentially powerful alternative research strategy" (p. 222). But multivariate techniques are not without problems themselves, inasmuch as large samples are required and interpretation of results can be difficult.

Although relational data provide more information about the family than do individual level data, interpretations should be made with caution, inasmuch as these data represent arbitrary mathematical combinations of scores from individuals, rather than data from measurement of actual family relationships and interactions. Interpretations are aided by presentation of both the original individual level data and the generated relational data. An example of a report containing both types of data is the symptoms study conducted by Drake, Verhulst, and Fawcett (1988). Here, symptoms reported by each spouse and those reported by both spouses were presented. Summary data included the numbers and kinds of symptoms most frequently reported by individuals as well as the numbers and kinds of symptoms most frequently reported by the couples.

Transactional Data

Transactional measurement strategies yield data that "reflect some product of the [family] system or behavioral interchange among system members that indicates the transactional unification of the system's whole that is significantly different from the sum of its parts" (Fisher and associates, 1985, p. 215). Transactional data are derived from the family unit functioning as a whole and do not reflect the individual members' contributions solely or in combined form.

GENERATING TRANSACTIONAL DATA

Although instruments that yield individual data can be used to generate relational data, they cannot be used to generate transactional data. Transactional data, as defined by Fisher and his associates (1985), can be generated only by means of naturalistic inquiry or observations of structured interactions among family members. Both quantitative and qualitative strategies may be used.

The most frequently cited quantitative methods for generation of transactional data are formal coding or ratings systems. Thirteen coding schemes and eight rating scales were analyzed and evaluated by Grotevant and Carlson (1989). Examples of coding systems include Straus and Tallman's (1971) Simulated Family Activity Measure (SIMFAM), Mishler and Waxler's (1968) interaction code, Wynne and associates' (1977) communication techniques, Reiss's (1981) observational methods of family study, and Watzlawick's (1966) Structured Family Interview. The following discussion of the SIMFAM exemplifies the major features of quantitative methods of transactional data generation.

The Simulated Family Activity Measure (SIMFAM) was developed by Straus and Tallman (1971) to assess five aspects of family functioning, including power, support, communication, problem solving, and creativity. The SIMFAM uses direct observations and tape recordings of family interaction under standardized conditions that require family members to engage in a task of discovering the rules to a shuffleboard-type game or a beanbag toss game.

The game is divided into innings separated by rest periods during which the family members may discuss strategy. The number of players usually is set at three — typically the mother, father, and a child. The family's task is to discover the rules of the game by observing the patterns of red and green lights they receive as feedback to the different scoring strategies they employ. A green light indicates that a participant has followed a rule and a red light indicates that a rule has been violated.

The SIMFAM is regarded as an atheoretical device (Forman and Hagan, 1984). It has, however, been used to operationalize the Circumplex model of family systems (Olson, Sprenkle, and Russell, 1979), and evidence supports the content, concurrent, and construct validity of the SIMFAM, which implies some theoretical base.

Qualitative approaches also may be used to generate transactional data. Lincoln and Guba (1985) regard naturalistic inquiry as an "alias" for several qualitative methods, including ethnography, phenomenology, and hermeneutics. Another qualitative approach is grounded theory

(Glaser and Strauss, 1967). All of the methods may, of course, be used to ask any number of questions about individuals, groups, situations, and events. For the purposes of this chapter, the questions would focus on family phenomena. In particular, the questions would deal with the family unit as a whole.

Naturalistic inquiry, as an encompassing term for several qualitative approaches, is characterized first by the human being as the instrument for data collection. According to Lincoln and Guba (1985), "the instrument of choice in naturalistic inquiry is the human . . . the human is the initial and continuing mainstay" (p. 236). Given the typical broad scope of a naturalistic inquiry, Lincoln and Guba recommend using teams of what they called *human instrumentation.*

The second characteristic of naturalistic inquiry is the indeterminate nature of the situation, that is, "not knowing what is not known" (Lincoln and Guba, 1985, p. 240). The indeterminate situation leads to the third characteristic, which is the initial use of open-ended interviews, followed by more structured techniques, such as selected observation, unobtrusive measures, document and record analysis, and recording of nonverbal cues, as understanding of the phenomenon being investigated increases.

The fourth characteristic of naturalistic inquiry is the continuous interplay of data collection and analysis. In contrast to quantitative methods that typically begin data analysis only after a considerable amount of data has been collected, naturalistic inquiry requires analysis of data from the onset of the study. Lincoln and Guba (1985) explained, "Data analysis must begin with the very first data collection, in order to facilitate the emergent design, grounding of theory, and emergent structure of later data collection phases" (p. 242).

ADVANTAGES AND DISADVANTAGES OF TRANSACTIONAL DATA

The major advantage of transactional data is that this type of data is the only type that actually yields comprehensive family system data. The Structured Family Interview, for example, permits holistic assessment of family system patterns (Whall, 1984). Another advantage is that observation of several family members yields "rich" data with a known context. The SIMFAM, for example, permits basic procedures to be systematically varied and provides a wide variety of ratings and scores from the repertoire of observed family behaviors (Forman and Hagan, 1984).

Another advantage is that the family interactions required by transactional data generating techniques can be tape recorded, often on videotape. Videotaping is viewed as a special advantage in transactional data generation because it provides opportunities to capture nonverbal behavior easily and to observe who is speaking to whom, which is particularly advantageous when family members have similar voices (Grotevant and Carlson, 1987).

One disadvantage of transactional data is the label for this type of data. Fisher (1982) acknowledged the disadvantage of labeling transactional data as such, citing the potential confusion with the use of the term *transactional* in the family therapy literature. He pointed out that his use of the term *transactional* is similar to that of the term *interactional* by many family therapists and researchers. For example, Cousins and Powers (1986) defined interactional data as those data resulting from the observation and analysis of behavior sequences for understanding family processes. And Grotevant and Carlson (1987) referred to "circular interaction processes [and] mutually dependent parts" (p. 49) in their discussion of family interaction. Both of these descriptions of interactions are essentially the same as Fisher's definition of transactional data.

Another disadvantage is, paradoxically, tape recording (Grotevant and Carlson, 1987). Equipment problems occur even with the most careful planning, and any kind of recording is intrusive. Furthermore, video recording equipment is bulky and expensive. An additional disadvantage deals with observation that encompasses nonverbal behavior. In this case, difficulties often arise in developing and using coding schemes for that kind of behavior.

Still another disadvantage is the need for a space large enough to accommodate the entire family and, in some cases, the need for a specially equipped location for the interaction task. The SIMFAM shuffleboard game, for example, requires a specially equipped room, although the beanbag task can be accomplished in the family's home. The latter, of course, requires the investigator(s) to travel to where the family lives. And yet another disadvantage of transactional level data is the considerable effort required to obtain the consent and continued cooperation of all family members. As Uphold and Strickland (1989) pointed out, "Bias . . . may be created when the researcher cannot obtain data from the entire family unit because one or more family members choose not to participate" (p. 408).

CONCLUSION

Several compendia of instruments that have been developed to measure family phenomena are now available (Grotevant and Carlson, 1989; Johnson, 1976; McCubbin and Thompson, 1987; Straus and Brown, 1978; Touliatos et al; 1990). Most of the instruments were originally designed to yield individual level data that do not adequately measure the family unit as a whole (Cousins and Powers, 1986; Fisher, 1982; Fisher and colleagues, 1985). Thus, the individual level data that are generated from use of these instruments must be combined to develop relational data. But even relational data do not capture whole family phenomena in the same way that transactional data do.

The challenge of generating relational and transactional data has occurred most appropriately at a time when the field of family nursing research and practice is in a period of rapid expansion. Use of relational and transactional data, as well as appropriate use of individual level data, may contribute to a fuller understanding of the characteristics of family units and help researchers and clinicians achieve their goal of dealing with the family as a whole. Indeed, although "family phenomena are the most difficult to capture in scientific terms [they] are also the most exciting and most fruitful to pursue" (Moriarty, 1990, p. 13).

Furthermore, the generation of data that are truly about the family and of the family should lead to formal middle-range family nursing theories. Contributions to formal family theory development certainly can come from quantitative methods. These contributions would be enhanced if researchers would state explicit hypotheses. Nye (1988) explained, "If researchers can formulate a number of hypotheses, . . . they may find that they can state a middle-range theory . . . for the guidance of their analysis and report" (p. 313).

The potential for formal theories is especially promising when naturalistic inquiry is used to generate transactional data. This is because most of the methods encompassed by naturalistic inquiry are designed to yield one or more clearly defined concepts and explicit propositions about the concepts. Using the classification system presented by Feetham in Chapter 4 of this book, the conclusion may be drawn that the resulting theories are truly family theories, rather than family-related theories, which would emerge from formalization of the findings of studies that yield individual or relational data.

REFERENCES

Andrews, M. P., Bubolz, M., & Paolucci, B. (1980). Ecological approach to study of the family. *Marriage and Family Review, 32*(1), 29–49.

Ball, D., McKenry, P. C., & Price-Bonham, S. (1983). Use of repeated-measures designs in family research. *Journal of Marriage and the Family, 45*, 885–896.

Barnhill, L. (1979). Healthy family systems. *Family Coordinator, 28*, 94–100.

Beck A. T., Ward, C. H., Mendelson, M., Mock, J., & Erbaugh, J. (1961). An inventory for measuring depression. *Archives of General Psychiatry, 4*, 561–571.

Bozett, F. W., & Hanson, S. M. H. (Eds.). (1990). *Cultural Variations in American fatherhood.* New York: Springer.

Brown, M. A. (1988). A comparison of health responses of expectant mothers and fathers. *Western Journal of Nursing Research, 10*, 527–542.

Clinton, J. F. (1987). Physical and emotional responses of expectant fathers throughout pregnancy and the early postpartum period. *International Journal of Nursing Studies, 24*, 59–68.

Cousins, P. C., & Powers, T. G. (1986). Quantifying family processes. Issues in the analysis of interaction sequences. *Family Process, 25*, 89–105.

Drake, M. L., Verhulst, D., & Fawcett, J. (1988). Physical and psychological symptoms experienced by Canadian women and their husbands during pregnancy and the postpartum. *Journal of Advanced Nursing, 13*, 436–440.

Drake, M. L., Verhulst, D., Fawcett, J., & Barger, D. (1988). Spouses' body image changes during and after pregnancy: A replication in Canada. *Image, Journal of Nursing Scholarship, 20*, 88–92.

Fawcett, J. (1978). Body image and the pregnant couple. *American Journal of Maternal Child Nursing, 3*, 227–233.

Fawcett, J., Bliss-Holtz, V. J., Haas, M. B., Leventhal, M., & Rubin, M. (1986). Spouses' body image changes during and after pregnancy: A replication and extension. *Nursing Research, 35*, 220–223.

Fawcett, J., & York, R. (1987). Spouses' strength of identification and reports of symptoms during pregnancy and the postpartum. *Florida Nursing Review, 2*(2), 1–10.

Feetham, S. L. (1984). Family research: Issues and directions for nursing. In H. H. Werley & J. J. Fitzpatrick (Eds.), *Annual review of nursing research* (Vol. 2, pp. 3–25). New York: Springer.

Ferketich, S. L., & Mercer, R. T. (1989). Men's health status during pregnancy and early fatherhood. *Research in Nursing and Health, 12*, 137–148.

Fisher, L. (1982). Transactional theories about individual assessment: A frequent discrepancy in family research. *Family Process, 21*, 313–320.

Fisher, L., Kokes, R. F., Ransom, D. C., Phillips, S. L., & Rudd, P. (1985). Alternative strategies for creating "relational" family data. *Family Process, 24*, 213–224.

Forman, B. D., & Hagan, B. J. (1984). Measures for evaluating total family functioning. *Family Therapy, 11*, 1–36.

Glass, J., & Polisar, D. (1987). A method and metric for assessing similarity among dyads. *Journal of Marriage and the Family, 49*, 663–668.

Glaser, B. G., & Strauss, A. L. (1967). *The discovery of grounded theory: Strategies for qualitative research*. Chicago: Aldine.

Glazer, G. (1989). Anxiety and stressors of expectant fathers. *Western Journal of Nursing Research, 11*, 47–59.

Grotevant, H. D., & Carlson, C. I. (1987). Family interaction coding systems: A descriptive review. *Family Process, 26*, 49–74.

Grotevant, H. D., & Carlson, C. I. (1989). *Family assessment: A guide to methods and measures*. New York: Guilford Press.

Johnson, O. G. (1976). *Tests and measurements in child development: Handbook II* (Vols. 1 and 2). San Francisco: Jossey-Bass.

Lasky, P., Buckwalter, K. C., Whall, A. L., Lederman, R., Speer, J., McLane, A., King, J. M., & White, M. A. (1985). Developing an instrument for the assessment of family dynamics. *Western Journal of Nursing Research, 7*, 40–52.

Lazowick, L. M. (1955). On the nature of identification. *Journal of Abnormal and Social Psychology, 51*, 175–183.

Lincoln, Y. S., & Guba, E. G. (1985). *Naturalistic inquiry*. Beverly Hills: Sage.

McCubbin, H. I., & Thompson, A. I. (Eds.). (1987). *Family assessment inventories for research and practice*. Madison: University of Wisconsin.

Mishler, E. G., & Waxler, N. E. (1968). *Interaction in families*. New York: Wiley.

Moriarty, H. J. (1990). Key issues in the family research process: Strategies for nurse researchers. *Advances in Nursing Science, 12*(3), 1–14.

Nye, F. I. (1988). Fifty years of family research, 1937–1987. *Journal of Marriage and the Family, 50*, 305–316.

Olson, D. H., Portner, J., & Lavee, Y. (1985). *FACES III*. St. Paul: University of Minnesota.

Olson, D. H., Russell, C. S., & Sprenkle, D. H. (1983). Circumplex model of marital and family systems: VI. Theoretical update. *Family Process, 22*, 69–83.

Olson, D. H., Sprenkle, D. H., & Russell, C. S. (1979). Circumplex model of marital and family systems: I. Cohesion and adaptability dimensions, family types, and clinical applications. *Family Process, 18*, 3–28.

Paolucci, B., Hall, O. A., & Axinn, N. W. (1977). *Family decision making: An ecosystem approach.* New York: Wiley.

Reiss, D. (1981). *The family's construction of reality.* Cambridge: Harvard University Press.

Roberts, C. S., & Feetham, S. L. (1982). Assessing family functioning across three areas of relationships. *Nursing Research, 31,* 231–235.

Straus, M. A., & Brown, B. W. (1978). *Family measurement techniques. Abstracts of published instruments, 1935–1974* (rev. ed.). Minneapolis: University of Minnesota Press.

Straus, M. A., & Tallman, I. (1971). SIMFAM: A technique for observational measurement and experimental study of families. In J. Aldous, T. Condon, R. Hill, M. Straus, & I. Tallman (Eds.), *Family problem solving: A symposium on theoretical, methodological, and substantive concerns* (pp. 379–438). Hynesdale, IL: Dryden Press.

Strickland, O. L. (1987). The occurrence of symptoms in expectant fathers. *Nursing Research, 36,* 184–189.

Thomas, R. B. (1987). Methodological issues and problems in family health care research. *Journal of Marriage and the Family, 49,* 65–70.

Thompson, L., & Walker, A. J. (1982). The dyad as the unit of analysis: Conceptual and methodological issues. *Journal of Marriage and the Family, 44,* 889–900.

Thomson, E., & Williams, R. (1984). A note on correlated measurement error in wife-husband data. *Journal of Marriage and the Family, 46,* 643–649.

Touliatos, J., Perlmutter, B. F., & Straus, M. A. (Eds.). (1990). *Handbook of Family Measurement Techniques.* Newbury Park, CA: Sage.

Uphold, C. R., & Harper, D. C. (1986). Methodological issues in intergenerational family nursing research. *Advances in Nursing Science, 8*(3), 38–49.

Uphold, C. R., & Strickland, O. L. (1989). Issues related to the unit of analysis in family nursing research. *Western Journal of Nursing Research, 11,* 405–417.

Watzlawick, P. (1966). A structured family interview. *Family Process, 5,* 256–271.

Whall, A. L. (1984). In search of holistic family assessment: An investigation of a clinical instrument. *Issues in Mental Health Nursing, 6,* 105–115.

Whall, A. L. (1986). *Family therapy theory for nursing: Four approaches,* Norwalk, CT: Appleton-Century-Crofts.

Wynne, L. C., Singer, M. T., Bartko, J. J., & Toohey, M. L. (1977). Schizophrenics and their families: Research on parental communication. In J. M. Tanner (Ed.), *Developments in psychiatric research* (pp. 254–286). London: Hodder and Stoughton.

PART

II

AN ANTHOLOGY OF NURSING PERSPECTIVES ON THE FAMILY

INTRODUCTION

In 1957, Hill, Katz, and Simpson began to classify the literature of family sociology into substantive categories. The goals of their classification of the literature were to identify gaps in existing knowledge and to facilitate the development of a systematic theoretical base for future work.

With similar goals in mind, the editors of this text offer a classification of the literature of family nursing along with reprints of representative publications in each category and a commentary on each reprinted paper. The classification used for the anthology is based on categories formulated by Meister (1985) and Murphy (1986). Meister's categories were

1. theoretical perspectives on the family
2. natural transitions and the family
3. health and the family
4. illness and the family
5. health policy and its impact on the family

Murphy's categories encompassed

1. health maintenance and successful coping in healthy families
2. family response to illness
3. family transitions and new family structures
4. family interface with societal institutions and environments, including health care settings
5. public policy and the family
6. cross-cultural family research.

The categories used in this anthology are
- changes in family structure
- healthy families
- the impact of illness on the family

The editors did not include Meister's category of theoretical perspectives but, rather, selected publications for the anthology that illustrate various aspects of family nursing theory development. Theoretical perspectives, then, pervade the categories. Furthermore, the policy category included in Meister's and Murphy's classifications was not used because the emphasis in this text is on theory development per se, rather than on the utilization of theory in the formulation of policies that have an impact on the family. Murphy's categories dealing with family interactions with the larger society and with cross-cultural research were not included here because the literature review revealed few available publications in these areas that fit the purpose of the anthology.

The categories for the anthology are admittedly quite broad, which is to be expected in the early stages of knowledge development in any field of study. Subdivisions in the categories, as well as new categories, most likely will appear as nurse scholars build upon the work already done.

The reprinted papers were selected after an extensive review of printed cumulative indexes of nursing literature, printouts from computer searches, and the editors' personal files. Each paper included in the anthology illustrates a particular point with regard to middle-range family nursing theory development. The editors recognize that the function of virtually all scholarly work is to advance knowledge. Unfortunately, however, the literature review yielded relatively few publications that include an explicit conceptual or theoretical perspective. Indeed, the outcome of the literature review for the anthology was similar to Lewis's (1986) conclusion that most studies of the effects of cancer on the family were atheoretical assessments of needs or problems. The editors also recognize that much of what appears to be atheoretical has theory embedded in an implicit manner. However, considering the focus of this text, the papers selected for the anthology reflect a more explicit than implicit emphasis on theory development. Finally, the editors recognize that the page limitations of the book precluded inclusion of many fine papers. What is included, then, is a representative sample of the family nursing literature emphasizing theory development.

The commentary preceding each paper focuses on its contribution to family nursing theory development. An attempt has been made to tie the new work that appears in Part I of the book of the previously published works reprinted in Part II by means of the commentaries. Toward that end, each commentary was guided by the following questions:

1. What is the composition of the family being considered?
2. Does the paper emphasize individuals within the context of their families or the family as a unit? That is, does the work represent a family-related or a family focus?
3. What contribution does the paper make to middle-range family nursing theory development?
   - What conceptual perspective is advanced?
   - What theory was generated or tested? Do the findings of theory-testing work support or refute the theory?
   - What are the methodological implications of the work?

The distinctions between conceptual models and middle-range theories and the meaning given to formal theory development that were presented in the Introduction to Part I of the book are continued in the Part II commentaries, as is the interest in formal theory development.

Briefly, a conceptual model is an abstract and general set of concepts and propositions that presents a global perspective of phenomena of interest to a field of study. A middle-range theory is a relatively specific and concrete set of concepts and propositions that describes, explains, or predicts a phenomenon. A formal theory is a middle-range theory articulated as an explicit set of concepts and propositions that may be presented as an equation or a diagram.

In each case in which the author of the reprinted publication did not ascribe the same meaning to a term as that used in this book, the difference is noted in the commentary. The editors hope that continued emphasis on the differences in levels of abstraction of knowledge will facilitate appreciation of what already has been accomplished in family nursing theory development and identification of directions for future work.

In keeping with the schema included in Part I, the editors elected to label the papers as family-related or family focused. Both types of theory development are regarded as equally valuable and needed for advancement of family nursing science and family nursing practice.

The commentaries are purposefully brief, so as not to detract from the reprinted papers. The editors hope that their comments will, however, foster further discussion of the contribution of the papers, separately and collectively, to the field of family nursing.

In conclusion, the work on classification of knowledge about the family was begun by Hill, Katz, and Simpson (1957), continued with Hill and Hansen's (1960) and Nye and Berardo's (1966, 1981) classifications of conceptual frameworks for the family, and culminated in Burr and associates' (1979) two volumes on contemporary family theories. Despite these sustained and concerted efforts by family sociologists to explicate the foundation for middle-range theory, Nye (1988) found that less than 25 percent of the family research published in sociology and interdisciplinary journals in 1987 included an explicit theoretical statement. The reasons for this essentially atheoretical approach to research, according to Nye, are "lack of interest and concern on the part of researchers, [as well as] lack of useful theory available to them" (p. 313).

The editors of this book firmly believe that the same situation does not have to prevail in the field of family nursing. The community of family nurse scholars already is sensitized to the need for explicit theory (Lobo, 1985), and many members of this community seem ready to formalize their findings. Furthermore, the utility of conceptual models and theories available to family nurse scholars is becoming more obvious. The success of this book, then, can perhaps be best judged not only by the amount of discussion it provokes in the community but also by the number of future family nursing publications that include an explicit and formal theoretical statement.

REFERENCES

Burr, W. R., Hill, R., Nye, F. I., & Reiss, I. L. (1979). *Contemporary theories about the family* (Vols. 1 and 2). New York: The Free Press.

Hill, R., & Hansen, D. A. (1960). The identification of conceptual frameworks utilized in family study. *Marriage and Family Living, 22,* 299–311.

Hill, R., Katz, A. M., & Simpson, R. L. (1957). An inventory of research in marriage and family behavior: A statement of objectives and progress. *Marriage and Family Living, 19,* 89–92.

Lewis, F. M. (1986). The impact of cancer on the family: A critical analysis of the research literature. *Patient Education and Counseling,* 8, 269–289.

Lobo, M. L. (1985, May). *Implementation of an invitational conference.* Paper presented at the Eighteenth Annual Communicating Nursing Research Conference, Western Council on Higher Education for Nursing, Seattle, WA.

Meister, S. (1985, May). *Identification of family research problems.* Paper presented at the Eighteenth Annual Communicating Nursing Research Conference, Western Council on Higher Education for Nursing, Seattle, WA.

Murphy, S. (1986). Family study and nursing research. *Image: Journal of Nursing Scholarship, 18,* 170–174.

Nye, F. I. (1988). Fifty years of family research, 1937–1987. *Journal of Marriage and the Family, 50,* 305–316.

Nye, F. I., & Berardo, F. M. (1966). *Emerging conceptual frameworks in family analysis.* New York: Macmillan.

Nye, F. I., & Berardo, F. M. (1981). *Emerging conceptual frameworks in family analysis.* New York: Praeger.

CHANGES IN
FAMILY STRUCTURE

CHAPTER

6

Nursing, the Family, and the "New" Social History

WANDA C. HIESTAND

A GROWING BASE of chronological descriptive studies in nursing coincides with growing interest in interpretive nursing history. Historians and sociologists are developing an extensive and rapidly expanding body of literature about nursing that is waiting to be examined and possibly integrated by scholars of nursing history.

Several models taken from the literature of social history and sociology seem particularly relevant for the interpretation of nursing history. These models deal with historical changes in the family, childhood as a modern idea, and the emergence of modern professions as a mechanism for social control. Each of these scholarly areas deals with the process of social change and attempts to explain the transformations of social forms into institutions.

This research was conducted under the auspices of the Nursing Research Emphasis Grant: Families and Parenting, Contract No. NU-00833, New York University, School of Education, Health, Nursing and Arts Professions, Division of Nursing. Appreciation is expressed to the anonymous reviewers and to Paul Mattingly for their suggestions in the development of this article.
Reprinted from *Advances in Nursing Science, 4*(3), 1–12, 1982.

CHILDHOOD AS A MODERN IDEA

Within the last 20 years social historians, stimulated by the interpretations of Phillipe Aries, have tended to agree that childhood is a modern idea that had no genuine counterpart prior to the 19th century. However, not all historians agree on the social consequences of this change in attitude with regard to children.

Some hold that a separate social category of "childhood" is detrimental, and that it contributes to a separation and alienation of children from an active part in the society as a whole.[1] Others hold that the quality of life has been greatly improved because children are recognized as a separate group with special needs.[2] Nursing has given considerable attention to the problems of children, as well as attempting to foster good parenting and preventive nursing intervention in promoting the welfare of the child. Can the new historical views regarding childhood provide a valid point from which to interpret the historical development of nursing goals?

Historians of the family report that after 1790 a range of demographic and economic factors altered social relationships within the family as well as in the larger American society. Kett identifies several demographic factors reflecting structural change in the family: a doubling of the median age for the total population, families with fewer children, and a narrowing of the age range between siblings. These structural changes meant that parents lived longer lives with fewer children closer together in age, possibly all teen-aged. After the mid-19th century, children increasingly stayed in parental homes until marriage, and parents increasingly lived to see their children reach maturity.[3(pp232-233)]

As a dominant affluent middle class blossomed during the 19th century, parents evolved new perspectives on the nature of children and their nurturing needs. In turn, the heightened value of nurture provided an avenue for women of the dominant class to establish child nurture as having unprecedented social importance. Eventually, the dynamics that transformed the view of childhood spurred the establishment of child-centered institutions for education, health, and welfare.

> Eventually, the dynamics that transformed the view of childhood spurred the establishment of child-centered institutions for education, health, and welfare.

Perspectives on the nature and needs of children, as parents prepared them for adulthood, changed as the economic system of industrial capitalism became established. This new economic system generated new social roles and avenues for social mobility. Capitalism used mobile wage earners in a more or less interchangeable manner and stimulated large waves of migration. At the same time, recognition grew among middle-class Americans that children must be prepared for life styles and work different from those of their parents.

As Katz points out, demographic shifts and transformations in economic order and family structure created heightened parental anxiety and new strategies of child nurture to ensure satisfactory transmission or improvement of status from parents to children.[4(pp390-399)] This was greatly influenced by the uncertainties of a shifting economic order. The socialization of children, particularly in the middle class, emphasized the importance of self-discipline, rationality, morality, and order as qualities to be internalized by the development of character.[5-8]

HISTORICAL ROLE OF FAMILY AND CLASS

The historical study of the family is at the center of the new socio-historical views. One influential interpretation is that the family changed from a self-sufficient working social unit made up of kin and nonkinship members to a small child-centered nuclear unit with the primary task of satisfying the emotional needs of its members. Inherent in this view is the belief that changes in form and function of the family have led to changes in internal family dynamics. Some historians interpret these changes as destructive; others see them as liberating for family members.[5,9,10]

The notion of the family as an agency of repression is consistent with the opinions of Florence Nightingale, who in 1852, at the age of 32, was chafing under the sexist restraints of her time and class (ie, upper class British Victorian women).

> The family? It is too narrow a field for the development of an immortal spirit, be that spirit male or female. The family uses people *not* for what they are, not for what they are intended to be, but for what it wants them for—for its own uses . . . This system dooms some minds to incurable infancy, others to silent misery.[11(p37)]

The influence of these ideas on the way modern nursing emerged under the influence of Nightingale must be a significant theme of nursing history. To what extent did the changing dynamics of family, child rearing, and ethnic/class values condition the role of nursing in America?

Along with changing perceptions of childhood in relationship to the family, there has been a change in the view of women's role in society. Lasch argues that the American family reached a peak state of crisis between 1870 and 1920. This crisis was precipitated by a dramatic rise in divorce, a lowered birth rate, the changing position of women, and the so-called "revolution in morals."[10] The striking conjunction in time between these developments and the rise of professional nursing, along with the facts that most nurses are women, that nursing was women's work, and that the family was the traditional focus for practice by visiting nurses, suggests that family history can be a fruitful context in which to explore the development of professional nursing.

Consideration of nursing history in relation to the changing American family, recognizing class and cultural differences, leads to different questions and suggests different interpretations from the usual view of nursing as a steady march of progress or as shaped completely by the rise of hospitals and the professionalization of medicine. One historical question might deal with the way nurses became a special occupational group involved in institutionalizing the social need for nurturance at various times throughout the life cycle, during both sickness and health. What were the family origins of nurses over time? How did nursing relate to the family to justify development of nursing as women's work? How did nursing intervention in families change over time? How were notions of family used in nursing practice and for the establishment of a women's occupation or profession?

PROFESSIONALISM

Social Control

Professions have frequently been studied as mechanisms for social control by elites over the underprivileged. In this view, the professional group consciously delineates an area of expertise based on educational criteria. With knowledge and skills identified, a public demand for the service of the professional or expert is generated at the same time that selective access to the profession prevents an oversupply and a system of legal licensure provides sanctions. This system depends on the existence of an economy based on markets and money.[12]

This view is presented by Larson to explain the rise of medicine as a modern profession. Medicine offers the most successful application of a model of social manipulation aimed at domination and exclusively to control a market for expertise.[12] Does nursing history reveal that this view is applicable to the long struggle to professionalize nursing?

Even though Larson's proposition may have historical validity as a sociological explanation for the successful development of modern medicine as a profession, this does not mean that the same sociological model can become the standard for all professional groups throughout history.[13] To be genuine, a history of professionalization must take into account the changing meaning of the term over time for each professional group.

The professionalization of medicine took place around the turn of the century as nursing leaders attempted to professionalize nursing in this country. How applicable is Larson's model to nursing? Can the same criteria be used to judge the degree to which nursing can be said to have succeeded or failed?

Institutionalization

Nursing offers a unique vantage point from which to examine the conflicting views of the structural-functional sociologists and the social historians with regard to the way institutions emerge. Sociologists of the Parsonian school view the process of emerging institutions as a logical progression toward a rational way to meet human needs—a process that is both inevitable and an improvement over older methods.[14,15] Critics argue that this view of the process of social change "devalues the role of ideas, discounting their power to challenge and change organizational arrangements."[16(p450)] It denies the real experiences of institutions, where conflict is usually inevitable. Rather than sociological theory, historical study of how an institution responds to varied dissonance may offer genuine understanding.

Nursing as an occupational group of institutionalized and professionalized caregivers thus has a special contribution to make toward understanding the historical process manifest in today's institutions and professions. This aspect is particularly relevant, since some historical research has presented the argument that traditional responsibilities of families, such as health maintenance and care of the sick and disabled, have been transferred to professional and community agencies with disastrous consequences.[10(pp3–21)]

The concept of professionalism has changed over time, yet the current definition of profession tends to be applied and thereby creates confusion in the exploration of nursing history. Although it is not appropriate to apply this static 20th-century construct to the dynamics of occupational transformations in nursing history, the often stated goals of professionalism can offer a focus for discussion of conflicts and debates of the values associated with differing views on this subject. Disagreement and discussion about the meaning of professionalization have been more or less continuous and reached the stage of public debate after only one generation of leadership.[18,19]

> The concept of professionalism has changed over time, yet the current definition of profession tends to be applied and thereby creates confusion in the exploration of nursing history.

Standards

For example, in 1893 a national organization of American nurses was initiated to establish standards of education and practice. The same year also witnessed the creation of secular public health nursing with the foundation of the Henry Street Settlement. These two significant developments represent an ideological shift away from religious orientation and toward modern professionalization with confrontation of modern economic realities.

The meaning of the term *profession* became an issue for debate and interpretation by nurses of the time. As nurses struggled to resolve their work-related problems through organization and improved educational preparation, Florence Nightingale (now 73 years old) was still arguing her religious elitist British view of nursing as a "high holy calling" and regarded concerns about money by nurses as somehow distasteful. Although she equated the intellectual motive with the professional motive (ie, "the desire and the perpetual effort to do the thing as well as it can be done")[17(p32)] and firmly believed in sound educational preparation for practice, Nightingale nevertheless viewed as one of the "dangers . . . making nursing a profession and not a calling."[17(p32)]

The personal ambiguities of significant leaders are an important aspect of interpretive history. The family and women's role were prominent issues in Victorian society. They produced ambiguous responses from women of the time, Nightingale being no exception.

A link between professional nursing and concern with family health was forged by Nightingale herself based on her views about hygiene and ideas relating to health care for women and children, especially during the crisis of childbirth. In spite of her personal sense of family-induced constraint, Florence Nightingale firmly believed that the family was the one supportive institution to follow us from cradle to grave. She wanted to "strengthen and enlarge ties"[20(p221)] to help women and children toward good health by providing midwifery and nursing services in the home. In her words, "While devoting my life to hospital work, to this conclusion I have always come, *viz*, that hospitals are not the best place for the sick poor except for severe surgical cases."[21] In establishing a new educational system for women, she intended not to force daughters "out of the family, we only wish them to be where their faculties will be best exercised, *wherever that is*."[20(p221)]

Conflict

Group tension and conflict is another crucial dimension for historical study. An example is the integration of midwifery functions into nursing. This process was an important professional issue for American nursing after 1912, echoing Nightingale's activities. As part of the Nightingale Fund, Nightingale established hospital-based apprenticeship education for nurses in 1860 and the Training School for Midwives in 1862. Although Nightingale saw nursing as a calling, midwifery held professional possibilities as a career for educated women.[22,23] Both fields focused on health promotion and were viewed as a way for women to provide health services to other women and their children in sickness and in health. Both fields prepared women to practice in the home after learning their respective specialties in a hospital associated with a school.

It is the task of the historian to explore such differences over genera-

tions and among classes and groups, as well as the personal ambivalences
of significant leaders, to assess their meaning in history.

AMERICAN NURSING AFTER 20 YEARS

Americans did not accept all of the Nightingale educational methods, yet
they shared her ambivalence toward professionalization. In spite of the
usual statement in nursing histories that the Nightingale system was
instituted in America in 1873, the Nightingale system as originally conceived was never established here. It was, in fact, nontransferable, partly
because of the difference between American and British class structures,
but also because money from the Nightingale Fund financed British
scholars.

Another significant difference no doubt stems from the fact that
American nursing was first established by wealthy American women,
philanthropist sponsors of training schools. The earliest founders did not
themselves become nurses. This contrasts with Nightingale, who prepared for nursing, practiced nursing, and also instituted education for
women of the upper class to become nurses with leadership roles.

Educational System

Among the issues faced by American nursing in 1895 was one which
illustrates some of these differences between the Nightingale educational
system and the American version (which at the same time expressed a
Nightingalian view of professionalism). The question was whether student nurses should pay for their education or be paid by the hospital. This
would allow them some income while they acquired their education.

In England special probationers, who were from the upper classes,
paid tuition, lived in special quarters, and were prepared to assume
administrative and leadership roles. Graduates of British hospital schools
attempted to establish the Nightingale system in America. For example,
L. Walker, directress of nurses at Presbyterian Training School for Nurses
in Chicago, was a graduate of St. Bartholomew's Hospital in London.
Voicing support for tuition charge and opposition to payment of students, Walker argued that

> it was a very good thing, for we got educated women who would not
> have come in if they had had to receive money from the outset. I
> should not have studied under these circumstances. I went in think-
> ing I was doing something for other people and paying my way, and
> when I was once in I wanted to remain. We get our best nurses that
> way, and we found it a good plan. We had a special probationer for
> each ward.[24(p29)]

American Louise Darche, superintendent of the school of nursing and matron of City Island Maternity Hospital in New York City, responded:

> I think it is a pity to compare women of wealth and leisure in England to our American women. That system is not possible in this country. I do not see the objection to giving people money to help them along when they are in schools. The work is not altogether scholastic; there is a great deal of repetition and of hard work. The monthly allowance is not objectionable to us in our training. In our own school we would exclude many of our best pupils by cutting off the allowance. I feel as if we should be making it unnecessarily hard for some women to work their way.[24(p29)]

Structure

Veneration of "the Founder" and failure of nursing to confront the generational and class differences inherent in Nightingale's views blurred class conflict and cultural differences. There seems to be a lack of perspective in the understanding of some of American nursing history. There is still a transformed American version of the necessity for hierarchy in nursing that is rooted in the militaristic Nightingale system. As Stewart wryly put it, modern nursing has been presented as "a steady onward and upward march with flags flying and grateful multitudes cheering the rapidly growing army that served under the Nightingale banner."[25(p286)]

> Veneration of "the Founder" and failure of nursing to confront the generational and class differences inherent in Nightingale's views blurred class conflict and cultural differences.

Precisely because larger social factors profoundly affected the emergence of nursing as a profession, modern nursing history cannot be understood by narrow studies of Nightingale's influence or specific institutions that pledged her allegiance. Broader questions about professional transformations must be asked in the study of nursing history.

HISTORICAL ROOTS OF SPECIALIZATION IN NURSING

Hospital and Family Nursing

The historical experience of nursing has contributed to confusion at another level. After only one generation, by 1893, specialization of nurses had become a problem for the profession.[26] Nightingale viewed hospital nursing as a specialty, emphasizing that it was not at all the same thing as medicine. She believed that the district nurse must be even more skilled and more broadly prepared for health teaching than the hospital nurse. The American profession at the turn of the century strongly reflected the tendency to specialize. There were infant nurses, district nurses for the sick poor, public health nurses in the community doing social nursing, tuberculosis nurses, contagious disease nurses, and school nurses.

In spite of this long history of nursing practice outside hospital walls and in responsible administrative posts, the stereotype of the nurse continues to be at the bedside in a hospital carrying out physicians' orders, although increasingly often in an intensive care unit with jumbles of wired machines in the background. This points out one important aspect of professional nursing that needs to be stressed. The specializations involve but a portion and not the whole of professional nursing. Historical questions should be asked as to what the relationship between these different nursing groups has been over time, what the nature of their conflicts has been, and the conditions under which they have failed or succeeded in implementing their professional values.

Midwifery

A historical study of the merger of nursing with midwifery during the early part of this century would be especially revealing. The practice of the midwife was necessarily involved in the family and in child nurture. Nursing leaders realized this and attempted to promote an integrated system of maternity care and midwifery service. Nurses in New York City assisted and supervised midwives in their work and encouraged development of a system of midwifery education for both midwives and nurses in midwifery. However, midwives and nurses faced competition from obstetricians who were themselves attempting to professionalize. The overlapping interests centering on childbirth were publicly expressed in debate of "the midwife question."[27-29] Nursing, particularly public health nursing, was intimately involved in this struggle over the institutional arrangement of a major health care service.

During the 19th century, nearly all European countries established control over lay-midwifery education and practice, monitoring its effectiveness by vital statistics. The figures demonstrated that prepared midwives who were neither physicians nor nurses provided safe effective care. The United States and Britain both had appallingly high mortality rates compared to other western countries. Between 1901 and 1910, the number of American-born infants who died before reaching the first birthday was 2,500,000 — a number equal to the total population of Chicago, America's second largest city.[29(pp4-5)] The death rate was estimated to range between 38.3 and 197.9 per 1,000 live births and was closely associated with the father's income: the lower the income, the higher the mortality rate.[29(pp87-88)] One public health official noted that simply being a baby could be called an extra-hazardous occupation.

In 1905, 42% of the total number of births in New York City were attended to by midwives; in Chicago it was 47%. Even though the percentages did not change between 1891 and 1905, the actual numbers doubled. The numbers were indeed staggering — 48,830 babies were delivered by lay midwives in New York City in 1905.[30,31] Little was known about the practice of rural midwives, who were completely without preparation in contrast to many urban midwives.

In 1902 midwifery came under national regulation for education and practice in Britain after a long bitter struggle to legitimize midwifery as part of the health care system. British midwives were supervised by British nurses, many of whom themselves became nurse midwives. Influenced by Nightingale and the British model, American nursing leaders attempted to integrate midwifery functions into nursing and to assume supervision over midwifery for normal maternity cases.

Completely ignored until the turn of the century, the midwife was held to no standards for practice or educational preparation. There ensued an intensive campaign in concert with the public health movement to raise national consciousness of maternal and infant health issues. Finally midwifery functions were assumed and nearly eliminated by the professionalizing of obstetricians instead of nurses.

The failure to establish nurse midwifery as a major component of the health care system stemmed from prejudice against those large numbers of immigrants who used midwifery services and from the fact that childbirth was translated into a pathological condition by obstetricians and accepted as such by the public. The majority of nurses failed to support the attempt to integrate midwifery into nursing. The reasons why this divergence occurred when it did are yet to be explored historically within nursing. The recent and dramatic public interest in midwifery thus links its history to a series of vital social questions.

CONTEMPORARY INTERPRETATIONS OF NURSING HISTORY

Ehrenreich and English in their book *For Her Own Good: 150 Years of Experts' Advice to Women* provide a sweeping review of the destructive, repressive aspects they see in scientific expertise and the profound need for "'womanly' values of community and caring . . . as the *only human* principle" for guiding social institutions.[32(p292)] *Exorcising the Midwives, The Rest Cure, "Right-Living" in the Slums*, and the *"Child Question"* are titles that head segments of this book and give a flavor of its tone.

Strikingly, it itemizes the same areas of life prominent in the early practice of the public health nurse. Did public health nursing align itself with the scientific experts and become a tool to implement social control intended to extend government through the family and to obliterate family privacy and self-confidence in child care? At what point in nursing history does child nurture assume importance as a professional concern? How is this concern expressed in nursing practice and literature? Does this change over time? How does it differ among various nursing groups?

PUBLIC HEALTH NURSING AS A FOCUS FOR RESEARCH

Public health nurses form one obvious and crucial group for historical study. Public health nursing practice confronts a range of professional issues meeting at the interface of new scientific knowledge stemming from the germ theory, Darwinism, and child psychology. It deals with professionalization in itself and other allied groups and is involved in implementation of health-promoting social policy. These early nurses interacted with a clientele made up of new, mainly poor, immigrants as well as rural poor. Both groups were viewed by the dominant culture as requiring modern socialization or Americanization. Nursing rhetoric, representing one part of the dominant American culture, reinforced the idea that nursing practice was centered on "the treatment of families in which there is sickness."

Illustrating these points, Wald wrote a series of three articles in 1904 for the *American Journal of Nursing*. It begins as follows:

> The treatment of disease among the poor assumes grave importance when regarded from its social, economic and moral aspects as well as its purely therapeutic ones. . . . Interference by the State with child labor, provision for play and outdoor exercise, and vigilant inspection of food supplies . . . are examples of general recognition of the social significance of having a well community.[33(p427)]

On another occasion, in speaking of ill children, she wrote:

> The child in the tenement house may perhaps have unwise attention when the mother is left to herself without professional supervision, but with careful technical care from the nurse, and her wise direction of the mother's efforts that result must operate to the advantage of the child.[34]

Ehrenreich asserts that social nurses like Wald imposed the manipulative scientific strategies of the expert on disorderly immigrant families, creating within-group snobbery and promoting corrupt capitalistic values.[32(pp158,186)] Yet Wald's writings suggest that a more "socialistic" interpretation is also possible. Wald sees the nurse as being socialized, "harmonized with the powers which aim at care and prevention rather than police power and punishment (forming) part of the great policy of bringing human beings to a higher level."[35(p60)] The Henry Street nurses maintained a farm in New Jersey open during the summer months as "a vacation house for mothers with little babies who need the restorative of country air."[36] One gets out of these sources a sense of the failure of one kind of professional vision of practice rather than a diabolical plot to entrap women or destroy families.

FAMILY CENTEREDNESS AND THE EMERGENCE OF PROFESSIONAL PRACTICE

Family has been a central theme throughout modern nursing, expressed in different ways by different groups over time. Today the American nursing profession maintains a strong commitment to family centeredness. Nursing practice viewed as professional in its own time has consistently made a point to include some understanding that the family has a participatory role in the health and sickness care of its members. Nightingale's most influential book, addressed to women as health care givers in their own families, viewed health promotion and nursing as "in reality the same."[37] For the first 60 years of American nursing (1873–1933), the trained professional nurse served mainly within families. Hospitals were heavily staffed not by professionals but by student nurses. Since the turn of the century, when the *American Journal of Nursing* began, the professional literature has consistently addressed the family's role.

> For the first 60 years of American nursing the trained professional nurse served mainly within families. Hospitals were staffed not by professionals but by student nurses.

Lasch has charged that the entire society has become "medicalized," swept along by a religion of health.[10,38] Medicalization and professional expertise are said to have subverted the family's self-confidence. Is nursing a participant or a victim of "life in the therapeutic state?" As one of the helping professions, perhaps in the guise of the nurturing parent, has nursing served its own goal to professionalize along the lines of the Larson model by proselytizing this religion of health to justify governmental spending to support services for health, education, and welfare? How has the professional nurse accommodated familial values, especially when they clashed with his or her own best professional judgment?

Before the historian of nursing accepts these highly pejorative views as valid for the interpretation of nursing, perhaps the converse questions should be asked. Has nursing, instead, attempted to be a buttress against these possibilities? Has it made common cause with the family in the course of its own professional clash with doctors? Has it had as its goal the promotion of informed choice and support of family integrity (as the literature claims)?

If professionalism provides the path to the destruction of the family and, by extension, of society, then it is important for the historian to examine the meaning of professionalism as it was (and is) meant by nursing leaders, as well as by those they were attempting to lead. Their definition of a profession at each point should be confronted in context. For the historian, occupational practice as it changed over time is important to understanding the nurse's experience. Although sociological constructs may be useful as abstractions, their static quality must be recognized as the dynamic process of historical change is explored.

REFERENCES

1. Aries P: *Centuries of Childhood: A Social History of Family Life*, Baldick R (trans). New York, Random House, Vintage Books, 1962, pp 412–413.
2. deMause L: The Evolution of Childhood, in deMause L (ed): *The History of Childhood*. New York, Harper & Row, Harper Torchbooks, 1974, pp 1–73.
3. Kett JF: *Rites of Passage: Adolescence in America 1790 to the Present*. New York, Basic Books, 1977, p 5.
4. Katz MB: The origins of public education: A reassessment. *History of Education Quarterly* 16:398, 1976.
5. Degler CN: *At Odds: Women and the Family in America from the Revolution to the Present*. New York, Oxford University Press, 1980.
6. Demos J, Demos V: Adolescence in historical perspective. *Marriage and the Family* 31:632–638, 1979.
7. Mattingly PH: *The Classless Profession*. New York, New York University Press, 1975, pp *xii, xiii.*
8. Mattingly PH: The meaning of professional culture. *Rev Education* 3:439, 440, 1977.
9. Stone L: The rise of the nuclear family in early modern England: The patriarchal stage, in Rosenberg CE (ed): *The Family in History*. Philadelphia, University of Pennsylvania Press, 1975, pp 56, 57.
10. Lasch C: *Haven in a Heartless World: The Family Besieged*. New York, Basic Books, 1979.
11. Nightingale F: *Cassandra*. Westbury, NY, The Feminist Press, 1979, p 37.
12. Larson MS: *The Rise of Professionalism: A Sociological Analysis*. Berkeley, Calif, University of California Press, 1977.
13. Johnson WR: Professions in process: Doctors and teachers in American culture. *History of Education Quarterly* 2:185–198, 1975.
14. Parsons T: *The Social System*. New York, The Free Press, 1951.
15. Parsons T: The stability of the American family system, in Bell NW, Vogel EF (eds): *A Modern Introduction to the Family*, rev ed. New York, The Free Press, 1968, pp 97–101.
16. Bender T, Hall PD, Haskell TL, et al: Symposium: Institutionalization and education in the nineteenth and twentieth centuries. *History of Education Quarterly* 20:449–451, 1980.
17. Nightingale F: Sick nursing and health nursing, in Hampton I, et al: *Nursing of the Sick-1893*. New York, McGraw-Hill Series in Nursing, 1949, p 32.
18. Katz FE: Nurses, in Etzioni A (ed): *The Semi-Professions and Their Organization*. New York, The Free Press, 1969, pp 54–81.
19. Davis F (ed): *The Nursing Profession: Five Sociological Essays*. New York, John Wiley and Sons, 1966.
20. Stewart IM: Florence Nightingale — Educator. *Teachers College Record* 41:22, 1939.
21. Nightingale F: Quotation taken from a commemorative calendar prepared by Committee on Education, National League for Nursing Education, June 22, 1921.
22. Nightingale F: *Introductory Notes on Lying-In Institution together with a Proposal for Organising an Institution for Training Midwives and Midwifery Nurses*. London, Longmans, Green and Co, 1871.

23. Nightingale F: Midwifery as a Career for Educated Women. London, Longmans, Green and Co, 1871, pp 105–110.
24. Minutes of the American Society of Superintendents of Training Schools for Nurses, February 13, 1895, National League for Nursing Manuscript Collection, National Library of Medicine, Bethesda, Md.
25. Stewart IM: *The Education of Nurses: Historical Foundations and Modern Trends.* New York, The Macmillan Co, 1947, p 286.
26. Hampton IA: Educational standards for nurses, in Hampton I (ed): *Nursing the Sick 1893.* New York, McGraw-Hill Series in Nursing, McGraw-Hill, 1949, p 6.
27. Kobrin FE: The American midwife controversy: A crisis of professionalization. *Bull Med Hist* 40:350–363, 1966.
28. Devitt N: The statistical case for elimination of the midwife: Fact versus prejudice, 1890–1935. *Women and Health* 4:81–96, 1935.
29. *Birth Registration.* Misc. Series No. 2, Monograph 1, US Dept of Labor, Children's Bureau, 1913, p 5.
30. Crowell EF: The Midwives of New York. *Charities and Commons* 17:667–677, 1907.
31. Crowell EF: The Midwives of Chicago. *J Am Med Assoc* 50:1346–1350, 1908.
32. Ehrenreich B, English D: *For Her Own Good: 150 Years of Experts' Advice to Women.* Garden City, NY, Anchor Press/Doubleday, 1978.
33. Wald LD: The treatment of families in which there is sickness. *Am J Nurs* 4:427, 428, 1904.
34. Wald LD: The district nurses' contribution to the reduction of infant mortality, 12 November 1909. Lillian Wald Papers, (Box 34–35); Rare Books and Manuscripts Division, The New York Public Library, Astor, Lenox and Tilden Foundations.
35. Wald LD: *The House on Henry Street.* New York, Henry Holt and Co, 1915, p 60.
36. Wald LD: Teacher's College Lectures. Lillian Wald Papers, (Box 34–35), Reel #24.
37. Nightingale F: *Notes on Nursing: What It Is and What It Is Not.* New York, Appleton-Century Co Inc, 1938, p 9.
38. Lasch C: Life in the therapeutic stage. *New York Review of Books,* June 12, 1980, pp 24–32.

COMMENTARY

Hiestand's paper presents the results of her theory-generating work. She describes the family system in relation to various sociopolitical forces, including "childhood" as a modern idea made possible by the development of a middle class, as well as the professionalization of nursing, which introduces the idea of social control of the discipline. Hiestand's focus is clearly on family units within the context of the social-political scene.

In keeping with the discovery focus of theory generation, Hiestand offers an interpretive historical examination that led to advancement of several hypotheses that require testing by means of future empirical research. Moreover, the issues raised in the paper require further exploration by means of nonempirical methods such as historical and philosophic inquiries as well as hermeneutic techniques. And the questions raised with regard to health policy require data-based answers.

The paper represents a significant contribution to middle-range family theory development in nursing. The literature review underscores nursing's early and continued interest in families. A special feature of Hiestand's work is the use of the historical approach to family theory development in nursing. The paper clearly reveals the utility of this rarely used approach.

ANN L. WHALL

CHAPTER

7

Spouses' Experiences During Pregnancy and the Postpartum: A Program of Research and Theory Development

JACQUELINE FAWCETT

A program of nursing research was established to test a theory proposing that wives and husbands have similar pregnancy-related experiences. The research was guided by a conceptual framework of the family as a living open system. Findings were conflicting from three studies that investigated the relationship between spouses' strength of identification and similarities in changes in various body image components during and after pregnancy; taken together the findings suggested that spouses do not have similar patterns of change in their body images during pregnancy and the postpartum. Two other studies investigated the relationship between spouses'

Reprinted from *Image: Journal of Nursing Scholarship, 21,* 149–152, 1989.

strength of identification and similarities in their reports of physical and psychological symptoms during pregnancy and the postpartum. In these studies the spouses reported similar physical and psychological symptoms during pregnancy and the postpartum. There was no evidence, however, in any of the studies of a relationship between spouses' strength of identification and similarities in their pregnancy-related experiences. The validity of the theory of similar pregnancy-related experiences and the credibility of the conceptual framework +of the family as an open system are questioned.

• • •

A long-standing assumption underlying family-centered maternity nursing practice is that pregnancy is a family experience; that is, all family members are involved in a pregnancy. The validity of this assumption was never publicly challenged; nor was it tested empirically. The purpose of this paper is to outline the development of a conceptual-theoretical framework that characterizes spouses pregnancy-related experiences as similar and to summarize the results of a program of research designed to test the theory.

CONCEPTUAL-THEORETICAL FRAMEWORK

The conceptual framework of the family as a living, open system guided theory development and testing (Fawcett, 1975). The conceptual framework is an extension and interpretation of Martha Rogers' (1970) Life Process Model. Rogers described the human being as a four dimensional energy field, an open system characterized by wholeness, pattern and organization, sentience and thought. The human energy field, according to Rogers, is coextensive with the four dimensional environmental energy field. Rogers claimed that human and environmental energy fields are engaged in mutual and simultaneous interaction.

Fawcett's (1975) conceptual framework of the family was based on the assumptions that one environmental field in which human beings are embedded is the family, and that the family is an open-system energy field. It was reasoned that if the family were an open-system energy field, the characteristics attributed by Rogers (1970) to the human open-system energy field could be attributed to the family. This line of reasoning is consistent with Rogers' (1983) own conceptualization of the family.

Briefly, the conceptual framework of the family describes the family as a living open system, an integral, unified whole characterized by a unique and ever-changing pattern and organization. Alterations in pattern and organization are described as being continuous; they reflect the mutual and simultaneous interaction between the family system and the environment.

The theory of similarities in spouses' pregnancy-related experiences was derived from the following conceptual framework concepts: open family system, pattern and organization, and mutual and simultaneous interaction. Pregnant and postpartal women and their husbands represent the open family system, pregnancy-related experiences represent pattern and organization, and strength of identification represents mutual and simultaneous interaction.

The following two conceptual framework postulates guided the development of theoretical propositions: (a) change in the pattern and organization of one family member is associated with a similar change in pattern and organization of other family members; and (b) mutual and simultaneous interaction is related positively to similarity of change in pattern and organization. These postulates represent an interpretation, or modification, of Rogers' (1970) statements about human beings, in that the postulates specify similarity of change in pattern and organization and a directional relationship between mutual and simultaneous interaction and change in pattern and organization. The theory therefore proposes that (a) wives and husbands have similar pregnancy-related experiences during pregnancy and the postpartum, and (b) the similarities in spouses' pregnancy-related experiences are positively related to the strength of their identification.

REVIEW OF THE LITERATURE

A review of the literature was undertaken in an attempt to identify specific pregnancy-related experiences of both pregnant women and their husbands. The literature revealed that women typically experience a number of physical symptoms including heartburn, nausea and vomiting, constipation or diarrhea, hemorrhoids, food cravings, changes in appetite, increased urination, backache, dyspnea, sensitivity to odors, skin irritations and fatigue. Some physical symptoms, especially fatigue, continue into the postpartum (Pritchard, MacDonald, & Gant, 1985; Reeder, Mastroianni, & Martin, 1983). Pregnant and postpartal women also experience some psychological symptoms such as mood swings, anxiety and depression (Cox, Conner, & Kendall, 1982; Glazer, 1980).

The literature also revealed that the profound and obvious change in the form and appearance of the woman's body during pregnancy and the postpartum is associated with considerable change in her body image. Studies have documented changes in attitude toward and perception of the body (Fisher, 1973; McConnell & Daston, 1961), which are the two main dimensions of body image (Schilder, 1950).

Investigators also have reported the occurrence of various physical and psychological symptoms in the husbands of pregnant women including gastrointestinal disorders, abdominal bloating, appetite changes, backache, toothache, lassitude, skin rashes, syncope, weight gain, leg cramps, anxiety, depression, tension, insomnia, irritability, nervousness and mood swings (Clinton, 1986, 1987; Lipkin & Lamb, 1982; Munroe, Munroe, & Nerlove, 1973; Strickland, 1987; Trethowan & Conlon, 1965). Investigators have reported that husbands of pregnant women express concerns about body intactness and dream about changes in their bodies (Colman & Colman, 1971; Liebenberg, 1969), suggesting that men experience body image changes during the childbearing period.

Male pregnancy-related experiences are referred to as the couvade syndrome (Trethowan & Conlon, 1965). Couvade phenomena are thought to be an expression of a man's involvement in pregnancy and his identification with his wife. It has been proposed that the more a husband identifies with his wife, the more likely he is to experience physical and psychological symptoms and body image changes during pregnancy and the postpartum (Colman & Colman, 1971; Trethowan & Conlon).

Most research related to the couvade syndrome has focused solely on the male partner, rather than comparing men's symptoms with those of their wives. One study compared spouses' symptoms and indicated that 10 couples experienced similar physiological and psychological changes during the pregnancy but did not specify what the changes were (Deutscher, 1969).

THEORY TESTING

The review of the literature led to the design of five studies that have tested the theory of similarities in spouses' pregnancy-related experiences. Three studies tested the theory as particularized for body image changes, and two studies tested the theory as particularized for physical and psychological symptoms. Inasmuch as all five studies have already been reported in detail, a summary of each is given below.

The three studies that focused on body image investigated the relationship between wives, and husbands' strength of identification and similarities in changes in various components of body image during and after pregnancy. These studies tested the theoretical propositions that (a) wives, and husbands' body image changes are similar during pregnancy and the postpartum and (b) similarities in spouses' body image changes are positively related to the strength of their identification.

The first body image study (Fawcett, 1978) focused on perceptions of the body. Perceived body space was defined as the amount of space individuals think that their bodies occupy; it was measured by the Topographic Device. Articulation of body space was defined as the extent to which individuals perceive their bodies as being separate from the surrounding environment; it was measured by the Figure Drawing Test. Strength of identification was defined as the amount of semantic similarity between spouses for a set of concepts related to identification; this was measured by the Identification Scale. Complete longitudinal data were available for 40 couples. Data were collected during the eighth and ninth months of pregnancy and the first, second, and twelfth postpartal months (articulation of body space was not measured at the twelfth postpartal month).

The second body image study was designed as a replication and refinement of the first study (Fawcett, 1987; Fawcett, Bliss-Holtz, Haas, Leventhal, & Rubin, 1986). This study also focused on perceptions of the body, again using the variable, perceived body space; and on attitudes toward the body, using the variable, global body attitude. Global body attitude was defined as individuals' general attitudes about the outward form and appearance of their bodies; it was measured by the Body Attitude Scale. Strength of identification, again, was measured by the Identification Scale. Longitudinal data were available on 54 couples. Data were collected during the third, sixth, and ninth months of pregnancy and during the first and second postpartal months. The third body image study was a replication of the second study, using a sample of 20 couples (Drake, Verhulst, Fawcett & Barger, 1988).

Content validity and acceptable levels of reliability were established for the population of interest for all instruments used in the three body image studies. The links among conceptual framework concepts, concepts of the theory as particularized for body image, and empirical indicators are shown in Figures 1 and 2.

The two studies that focused on spouses' symptoms investigated the relationship between wives, and husbands' strength of identification and similarities in their reports of physical and psychological symptoms during pregnancy and the postpartum (Drake, Verhulst, & Fawcett, 1988; Fawcett & York, 1986, 1987). These studies tested the theoretical propo-

Conceptual model concepts	Open family system	Pattern and organization		Mutual and simultaneous interaction
Concepts of the theory	Pregnant and postpartal couples	Perceived body space	Articulation of body concept	Strength of identification
Empirical indicators	Couples in 8th, 9th months of pregnancy; 1st, 2nd, 12th postpartal months	Topographic device	Figure drawing test	Identification scale

SOURCE: *Fawcett, J. (1978). Body image and the pregnant couple.* **American Journal of Maternal Child Nursing, 3, 227–233.**

Figure 1.   Conceptual-theoretical-empirical structure for first study of spouses' body image changes during pregnancy and the postpartum.

Conceptual model concepts	Open family system	Pattern and organization	Mutual and simultaneous interaction
Concepts of the theory	Pregnant and postpartal couples	Perceived body space	Global body attitude	Strength of identification
Empirical indicators	Couples in 3rd, 6th, 9th months of pregnancy; 1st, 2nd post-partal months	Topographic device	Body attitude scale	Identification scale

SOURCES: *Fawcett, J., Bliss-Holtz, V. J., Haas, M. B., Leventhal, M., & Rubin, M. (1986). Spouses' body image changes during and after pregnancy: a replication and extension.* **Nursing Research, 35,** *220–223; Drake, M. L., Verhulst, D., Fawcett, J., & Barger, D. F. (1988). Spouses' body image changes during and after pregnancy: A replication in Canada.* **IMAGE: Journal of Nursing Scholarship, 20,** *88–92.*

Figure 2.   Conceptual-theoretical-empirical structure for second and third studies of spouses' body image changes during pregnancy and the postpartum.

sitions that (a) wives, and husbands' reports of physical and psychological symptoms are similar during pregnancy and the postpartum and (b) similarities in spouses' reports of physical and psychological symptoms are positively related to the strength of their identification.

Physical symptoms were defined as reports of pregnancy-related bodily symptoms (e.g., nausea, appetite changes, leg cramps) and were measured by 20 items on a Symptoms Checklist. Psychological symptoms were defined as reports of psychological changes associated with childbearing (e.g., anxiety, depression) and were measured by 3 items on the Symptoms Checklist. In the first study, psychological symptoms also were measured by the Beck Depression Inventory. Strength of identification was again measured by the Identification Scale. The first study included data from 70 couples including 23 couples in an early pregnancy group, 24 in a late pregnancy group, and 23 in a postpartum group. The second study included data from 20 couples. Data from these couples were collected during the third, sixth, and ninth months of pregnancy and the first and second postpartal months. Content validity and acceptable levels of reliability were established for the population of interest for the instruments used in the two symptoms studies. The conceptual-theoretical-empirical structures for these studies are illustrated in Figures 3 and 4.

The findings from the body image studies are conflicting. The results of the first study indicated that both spouses experienced changes in perceived body space and that these changes were similar. This finding was not replicated in the second and third studies, where the findings

Conceptual model concepts	Open family system	Pattern and organization		Mutual and simultaneous interaction
Concepts of the theory	Pregnant and postpartal couples	Physical symptoms	Psychological symptoms	Strength of identification
Empirical indicators	Early and late pregnancy groups, postpartal group	Symptoms checklist	Symptoms checklist; Beck Depression Inventory	Identification scale

SOURCES: *Fawcett, J., & York, R. (1986). Spouses' physical and psychological symptoms during pregnancy and the postpartum.* **Nursing Research, 35,** *144–148; Fawcett, J., & York, R. (1987). Spouses' strength of identification and reports of symptoms during pregnancy and the postpartum.* **Florida Nursing Review,** *2(2), 1–10.*

Figure 3. Conceptual-theoretical-empirical structure for first study of spouses' physical and psychological symptoms during pregnancy and the postpartum.

indicated that although wives experienced changes in perceived body space, husbands did not. Thus there was no evidence of similarities in spouses' perceived body space changes. Neither wives nor husbands demonstrated any changes in articulation of body concept in the first study, obviously resulting in no evidence of similarities for spouses in this variable. Wives in the second and third studies experienced statisti-

Conceptual model concepts	Open family system	Pattern and organization		Mutual and simultaneous interaction
Concepts of the theory	Pregnant and postpartal couples	Physical symptoms	Psychological symptoms	Strength of identification
Empirical indicators	Couples in 3rd, 6th, 9th months of pregnancy; 1st, 2nd post-partal months	Symptoms checklist	Symptoms checklist	Identification scale

SOURCE: *Drake, M. L. Verhulst, D., & Fawcett, J. (1988). Physical and psychological symptoms experienced by pregnant Canadian women and their husbands.* **Journal of Advanced Nursing, 13,** *436–440.*

Figure 4. Conceptual-theoretical-empirical structure for second study of spouses' physical and psychological symptoms during pregnancy and the postpartum.

cally significant changes in global body attitude. Husbands in the second study experienced no changes in global body attitude and those in the third study exhibited a tendency toward changes in this variable. There was therefore no evidence of similarities in spouses' global body attitude changes in either study. Furthermore, there was no evidence in any of the studies of a relationship between spouses' strength of identification and similarities in their body image changes.

The findings from the two symptoms studies indicated that spouses report similar physical and psychological symptoms during pregnancy and the postpartum. However, there was no evidence in either study of a relationship between spouses' strength of identification and similarities in their reports of symptoms.

DISCUSSION

Taken together, the findings of the five studies provide minimal support for the theory of similarities in spouses' pregnancy-related experiences. It is unlikely that the conflicting findings were the result of methodological flaws, since the instruments used in the studies were valid and reliable measures of the theory level concepts, and the sample sizes were adequate. Initial findings for the theoretical proposition asserting similarities in spouses' patterns of change in perceived body space during pregnancy and the postpartum were not upheld in two replication studies. There was no evidence of change in articulation of body concept for either spouse, suggesting that this component of body image may be more stable than previously thought. Although the wives experienced global body attitude changes, their husbands did not. Thus there was no evidence of similarities in wives and husbands' changes in this variable.

Given the results of the body image studies, the findings for similarities in spouses' reports of physical and psychological symptoms must be interpreted with caution. Further replication of this research is warranted.

The lack of evidence for the theoretical proposition asserting a positive relationship between spouses' strength of identification and similarities in their pregnancy-related experiences may be because of a disparity between the definition of identification, as measured by the Identification Scale, and that implied by investigators, who claimed that identification is responsible for similarities in spouses' pregnancy-related experiences (Colman & Colman, 1971; Trethowan & Conlon, 1965). It is recommended that other definitions of identification such as imitation (Schilder, 1950) be considered in future research.

The collective findings of the five studies raise questions about the credibility of the conceptual framework of the family as a living open system. The results of the research provide inconsistent support for the postulate that change in pattern and organization of one family member is associated with a similar change in another member. No support is provided for the postulate that mutual and simultaneous interaction is related positively to similarity of change in pattern and organization. This could be because of an inappropriate choice of theoretical representatives for conceptual framework concepts. The conceptual framework concept, pattern and organization, might be better represented theoretically by pregnancy-related experiences other than body image and symptoms. Furthermore, the conceptual framework concept, mutual and simultaneous interaction, might be better represented theoretically as the quality of the marital relationship, the couple's desire for a child, the man's involvement in the pregnancy, intimacy, or empathy.

The findings also could be the result of flaws in the conceptual framework. A major flaw seems to be in the postulate of *similar* changes in pattern and organization of family members. The inclusion of this postulate may be a faulty interpretation of Rogers's (1970) work or a faulty modification of traditional open systems formulations, which assert that change in one component of a system is associated with change in another component of that system (Bertalanffy, 1968).

A serious threat to the credibility of the conceptual framework and to traditional open systems formulations is the finding that husbands did not always demonstrate observable pregnancy-related experiences. Thus, even a revised conceptual framework postulate stating that a change in pattern and organization of one family member is associated with a nonsimilar change in pattern and organization of another family member would not have consistent empirical support.

Perhaps it is too early to question the credibility of the conceptual framework. However, conceptual frameworks must be open to constant criticism or they will become ideologies rather than starting points for scientific work.

This program of research, derived from one conceptual framework of the family, provides mixed evidence regarding the assumption that pregnancy is a family experience. It remains for other research programs derived from other conceptual frameworks to yield the much-needed empirical data that will support or refute the assumption of family involvement in pregnancy.

REFERENCES

Bertalanffy, L. (1968). **General system theory**. New York: George Braziller.

Clinton, J. F. (1986). Expectant fathers at risk for couvade. **Nursing Research, 35,** 290–295.

Clinton, J. F. (1987). Physical and emotional responses of expectant fathers throughout pregnancy and the early postpartum period. **International Journal of Nursing Studies, 24,** 59–68.

Colman, A. D., & Colman, L. L. (1971). **Pregnancy: The psychological experience.** New York: Herder and Herder.

Cox, J. L., Connor, Y., & Kendall, R. E. (1982). Prospective study of the psychiatric disorders of childbirth. **British Journal of Psychiatry, 140,** 11–17.

Deutscher, M. (1969). First pregnancy and the origins of family: A rehearsal theory. **American Journal of Orthopsychiatry, 39,** 319–320.

Drake, M. L., Verhulst, D., & Fawcett, J. (1988). Physical and psychological symptoms experienced by pregnant Canadian women and their husbands. **Journal of Advanced Nursing, 13,** 436–440.

Drake, M. L., Verhulst, D., Fawcett, Jr., & Barger, D. F. (1988). Spouses' body image changes during and after pregnancy: A replication in Canada. **IMAGE: Journal of Nursing Scholarship, 20,** 88–92.

Fawcett, J. (1975). The family as a living open system: An emerging conceptual framework for nursing. **International Nursing Review, 22,** 113–116.

Fawcett, J. (1978). Body image and the pregnant couple. **American Journal of Maternal Child Nursing, 3,** 227–233.

Fawcett, J. (1987). Re: Spouses' body image changes during and after pregnancy: A replication and extension (Letter to the editor). **Nursing Research, 36,** 220, 243.

Fawcett, J., Bliss-Holtz, V. J., Haas, M. B. Leventhal, M., & Rubin, M. (1986). Spouses' body image changes during and after pregnancy: a replication and extension. **Nursing Research, 35,** 220–223.

Fawcett, J., & York, R. (1986). Spouses' physical and psychological symptoms during pregnancy and postpartum. **Nursing Research, 35,** 144–148.

Fawcett, J., & York, R. (1987). Spouses' strength of identification and reports of symptoms during pregnancy and the postpartum. **Florida Nursing Review, 2**(2), 1–10.

Fisher, S. (1973). **Body consciousness: You are what you feel.** Englewood Cliffs, NJ: Prentice-Hall.

Glazer, G. (1980). Anxiety levels and concerns among pregnant women. **Research in Nursing and Health, 3,** 07–113.

Liebenberg, B. (1969). Expectant fathers. **Child and Family, 8,** 265–278.

Lipkin, M., & Lamb, G. S. (1982). The couvade syndrome: An epidemiologic study. **Annals of Internal Medicine, 96,** 509–511.

McConnell, O. L., & Daston, P. G. (1961). Body image changes in pregnancy. **Journal of Projective Techniques, 25,** 451–456.

Munroe, R. L., Munroe, R. H., & Nerlove, S. B. (1973). Male pregnancy symptoms and cross-sex identity: Two replications. **Journal of Social Psychology, 89,** 147–148.

Pritchard, J. A., MacDonald, P. C., & Gant, N. F. (1985). **Williams' obstetrics** (17th ed.). Norwalk, CT: Appleton-Century-Crofts.

Reeder, S. R., Mastroianni, L., & Martin, L. L. (1983). **Maternity nursing** (15th ed.). Philadelphia: Lippincott.

Rogers, M. E. (1970). **An introduction to the theoretical basis of nursing.** Philadelphia: F. A. Davis.

Rogers, M. E. (1983). Science of unitary human beings: a paradigm for nursing. In I. W. Clements & F. B. Roberts, **Family health. A theoretical approach to nursing care** (pp. 219–227). New York: Wiley.

Schilder, P. (1950). **The images and appearances of the human body.** New York: International Universities Press.

Strickland, O. L. (1987). The occurrence of symptoms in expectant fathers. **Nursing Research, 36,** 184–189.

Trethowan, W. H., & Conlon, W. F. (1965). The couvade syndrome. **British Journal of Psychiatry, 111,** 57–66.

COMMENTARY

This article reports the findings of a program of research that sought to develop middle-range family theory from a conceptual model of nursing. As such, it is one of only a few research programs focused on family theory development within the context of a nursing model.

The emphasis here is on the family system, with pregnant women and their husbands making up the system. Descriptions and diagrams of the linkages between the middle-range theories dealing with changes in body image and reports of physical and psychological symptoms and the conceptual model facilitate understanding of the process of theory derivation from a nursing model. Results of several theory-testing studies, however, raise doubts about the validity of the theories and, therefore, the credibility of the parent conceptual model.

A methodological point of interest is the creation of relational data by means of computation of "similarity scores" for wives' and husbands' body image changes and symptoms reports, as well as by computation of the strength-of-identification score. Another methodological point is the investigator's suggestions for further research that takes potentially intervening variables into account.

ANN L. WHALL

CHAPTER

8

Effect of Stress on Family Functioning During Pregnancy

RAMONA T. MERCER
SANDRA L. FERKETCH
JEANNE DeJOSEPH
KATHARYN A. MAY
DEANNA SOLLID

A theoretical model hypothesized to predict family functioning was tested in four groups of expectant parents, followed by exploratory model building. The groups studied during the 24th to 34th weeks of pregnancy included 153 high-risk hospitalized women, 75 of their partners, 218 low-risk women from the general obstetric clinic, and 147 of their partners. Both partners in the high-risk situation reported greater discrepancy in family functioning than partners in the low-risk situation. The hypothesized models proved to have low explanatory power, accounting for 13% to 15% of the variance. The final empirical models developed explained 33% of the variance in family functioning among high-risk women and 48% among their

Reprinted from *Nursing Research, 37,* 268–275, 1988.

partners, 23% among low-risk women, and 32% among their partners. The empirical models differed from the hypothesized models in that variables postulated to have only indirect effects were shown to have direct effects on family function and intergenerational variables significantly expanded the theoretical model.

Family functioning is influenced by many forces inside and outside the family. All pregnant families experience a degree of stress, anticipation, and change involving intrapersonal, interpersonal, and intrafamily boundaries and relationships. Stressors during pregnancy, such as obstetric risks and unanticipated events, reduce the predictability of the outcomes for both mother and infant and have the potential to increase anxiety and depression to the extent that interpersonal and family relationships are affected.

The purpose of this study was to determine the effect of antepartum stress on family functioning. *Stress* was defined as undesirable events, negative life events, and at-risk conditions (pregnancy risk) that challenge the family's resources for dealing with the events. Families who were experiencing a pregnancy in which the woman was considered low-risk and was attending the general obstetric clinic and families who were experiencing a more stressful pregnancy in which the woman was high-risk and hospitalized were studied. The overall goal was to search for information that would aid in providing more salient nursing intervention for childbearing families facing the normative stress of pregnancy and those facing more acute stress.

The *family* was defined as a dynamic system that functions as a whole, made up of subsystems of individuals and dyads. Individuals included the expectant mother, expectant father, unborn infant, and dyads included the mother-father, mother-unborn infant, and father-unborn infant. It was assumed that stress experienced by an individual or dyad in the family system would affect the function of the total system.

Data reported here are from a larger study in which family developmental theory provided the overarching theoretical framework. This framework emphasizes the interrelatedness of family parts and allows focus on process occurring over time, with potential for family development to occur with adaptation to stress (Mercer, May, Ferketich, & DeJoseph, 1986).

RELEVANT LITERATURE

Although stressful life events related to childbirth and early parenthood have been studied (Bloom, 1985), little research has focused on stress as it affects overall family functioning during pregnancy. Stress from negative life events has been observed to contribute to emotional disequilibrium during pregnancy (Tilden, 1983) and to gestational complications

(Norbeck & Tilden, 1983), both of which may affect the family subsystems and the family as a system. Stressful life events experienced during pregnancy were found to be negatively related to family functioning (Smilkstein, Helsper-Lucas, Ashworth, Montano, & Pagel, 1984). Curry and Snell (1985) reported that higher stress from negative life events was associated with less progression in maternal role behaviors.

Obstetric problems and maternal health concerns have also been identified as contributing to maladaptation to pregnancy and the neonatal period (Cohen, 1979). The risk assessment of the pregnant woman can have a profound impact on the course of her pregnancy, the options she may select for birth, and her infant's mortality rate (Committee on Assessing Alternative Birth Settings, 1982). Although risk scores from complications scales are useful in predicting neonatal and infant outcome (Molfese & Thomson, 1985), the change in intensity of antepartal care and the restriction of choice of type of birth all have the potential to increase stress for the pregnant woman, her mate, and the total family system.

In high-risk situations requiring hospitalization, the pregnant woman faces unique stressors, including both normative stress from pregnancy and more acute stressors (Dore & Davies, 1979; Penticuff, 1982; Perry, Parer, & Inturrisi, 1986). There is consensus that hospitalization disrupts a pregnant family's functioning (Kemp & Page, 1987; Merkatz, Budd, & Merkatz, 1978; Williams, 1986).

Concern that antepartal hospitalization may impede the achievement of the usual tasks of pregnancy was the focus of several who studied the hospitalized pregnant woman (Curry & Snell, 1985; Merkatz, 1978; White & Ritchie, 1984). A finding common to all studies was the intense stressor of separation from family and home imposed by the hospitalization. Hospitalized women who had children at home reported greater stress than those without children. Lack of control, mood swings, and worry about their partners were also identified as stressors (Curry & Snell). In addition, an intergenerational influence on family functioning was suggested; the hospitalized woman's relationship with her mother was positively related to her maternal role behaviors (Curry & Snell). Intergenerational influences on the course of pregnancy and on the family have been reported aside from stress or risk situations; a woman's positive relationship with her father was associated with a satisfying pregnancy experience, as was an affectionate relationship with her husband (Gladieux, 1978).

In a prospective study, family functioning was found to account for 7% of the variance in infant birthweight (Ramsey, Abell, & Baker, 1986). Richardson (1987) argued that poor marital relationships within the family frequently lead to premature birth. In one study, families with high-risk infants reported less agreement on family matters, sexual activity, celebrations, and less closeness to their infants than families with

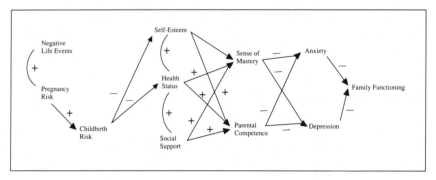

Figure 1. Hypothesized Theoretical Model: Effects of Antepartum Stress on Family Functioning

low- or moderate-risk infants (White & Dawson, 1981). Fathers in families with high-risk infants were least likely to help with infant care yet reported having their patience tested the most by the infant. The findings for families with high-risk infants were, however, confounded by lower socioeconomics status, less help, and younger mothers. Blackburn and Lowen (1986) found that mothers reported more intense emotional responses to a premature birth than fathers. This finding raises questions as to whether expectant mothers also have a more intense emotional response to premature labor.

Thus, although few studies have focused on family functioning during pregnancy, social, psychological, and coping resources have been found to influence the outcome of stress (Pearlin & Schooler, 1978). In an extensive review of the literature, major variables were identified as a basis for a theoretical causal model: Stress from negative life events and pregnancy risk were predicted to have direct negative effects on self-esteem and health status; self-esteem, health status, and social support were predicted to have direct positive effects on sense of mastery; sense of mastery was predicted to have direct negative effects on anxiety and depression which in turn have direct negative effects on family functioning (Mercer et al., 1986). (See Figure 1.) Because family functioning in the childbearing period has been studied largely from the woman's point of view, it was critical to study family functioning from the man's perspective as well. Findings that focused on early parenthood showed that men experience fewer life changes with the addition of a child than women (Belsky, Lang, & Rovine, 1985; Grossman et al., 1980; Harriman, 1983). Thus, the theoretical model was tested among four groups of expectant parents to determine whether there were differences in predictors among men and women as well as in the situational stress of high-risk pregnancy and low-risk pregnancy.

HYPOTHESES

I. High-risk women experiencing antenatal hospitalization and their partners will report less optimal family functioning than low-risk women and their partners.

II. Expectant partners will report similar levels of family functioning.

METHOD

Sample: This study of 593 subjects was designed to test for differences between expectant couples, in both high-risk and low-risk situations and to test causal models predicting family functioning in both situations. Subjects included 153 high-risk hospitalized women (HRW), 75 expectant father partners of high-risk women (HRM), 218 low-risk women (LRW), and 147 partners of low-risk women (LRM) who were interviewed during the 24th to 34th weeks of the woman's pregnancy.

All subjects were 18 or older, fluent in English, and, if unmarried, were living together and planning to parent together. The low-risk sample of expectant mothers attended the general obstetric clinic, had no chronic disease, had only mild symptoms of pregnancy-induced disease, if any, and responded to routine management.

The groups did not differ significantly by socioeconomic status (Hollingshead, 1975), race, or marital status, $\chi^2 > .05$. Ages of women ranged from 18 to 45 years ($M = 29$ years); of men, from 19 to 61 ($M = 31$ years). Three-fourths of the high-risk groups and two-thirds of the low-risk groups (70% of the total sample) were white; other ethnic groups included 11% Asian, 10% Hispanic, 4% black, and 4% other. Partners of low-risk women had more graduate and/or professional education, $\chi^2(12) = 27.07$, $p = .008$. Over one-third (35%) of the total sample had some college education, 23% had a baccalaureate degree, and 20% had a graduate or professional degree.

Partners of high-risk women had more children than men in the low-risk group, but the two groups of women did not differ significantly from one another or from the groups of men, $F(3,581) = 3.59, p < .02$, Tukey B multiple range test. Fifty-two percent of those expecting their first child were HRW, 46% were HRM, 56% were LRW, and 56% were LRM. Children from previous marriages accounted for differences between mates. Over half (54%) of the total sample were expecting their first child; 30% had one child, 11% had two children, and 5% had three or more children.

Among HRW, reasons for hospitalization included: preterm labor and/or premature rupture of the membranes 72%, pre-eclampsia or hypertension 8%, bleeding or placenta previa 4%, diabetes 3%, Rh incompatibility 3%, asthma 2%, and 1% each upper respiratory infection, thyroid problem, renal disease, surgery, thrombitis, and back injury. Pregnancy-risk scores among HRW were $M = 35.78$, $SD = 19.19$, range 10 to 102, with 39% scoring < 26, the cut point for high-risk status; among LRW, $M = 10.13$, $SD = 8.47$, range 0 to 49, with 6% scoring > 26. Factors that contributed to the 6% of LRW's scores that were > 26 included previous pregnancies such as low birth weight or postterm infants, previous cesarean births, viral infections, and substance intake such as cigarette smoking, alcohol, or drugs. High-risk hospitalized women with a score of 10 had no risk factor other than preterm labor or premature rupture of membranes.

Instruments: Family functioning was measured by the 21-item Feetham Family Functioning instrument (Feetham & Humenick, 1982; Roberts & Feetham, 1982), which was constructed to measure three broad areas of family function. *Family functioning* was defined as the individual's view of the activities and relationships between the family and its subsystems (division of labor, housework), including the individuals (between mates, parent-child), and between the family and broader social units (school, work) (Feetham & Humenick). Respondents rated each item from 1 to 7 for the actual situation, then rated each item for what was desired, and a discrepant score between the two was derived with a possible range of zero to 126. Thus, cultural or family social value differences were accounted for. The smaller the score, the more optimal or less discrepant the family functioning. The Cronbach alpha for the discrepant score was .81 (Roberts & Feetham). Cronbach alphas for the discrepant scores among groups in this study ranged from .78 to .82.

Negative life events stress was measured by Norbeck's (1984) 82-item adaptation of Sarason, Johnson, and Siegel's (1978) Life Experiences Survey, in which items were regrouped by topic for clarity and items added for women. This better organized adaptation was preferred as items that related to women only were identified by adding (female) after the event. Respondents rated life events that had been experienced the previous year as positive or negative, and assigned a weight of *no effect*(0) to *great effect*(3). The test-retest reliability for the score was .78 (Norbeck, 1984).

The extent of pregnancy risk was assessed using a version of the instrument reported by Hobel, Hyvarinen, Okada, and Oh (1973) that was updated to reflect current diagnostic procedures and interventions. A panel of perinatal nurse specialists and a physician expert in obstetrics established content validity. Various prenatal risks such as family history of diabetes or drug allergy receive a value of 1, history of epilepsy or fetal anomalies are rated 5, and premature labor with betamimetic therapy, premature rupture of membranes, intrauterine transfusions, alcohol abuse, or emotional problems are rated 10. The cut point to separate high- from low-risk status is considered to be 26 as opposed to the earlier

10 (C. J. Hobel, personal communication, March 21, 1984). The Hobel et al. risk assessment scale has been used for prediction and multivariate analyses, and is considered one of the more robust risk assessment scales (Committee on Assessing Alternative Birth Settings, 1982).

Self-esteem, the level of self-acceptance or value placed on self, was measured by Rosenberg's (1979) 10-item scale, using a 1- to 4-point rating for each item. The possible range was 10 to 40 with a higher score indicating higher self-esteem. Cronbach alpha reliabilities for the four groups in this study ranged from .84 to .87.

Perception of health status was measured by the 22-item General Health Index (Davies & Ware, 1981). This measure is not focused on specific components of health (physiologic, physical, or mental), but allows respondents to indicate the objective information they have about their general health and how they feel about that information. Items measure the individual's perception of current health, prior health, health outlook, resistance to illness, health worry/concern, and sickness orientation. The measure shows variability in general populations. The stability of the measure contributes to precision in repeated-measures designs with consistent reliability (Cronbach alpha = .89) (Davies & Ware, 1981). Cronbach alpha reliabilities in this study ranged from .82 to .88.

Three dimensions of social support were measured: perceived, received, and the size of the social network. Barrera's (1981) 40-item Inventory of Socially Supportive Behaviors was used to measure help received during the past 4 weeks. Cronbach alphas ranged from .94 to .95. Perceived support was measured with an adaptation of the scale used by Wandersman, Wandersman, and Kahn (1980) and developed by McMillan (1976). The 6-item scale had alpha reliabilities in this study ranging from .73 to .80. The size of the network was measured by having subjects identify the number of persons for 19 categories (such as friends, family members, mate, and co-workers) who were helpful to them.

A 7-item Sense of Mastery Scale (Pearlin, Lieberman, Menaghan, & Mullan, 1981) was used to tap the extent that the respondent feels life's chances are under control as opposed to being under the rule of fate. Alpha reliabilities for the four groups ranged from .70 to .76.

State and trait anxiety were measured using the State-Trait Anxiety Inventory (Spielberger, Gorsuch, Lushene, Vagg, & Jacobs, 1983). Spielberger et al. differentiated between state anxiety as a situation-specific response and trait anxiety as a stable indicator of anxiety proneness. The measure has been used extensively and has robust reliabilities (.91 to .95) and construct validity. The test-retest correlations for the trait anxiety scale ranged from .73 to .76 for adults (Spielberger et al.). Cronbach alpha reliabilities ranged from .92 to .95 for state anxiety and from .90 to .93 for trait anxiety across the four groups.

The 20-item Center for Epidemiologic Studies Depression Scale designed to measure depressive symptomatology in the general population was used to measure depression (Radloff, 1977). It has a high degree of internal consistency (.89 to .90), construct validity, and concurrent validity when compared to clinical diagnostic criteria as well as with other self-report scales (Radloff). Reliabilities in this study ranged from .83 to .88.

Intergenerational relationships were determined by having respondents rate their relationships with each parent (or parental figure) as a child, as a teenager, and currently. The items were rated *very well* (1), *usually well* (2), *no parent figure or no contact* (3), *usually poorly* (4), and *very poorly* (5). Current contact with each parent was rated from *daily* or *almost daily* (1) to *never* (7).

Procedure: Data were collected through a semistructured interview and a booklet of self-completed standardized instruments. Hospitalized women were approached to determine their interest in participation in the project as soon as the nurse in charge of their care advised that their condition permitted contact. After informed consent, the interview was held in the hospital room for high-risk women and in the obstetric clinic for low-risk women. The women's partners were invited to participate either by the woman or by the interviewer. Because few men were encountered in the obstetric clinic, appointments for their interviews were scheduled by telephone.

Test booklets were left with the women to complete at their leisure and were either picked up the next day or returned by mail. Upon receipt of each completed test booklet, a $5.00 honorarium was mailed to the subject.

Data Analysis: Student's t or Smith Satterthwaite t tests for groups with unequal variances were used to determine differences between high- and low-risk groups and matched pairs t tests to determine differences between partners in high- and low-risk situations. Correlation matrices to test for multicollinearity of the theoretical model variables showed only two correlations that exceeded .65. These were between state anxiety and depression in low-risk women, $r = .69$, and their partners, $r = .67$. The theoretical model in Figure 1 was tested in each group with sets of structural equations (Turner & Stevens, 1971). Residual analysis was used to assess both mathematic and causal model assumptions (Verran & Ferketich, 1984, 1987; Ferketich & Verran, 1984). Model respecification was done with demographic and other variables that met model-building requirements (Ferketich & Verran). Models were augmented where appropriate and mathematic model assumptions were reassessed (Verran & Ferketich, 1984, 1987). Final models were compared across groups for unique and common predictors. The accepted level of significance for all analyses was $p \leq .05$.

RESULTS

Hypotheses: As hypothesized, high-risk women reported significantly less optimal family functioning than low-risk women, $t(348) = 2.15$, $p = .03$, and partners of HRW reported less optimal family functioning than low-risk partners, $t(118) = 2.43$, $p = .02$. The mean discrepant scores for family functioning were: HRW, 20.76, $SD = 12.86$; HRM, 18.51, $SD = 11.84$; LRW, 17.96, $SD = 11.37$; and LRM, 14.65, $SD = 9.35$.

The hypothesis that partners would report similar levels of family functioning held true only in the high-risk situation, $t(69) = 1.08$, $p = .29$. However, in the low-risk situation, low-risk men reported significantly less discrepant family functioning, $t(138) = 2.64, p = .009$, than the women.

Because all men did not participate in the study, one-half of the hospitalized women and one-third of the LRW were not tested in the matched pairs t tests; therefore, t tests for sex differences between high- and low-risk groups were done using the total sample. These findings agreed with the matched-pairs t tests. Differences were not observed in the high-risk situation, $t(216) = 1.25$, $p = .21$, but continued to be significant in the low-risk situation, $t(342) = 2.98$, $p = .003$.

Tests of Causal Models.   In testing the hypothesized theoretical model for direct links with the system of structural equations, only 13% to 15% of the variance in family functioning was directly explained by either anxiety or depression. Among HRW, state anxiety was the predictor; and among all other groups, depression was the predictor. The failure of both anxiety and depression to enter the theoretical model as had been hypothesized was probably due to the high correlation between the two variables. See Table 1 for a summary of model testing.

Figure 2 shows the direct and indirect links with standardized beta weights in the final respecified empirical model for HRW. Sense of mastery became the dominant predictor of family functioning as reported by these women, accounting for 17% unique variance in the empirical model. Self-esteem and stressors from negative life events accounted for 24% of the variance in sense of mastery. Trait anxiety, an indicator of anxiety proneness to perceive stressful situations as threatening and to respond to such situations with elevations in state anxiety (Spielberger et al., 1983), replaced the situation-specific response of state anxiety as a better predictor in the HRW's model. Of interest was the more positive relationship of children with their fathers, contributing 7% unique variance to their perceived family functioning to bring the total explained variance to 33%.

Only direct effects of variables on family functioning were found in the model for partners of HRW to explain 48% of the variance. Perceived

TABLE 1. Results of Causal Model Tests to Predict Family Functioning

Models	Variable	R^2	R^2	Unique Total Standardized Beta Weight	F	p
Hypothesized Theoretical Models						
High-risk women	State anxiety	.1316	.1316	.36	19.09	.000
Low-risk women	Depression	.1330	.1330	.36	27.92	.000
High-risk men	Depression	.1267	.1267	.36	10.01	.002
Low-risk men	Depression	.1487	.1487	.39	24.02	.000
Final Empirical Models						
High-risk women	Mastery	.1696	.1696	−.25	25.33	.000
	Trait anxiety	.0902	.2598	.33	14.99	.000
	Relationship father/child	.0696	.3294	.26	12.66	.001
Low-risk women	Depression	.1330	.1330	.27	27.92	.000
	Perceived support	.0973	.2303	−.33	22.88	.000
High-risk men	Perceived support	.3191	.3191	−.54	31.40	.000
	Relationship mother/teen	.1195	.4386	.32	14.05	.000
	Negative life events	.0444	.4830	.21	5.58	.021
Low-risk men	Perceived support	.1721	.1721	−.37	26.20	.000
	Health perception	.0462	.2183	−.15	7.38	.008
	Negative life events	.0778	.2961	.28	13.70	.000
	Contact with father	.0271	.3232	.17	4.93	.028

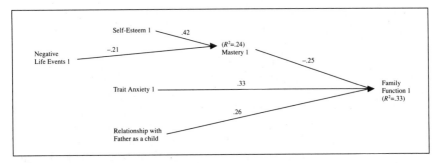

Figure 2.   Final Empirical Model for High-Risk Women

social support (beta = −.54) was the major predictor accounting for 32% unique variance. The less their perceived support the more discrepant their family functioning. A positive relationship with their mother as a teenager (beta = .32) predicted 12% of the unique variance for men in their family functioning. Negative life events (beta = .21) had direct effects rather than the hypothesized indirect effects on their family functioning, contributing 4% variance.

Although less variance was explained in the LRW's final empirical model (23%), their model was more complex, and more closely approximated the original theoretical model. See Figure 3 which also shows standardized beta weights. Depression was the major predictor of family functioning, explaining 13% of the variance. Perceived support had unhypothesized direct effects on family functioning, explaining 10% of the variance. Sense of mastery, negative life events, and health perception had indirect effects on family functioning through depression, explaining 32% of the variance in depression. Self-esteem, pregnancy risk, negative life events, and health perception explained 36% of the variance in sense

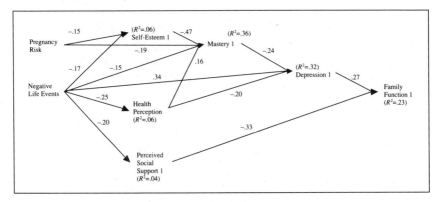

Figure 3.   Final Empirical Model for Low-Risk Women

of mastery. Negative life events had indirect effects on family functioning through sense of mastery, self-esteem, depression, health perception, and perceived support.

The men in the low-risk pregnancy situation who viewed their family functioning more optimally than either their partners or men in the high-risk situation had 32% explained variance in the final empirical model. As was the case with men in the high-risk situation, perceived support (beta $= -.37$) was the major predictor of family functioning, $R^2 = .172$. Negative life events (beta $= .28$) accounted for 8% of the variance in family functioning directly, and had indirect effects through health perception, $R^2 = .0477$, beta $= -.22$. Health perception (beta $= -.15$) explained 5% of the variance directly and the extent of current contact with their fathers (beta $= .17$) explained 3%. More optimal health status, less negative life events' stress, more frequent current contact with fathers, and greater perceived support were linked with more optimal family functioning.

DISCUSSION

High-risk women and their partners perceived a greater discrepancy in family functioning than low-risk women and their partners as was hypothesized. The mean scores of 20.76 for HRW, 18.51 for HRM, 17.96 for LRW, and 14.65 for LRM are all somewhat higher than the prepartum mean score reported by a sample of mothers and fathers who had infants with myelodysplasia ($M = 13.40$) (Feetham, Tweed, & Perrin, 1979). All of the means fell within the range of mean scores (9.00 to 25.78) cited by Feetham and Humenick (1982) for four samples of parents, including samples with normal and handicapped children. The lack of significant difference in scores of HRW and HRM suggests that either the immediacy of the stressors from the antepartal maternal hospitalization affected both partners' perceptions of family functioning similarly, or they were more congruent in their views initially. However, differences between women's and men's scores in both high- and low-risk pregnancies were not large, and the significance for low-risk couples may be an artifact of the larger sample sizes. The finding that men tended to have a more optimal view of family functioning than their partners may reflect that changes occurring with pregnancy affect women more acutely. Harriman (1983) reported that wives perceived greater overall life change, particularly in their personal lives, and negatively perceived change was more difficult for them than for their husbands.

The variables having direct effects on family functioning in the high-risk women's empirical respecified model were distinctly different from all other models. Sense of mastery was the major predictor of family functioning for this group, explaining 17% of the variance; mastery or control in the situation may be more critical when one is separated temporarily from family. However, the risk status with its uncertainty for infant outcome cannot be separated from the hospitalization experience in this study, so this is conjecture. Negative life events and self-esteem had direct effects on their sense of mastery. The HRW's anxiety proneness in responding to stress was also a unique predictor, explaining 9% of the variance. The question may be raised whether this proneness to anxiety may have also been a factor in their high-risk condition. The contribution of 7% of the variance by their relationship with their fathers as children, suggests that these early relationships with their fathers were important for later male-female relationships within their families. Gladieux (1978) reported that pregnant women's positive relationships with their fathers were linked to a satisfying pregnancy outcome and experience. Gladieux postulated that the woman's relationship with her father influences her value of femininity and comfort in heterosexual relationships. In another study the perceived quality of childhood relationships for both mother and father were found to be related to subsequent quality of adult social support systems (Flaherty & Richman, 1986). High-risk women who perceived more positive relationships with their fathers during childhood may also have perceived greater support from their partners and others during pregnancy.

That extent of pregnancy risk would not be a major stressor affecting HRW was unexpected. The Hobel et al. (1973) pregnancy risk scale is limited by the assigned values of 1, 5, or 10 for a risk situation; a better measure in which the risk items are more proportionate to one another and to the stress induced is needed. For example, if women had rated the amount of perceived stress for each item as was done for negative life events this may have led to different findings. Variables such as social support, age, socioeconomic status, education, or number of children also failed to have effects on family functioning in this group of high-risk women. The failure of extent of pregnancy risk to be predictive in the HRW's model and the uniqueness of their model suggest a need for further study in which HRW who are not hospitalized are studied along with those who are hospitalized.

The LRW's empirical model of direct and indirect effects is the most supportive of the theoretical models posed at the onset of the study. For the most part, stress from negative life events and pregnancy risk had negative effects on social support, self-esteem, and health perception, as expected. Direct links between stress from negative life events to self-esteem, health perception, mastery, depression, and perceived support were evident, as were links from pregnancy risk to self-esteem and mastery. Therefore, the impact of these two stress variables were not only direct, but also indirect, and had a fairly powerful influence. Self-esteem and health perception in turn affected mastery as was hypothesized, with health perception having an additional direct link to depression. Only depression of the two hypothesized variables affected family functioning, and perceived social support had an unhypothesized, but direct link to family functioning. Much of the literature base used to develop the hypothesized model was grounded in low-risk populations, and may help explain why this group's final empirical model more closely adhered to the hypothesized model.

The HRW's partners' final empirical model explaining family functioning was the least complex of all models, yet it explained the greatest percentage of variance (48%). Negative life events, perceived support, and relationship with their mothers as teenagers had direct effects on family functioning; no indirect effects were found. Perceived support contributed to more optimal family functioning and high stress from negative life events was linked to an increase in discrepant family functioning. Men tend to depend on their partners for their major support (Antonucci, 1985); therefore, with his mate in the hospital, external sources of support perhaps become more critical for family function. Others reported that men who identified more strongly with their mothers and who saw their mothers as nurturant coped better with pregnancy and felt better about themselves as fathers (Grossman et al., 1980). Thus, support exists for the empirically derived model for men in the high-risk situation.

Perceived support and negative life events also had direct effects on family functioning of men in the low-risk situation. Health perception and extent of current contact with their fathers also had direct effects. The men's current contact with their fathers as a predictor of family functioning is in contrast to the HRM's relationship with their mothers as teenagers. In the low-risk situation without the higher level of stress, the man's father may be a role model and a support for fatherhood.

Causal factors in the men's final empirical models differed substantively from the women's models. Perceived support accounted for much more variance in family functioning among men than among women (HRM, 32%; LRM, 17%; LRW, 10%; HRW, 0%). This finding suggests that during pregnancy, support is particularly critical for men, as the man's major source of support, his wife, is more preoccupied with events occurring within her body and may be somewhat less available to her partner at that time. Negative life events' stress also had direct effects on family functioning in the men's models, but only indirect effects through personal trait and resource variables in the women's models. This finding

Data for this paper are from the project, Antepartum Stress: Effect on Family Health and Functioning, supported by the National Center for Nursing Research, National Institutes of Health, under Grant Number R01 NR 01064, Ramona T. Mercer, principal investigator.
An adaptation of this paper was presented at the Sigma Theta Tau International Biennial Convention in San Francisco, CA, November 10, 1987.

suggests that men are not affected as personally by stress as women. Both pregnancy risk and negative life events' stress had direct negative effects on LRW's self-esteem and sense of mastery, but among HRW negative life events had direct negative effects on their sense of mastery. Johnson and Sarason (1979), in a review of moderators of life stress, suggested that persons who perceive themselves as having less control over their environment are more adversely affected by life stress. Pearlin and Schooler (1978) reported that men had a decided advantage over women in coping with stress; men's self-esteem, self-denigration, and mastery along with their responses to stress were more potent in controlling stress. Thus, although perceived support was a stronger predictor of family functioning among men, the finding that stress had direct effects on personality characteristics of women indicates that support is no less critical for them.

The failure of received support or the size of the support network to enter into the model-building phases at any point indicates that perceived support is more critical than other types of support to childbearing families. Barrera (1981) found that received support seemed to reflect the extent of stress experienced in a population of pregnant teenagers, and even when relatives were supportive, their support was ineffective if there was conflict in the relationship. One literature review indicated that it is the absence of support that interferes with adjustment, rather than the presence of support that facilitates it (Tucker, 1982). In this study perceiving that support was available if needed was more important than the extent of help received during the past month.

Intergenerational influences on men's perception of family functioning were different from the women's as well as from one another. Intergenerational influences were not found in the low-risk women's model. In the high-risk women's model, the intergenerational influence was at a younger age (as children) in contrast to high-risk partners when influences were during the teenage years, and low-risk partners when influences were current. Further explication of these links and tests in other populations is necessary. Exploration of how young childbearing families can be helped to strengthen both their family ties and relationships within their family systems is also needed.

REFERENCES

Antonucci, T. C. (1985). Social support: Theoretical advances, recent findings and pressing issues. In I. G. Sarason & B. R. Sarason (Eds.), *Social support: Theory, research and applications* (pp. 21–37). Norwell, MA: Martinus Nijhoff.

Barrera, M., Jr. (1981). Social support in the adjustment of pregnant adolescents. In B. H. Gottlieb (Ed.), *Social networks and social support* (pp. 87–89). Beverly Hills, CA: Sage Publications.

Belsky, J., Lang, M. E., & Rovine, M. (1985). Stability and change in marriage across the transition to parenthood: A second study. *Journal of Marriage and Family, 47,* 855 – 865.

Blackburn, S., & Lowen, L. (1986). Impact of an infant's premature birth on the grandparents and parents. *Journal of Obstetric, Gynecologic, and Neonatal Nursing, 15,* 173 – 178.

Bloom, B. L. (1985). *Stressful life event theory and research implications for primary prevention* (DHHS Publication No. ADM 85-1385). Washington, DC: US Government Printing Office.

Cohen, R. L. (1979). Maladaptation to pregnancy. *Seminars in perinatology, 3,* 15 – 24,

Committee on Assessing Alternative Birth Settings. (1982). *Research issues in the assessments of birth settings.* Washington, DC: National Academy Press.

Curry, M. A., & Snell, B. J. (1985). *Antenatal hospitalization: Maternal behavior and the family* (Final Report Grant No. R01 NU 00939, Division of Nursing, Bureau of Health Professions, Health Resources and Services Administration, U.S. Public Health Service). Portland, OR: Department of Family Nursing.

Davies, A. R., & Ware, J. E., Jr. (1981). *Measuring health perceptions in the health insurance experiment.* Santa Monica, CA: The Rand Corporation.

Dore, S. L., & Davies, B. L. (1979). Catharsis for high-risk antenatal inpatients. *MCN, American Journal of Maternal Child Nursing, 4,* 96 – 97.

Feetham, S. L., Tweed, H., & Perrin, J. S. (1979). Practical problems in selection of spina bifida infants for treatment in the USA. *Zeitschrift fur Kinderchirurgie und Grenzgebiete, 28* 301 – 306.

Feetham, S., & Humenick, S. S. (1982). The Feetham family functioning survey. In S. S. Humenick (Ed.), *Analysis of current assessment strategies in the health care of young children and childbearing families* (pp. 259 – 268). Norwalk, CT: Appleton-Century-Crofts.

Ferketich, S. L., & Verran, J. A. (1984). Residual analysis for causal model assumptions. *Western Journal of Nursing Research, 6,* 41 – 60.

Flaherty, J. A., & Richman, J. A. (1986). Effects of childhood relationships on the adult's capacity to form social supports. *American Journal Psychiatry, 143,* 851 – 855.

Gladieux, J. B. (1978). Pregnancy — the transition to parenthood: Satisfaction with the pregnancy experience as a function of sex role conceptions, marital relationship, and social network. In W. B. Miller & L. F. Newman (Eds.), *The first child and family formation* (pp. 275 – 295). Chapel Hill, NC: University of North Carolina, Carolina Population Center.

Grossman, F. K., Eichler, L. S., Winickoff, S. A., Anzalone, M. K., Gofseyeff, M. H., & Sargent, S. P. (1980). *Pregnancy, birth, and parenthood.* San Francisco: Jossey-Bass Publishers.

Harriman L. C. (1983). Personal and marital changes accompanying parenthood. *Family Relations, 32,* 387 – 394.

Hobel, C. J., Hyvarinen, M. A., Okada, D. M., & Oh, W. (1973). Prenatal and intrapartum high-risk screening. *American Journal of Obstetrics and Gynecology, 117,* 1 – 9.

Hollingshead, A. A. (1975). *Four factor index of social status.* New Haven, CT: Department of Sociology, Yale University.

Johnson, J. H., & Sarason, I. G. (1979). Moderator variables in life stress research. In I. G. Sarason & C. D. Spielberger (Eds.), *Stress and anxiety* (vol. 6, pp. 151 – 167). New York: Hemisphere Publishing Co.

Kemp, V. H., & Page, C. K. (1987). The psychosocial impact of a high-risk pregnancy on the family. *Journal of Obstetric, Gynecologic, and Neonatal Nursing, 15,* 232 – 236.

McMillan, D. (1976). [Alienation and environmental integration of adolescents]. Unpublished grant, R. Newbrough, principal investigator.

Mercer, R. T., May K. A., Ferketich, S., & DeJoseph, J. (1986). Theoretical models studying the effect of antepartum stress on the family. *Nursing Research, 35,* 339 – 346.

Merkatz, R. (1978). Prolonged hospitalization of pregnant women: The effects on the family. *Birth and the Family Journal, 5,* 204 – 206.

Merkatz, R. B., Budd, K., & Merkatz, I. R. (1978). Psychologic and social implications of scientific care for pregnant diabetic women. *Seminars in Perinatology, 2,* 373–381.

Molfese, V. T., & Thomson, B. (1985). Optimality versus complications. Assessing predictive values of perinatal scales. *Child Development, 56,* 810–823.

Norbeck, J. S. (1984). Modification of life event questionnaires for use with female respondents. *Research in Nursing & Health, 7,* 61–71.

Norbeck, J. S., & Tilden, V. P. (1983). Life stress, social support, and emotional disequilibrium in complications of pregnancy: A prospective, multivariate study. *Journal of Health and Social Behavior, 24,* 30–46.

Pearlin, L. I., & Schooler, C. (1978). The structure of coping. *Journal of Health and Social Behavior, 19,* 2–21.

Pearlin, L. I., Lieberman, M. A., Menaghan, E. G., & Mullan, J. T. (1981). The stress process. *Journal of Health and Social Behavior, 22,* 337–356.

Penticuff, J. H. (1982). Psychologic implications in high-risk pregnancy. *Nursing Clinics of North America, 17*(1), 69–78.

Perry, S. E., Parer, J. T., & Inturrisi, M. (1986). Intrauterine transfusion for severe isoimmunization. *MCN, American Journal of Maternal Child Nursing, 11,* 182–189.

Radloff, L. (1977). The CES-D Scale: A self-report depression scale for research in the general population. *Journal of Applied Psychological Measurement, 1,* 385–401.

Ramsey, C. N., Jr., Abell, T. D., & Baker, L. C. (1986). The relationship between family functioning, life events, family structure, and the outcome of pregnancy. *Journal of Family Practice, 22,* 521–527.

Richardson, P. (1987). Women's important relationships during pregnancy and the preterm labor event. *Western Journal of Nursing Research, 9,* 203–222.

Roberts, C. S., & Feetham, S. L. (1982). Assessing family functioning across three areas of relationships. *Nursing Research, 31,* 231–235.

Rosenberg, M. (1979). *Conceiving the self.* New York: Basic Books.

Sarason, I. G., Johnson, H. H., & Siegel, J. M. (1978). Development of the Life Experiences Survey. *Journal of Consulting and Clinical Psychology, 46,* 932–946.

Smilkstein, G., Helsper-Lucas, A., Ashworth, C., Montano, D., & Pagel, M. (1984). Predictions of pregnancy complications: An application of the biopsychosocial model. *Social Sciences Medicine, 18,* 315–321.

Spielberger, C. F., Gorsuch, R. L., & Lushene, R., Vagg, P. R., & Jacobs, G. A. (1983). *Manual for the State-Trait Anxiety Inventory.* Palo Alto, CA: Consulting Psychologists Press.

Tilden, V. P. (1983). The relation of life stress and social support to emotional disequilibrium during pregnancy. *Research in Nursing & Health, 6,* 167–174.

Tucker, M. B. (1982). Social support and coping: Applications for the study of female drug abuse. *Journal of Social Issues, 38,* 117–137.

Turner, M. E., & Stevens, C. D. (1971). The regression analysis of causal paths. In H. M. Blalock, Jr. (Ed.), *Causal models in the social sciences* (pp. 75–100). Chicago: Aldine Publishing Co.

Verran, J. A., & Ferketich, S. L. (1984). Residual analysis for statistical assumptions of regression equations. *Western Journal of Nursing Research, 6,* 27–40.

Verran, J. A., & Ferketich, S. L. (1987). Testing linear model assumptions: Residual analysis. *Nursing Research, 36,* 127–130.

Wandersman, L., Wandersman, A., & Kahn, S. (1980). Social support in the transition to parenthood. *Journal of Community Psychology, 8,* 332–342.

White, M., & Dawson, C. (1981). The impact of the at-risk infant on family solidarity. *Birth Defects: Original Article Series, 17*(6), 253–284.

White, M., & Ritchie, J. (1984). Psychological stressors in antepartum hospitalizations: Reports from pregnant women. *Maternal-Child Nursing Journal, 13,* 47–56.

Williams, M. L. (1986). Long-term hospitalization of women with high-risk pregnancies: A nurse's viewpoint. *Journal of Obstetric, Gynecologic, and Neonatal Nursing, 15,* 17–21.

COMMENTARY

The research reported here by Mercer and her colleagues reflects a family focus, with the family regarded as a unit or system. The family members of particular interest in this paper are the pregnant woman and her partner. Family developmental "theory" serves as the conceptual model for middle-range theory development. Note that Mercer and her colleagues refer to family developmental theory as the theoretical framework for their work. In keeping with the terminology used in this book, we regard the family developmental perspective as a conceptual model from which the more specific middle-range theory of stress and family functioning was derived for the study.

Methodologically, the study deviates from a focus on the family unit by using individual level data, with scores obtained from the pregnant women separated from those obtained from their partners. Thus, family functioning was the individual's view of family activities and relationships. No attempt was made here to create relational data by combining scores. Instead, similarities in family functioning were determined via comparison of group means (pregnant women versus their partners).

A special feature of this paper is the inclusion of a diagram of the hypothesized middle-range theory of the effects of antepartum stress on family functioning as well as diagrams of the modifications of that theory developed on the basis of the study results. Note that slightly different theories were developed for each of the study groups (low-risk women, high-risk women, partners of low-risk women, partners of high-risk women).

JACQUELINE FAWCETT

CHAPTER

9

Supportive Measures for High-Risk Infants and Families

KATHRYN E. BARNARD
CHARLENE SNYDER
ANITA SPIETZ

The experience of providing a 3-month nursing program of care to infants and their families with physical, health, and social-environmental risks is presented. An individualized case approach was used which first involved a nursing assessment of the family, infant, and environmental needs and then was followed by subsequent appropriate nursing intervention. Brammer's conceptual model about the helping process was used to assist the analysis of the success or failure experienced in assisting these high-risk families. The differences that emerged were in the mothers' involvement in the exploration phase which involves goal setting. Families with incomplete progression through the helping process not only participated in less mutual decision making, but they were also less open to the initial assessment phase and had higher social risk. The nurses had

Reprinted from K. E. Barnard, P. A. Brandt, B. S. Raff, & P. Carroll (Eds.), *Social support and families of vulnerable infants* (Birth Defects: Original Article Series, Vol. 20, No. 5, pp. 291–329). White Plains, NY: March of Dimes Birth Defects Foundation, 1984.

less total contact with the uninvolved families. A brief description of a subsequent approach to provide effective nursing to a socially high-risk group of pregnant women is given. The approach involves a more extended period of intervention and emphasizes the development of a therapeutic relationship.

This paper will describe our experience in supporting vulnerable families with one type of nursing intervention which was part of a larger research project to experimentally test three models of providing nursing services to families of newborns. The assumptions of the larger research project, "Models of Newborn Nursing Services," were that the parent-infant system is influenced by the individual characteristics of each member; and when the parent and infant are acting together in mutually dependent ways, there is optimal interaction and adaption in synchrony. We further assumed that in the development of the parent-child relationship, there is reason to believe that complex and competent functioning is extremely unlikely to occur in certain families. Some of these families include infants whose biological and physical status makes it difficult or impossible for the infants to send cues or to respond to their caregiver. Some of the families include parents who lack knowledge about infant behavior and development. Other families may not adapt because the parents' level of life stress is high, their level of support is low, and they are unable to apply the knowledge and skills they have.

We combined these assumptions into our selection criteria for the families where there were nonoptimal infant characteristics or nonoptimal parent characteristics. The nonoptimal characteristics of the infants were primarily biological factors including prematurity, low birth weight, and complications of pregnancy, labor, and delivery; while the characteristics of nonoptimal parents included those which interfere with adaptive behavior and are primarily social in nature. Although little research has been directed specifically at adaptive behavior as a function of social class or educational level, it is known that these variables are related to infant developmental test scores. Moreover, lower social class and educational level are both associated with higher levels of family disorganization.

Thus, the subjects we selected had what we termed double vulnerability, i.e., they had both biological complications during pregnancy, and they represented families with social problems. We hypothesized that if either partner in the parent-child interaction had nonoptimal characteristics, the chances for parent-child adaption, especially for synchrony, would be markedly decreased. This is most dramatically true for those families in which both the parents and the baby have nonoptimal characteristics. Several studies have shown that measures of general infant development are particularly low for children in these circumstances (McDonald, 1964; Werner, Bierman, & French, 1971; Willerman, Broman, & Fiedler, 1970).

The only empirically tested nursing approaches designed to facilitate adaptation that we are aware of have been relatively unstructured and generally supportive in nature. Most commonly, they have served as controls in research studies which tested the efficacy of other programs. Where nursing served as the control group, the children did not show any positive benefit; whereas in the experimental group which used the educational approach with the infant or parent, the infant showed cognitive gains. Before this study, no systematic study has been made of a program specifically designed to use nursing care as a facilitator of parent-child adaptation in synchrony.

In spite of the lack of research, thousands of nurses are offering care at times and in places where they might favorably influence parent-child adaptation. For example, in the newborn nursery, nurses are able to easily assess the biological characteristics of the infant which may contribute positively or negatively to adaptation in the parent-child dyad. Similarly, postpartum care nurses often have a chance to provide information to new mothers and fathers about infant care and development. The most promising service setting for the nurse to promote adaptation and synchrony, however, is in the patient's home. Whether these visits are for all new mothers or only selected ones, this entry into the home environment provides an unusually effective opportunity for promoting adaptive behaviors.

OVERVIEW

Since unstructured, general, supportive nursing programs in the home have been shown to be ineffective in producing gains in infant development, we sought to design and implement alternative nursing programs which could be used by public health nurses in home visits. We wanted to determine if nursing care programs designed to facilitate mutual adaptation between high-risk infants and their parents in the first months of life would, in fact, modify this process and improve subsequent development of the infant and the parent-child relationship. We tested three programs, all designed to be used from birth through 3 months postpartum. These programs were called the Nursing Parent and Child Environment (NPACE), Nursing Support Infant Bio-Behavioral (NSIBB), and Nursing Standard Approach to Care (NSTAC).

The NPACE, an acronym for a program conducted in the parent and child's environment, was a system for the provision of individualized nursing care to families with new babies. The NPACE program focused broadly on the whole spectrum of parent and infant needs during the first few months after birth, and it made extensive use of systematic screening and assessment.

The NSIBB, an acronym for Nursing Support of Infant Bio-Behavioral, was a program to provide more standardized nursing care to families with new babies. The NSIBB program focused specifically upon the mothers' and fathers' needs for parenting skills and their knowledge of child development, and it included explicit training for the parents in the assessment of their infant's behavior. It was based on information about the biological and behavioral course of development during the first 3 months of life and the influence that development has upon adaptive behavior on both the infant and the parent.

The NSTAC, an acronym for Nursing Standard Approach to Care, was a global designation for the general support services offered by the Seattle-King County Health Department, which are representative of many health department programs.

THE NPACE PROGRAM

The subject of the present paper is to describe more fully the process of nursing intervention with families in the NPACE program. The intent of this paper is to discuss the supportive nature of the nursing intervention in the NPACE program in relation to the characteristics of the sample population and the content of the nursing program. We will indicate the stresses these families were experiencing during the first 3 months of the postpartum period in relation to care of a newborn, the characteristics of these families, and how NPACE nurses were able to provide support to these vulnerable families during this transitional period. The NPACE program did provide support to the families.

It is important to note from the literature that support is viewed as a complex phenomenon. Cobb (1976) defines support as information leading one to believe that he is cared for, loved, esteemed, and a member of a network of mutual obligation. He further elaborates that information is a major product of support, information about self and resources. The mechanisms by which social support may negate the effects of a life stress, such as having a new baby, have not been determined. Bowlby (1977) spoke of persons being more effective when they are confident about their support system. Karen Lindner (1982) found a relationship between individuals' problem solving skills and high or low satisfaction with their support system. Individuals with low social support had a poorer quality of problem solving. She also found that when individuals with low social support were given social support during a test of their problem solving procedure, the low support individuals with supportive instructions did improve their scores on the quality of solution. The quality of solution was judged by whether the respondent had the protagonist in the story initiate action leading to the solution of the problem, or if the protagonist merely reacted to some action taken by others. A higher quality rating was given if the respondent initiated instrumental action. Therefore, there is evidence that support is potentially important in helping individuals adapt to problem situations.

METHOD

NPACE was an individualized program based upon a nurse's systematic assessment of family strengths and weaknesses. The key words are: individualized (because it was designed to meet the individual needs of family members), systematic (since it utilized a variety of assessments in a semistructured manner), and strengths (because the nurses attempted to build on the positive qualities and assets in the family rather than focusing on or working from a deficit model).

The NPACE program was designed and conducted by C. Snyder and A. Spietz, two nurses with M.S.N. degrees, for the purpose of providing services to a population of mothers and their infants who were extremely vulnerable due to biological reasons which placed them at risk during pregnancy or the intrapartum period, and because the mothers had a high school education or less. Due to lack of a sufficient number of subjects toward the end of the program, recruitment was initiated with a hospital OB clinic. Consequently, a few of those enrolled in the program achieved a higher educational level.

The program was carried out through the systematic use of approximately 15 assessment tools (see Table 1), which were developed and validated in the course of the Nursing Child Assessment Project (Barnard & Eyres, 1976) or adapted from the work of other researchers whose work was related to the early postpartum period. The assessments provided a semistructure to the NPACE approach which allowed the nurses to be flexible in meeting individual needs. The flexibility allowed the nurse to focus on either the mother, the infant, or both. The assessments

TABLE 1.   NPACE Program Assessments

Questionnaire
1. Neonatal Perception Inventory (NPI) (Broussard & Hartner, 1976)
2. Life Change Events (Holmes & Rahe, 1967)
3. Dudley-Welke Coping Scale Questionnaire (Dudley & Welke, 1977)
4. Temperament-Questionnaire (Carey, 1972)
Interviews
1. Database, mother (Seattle-King County Health Department)
2. Database, infant (Seattle-King County Health Department)
3. Developmental Expectations (NCAP) (Barnard & Eyres, 1979)
4. Psychosocial Assets (NCAP)
5. Father Involvement (NCAP)
6. Neonatal Perception Inventory (NPI)
7. Parent Mutuality Interview (NCAP)
8. Motherhood Feelings (NCAP)
9. Parent Concerns (NCAP)
Rewards
1. Nursing Child Assessment Sleep Activity Record (NCAP)
Observations
1. Nursing Child Assessment Feeding Scale (NCAFS) (Barnard, 1979)
2. Nursing Child Assessment Teaching Scale (NCATS) (Barnard, 1979)

used were: questionnaires that were filled out by the mothers, interviews by the nurses, records that the mothers were asked to keep of their own or their infant's behavior, and observations of behavior and interactions by the nurses. Each assessment assisted in determining the physical, supportive, psychosocial, and adaptive abilities of the families.

The use of assessments in the NPACE intervention program was important for the following reasons:

1. The assessments provided a framework for:
   a. giving feedback to the family.
   b. additional assessments.
2. The assessments:
   a. were stimuli for the parents, giving them ideas for teaching and interacting with their child.
   b. provided:
      (1) a structure and organization to the visit, as well as to the time spent with the parent.
      (2) a framework for resource materials.
      (3) an environment for building rapport and trust.
   c. promoted parent participation and subsequent parent involvement.
3. Assessment results provided a:
   a. framework to determine family strengths and weaknesses.
   b. guide for mutual goal setting with the parents.

NPACE was broadly focused on the many family needs that may emerge during the period following birth. More specifically, it was based on the philosophy that parenthood is a transitional period and that parents, especially those at risk, have special needs for support, validation, new information, and direction. The nurse was used to provide support, not only through frequent contact, but also by recognizing that parents have the need to talk about feelings and concerns. By assuming the role of an active listener, the nurse could help nurture the parents' growth and strengths. It was recognized that parents have the need to know that what they are doing is right, and validation aids them in becoming more confident about their own skills and successes. New parents generally are also eager to learn all they can about their newborn and, therefore, benefit from the new information a nurse is able to provide. During this time, parents often express a feeling of confusion and can benefit from any direction or organization the nurse can supply. Nursing support ranges from asking parents to keep a 7-day sleep-awake activity record of their infant to merely reminding mothers to drink 7-8 glasses of fluid daily to maintain lactation.

The NPACE program content is best described in reference to the Nursing Child Assessment Interactional Model (Barnard, 1979, p. 19), and the components are illustrated in Figure 1. The largest circle represents the environment of the child and parent(s). The smallest circle

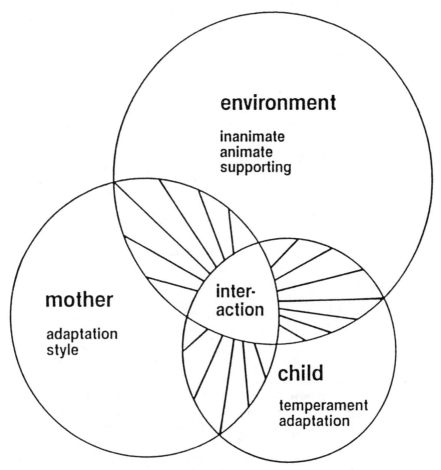

Figure 1.   The child health assessment interaction model. *Note.* From *Nursing Child Assessment Satellite Teaching Manual* by K.E. Barnard. Copyright 1979 by K.E. Barnard. Reprinted by permission.

depicts the child and the child's unique physical and behavioral characteristics. The remaining circle represents the characteristics of the mother or primary caregiver. The overlapping areas of the circle in this model represent the interactions that occur between the infant, mother, and environment.

SAMPLE

Marital Status.   Most of the mothers were married or living with a partner (62% at the time of delivery). The remainder of the mothers were living alone or had a partner who was emotionally unsupportive for a satisfactory relationship.

Parity. This was the first baby for 33 (55%). The remainder of the mothers (N = 27, 45%) had 2–5 children.

Age. The age distribution for the NPACE mothers at the time of delivery ranged from 17–35 years. There were 13 (22%) adolescents. The majority of the mothers (N = 43, 71%) were 20–29 years, and only 4 mothers (7%) were over 30 years.

Race. The majority of mothers (N = 46, 77%) were Caucasian. Sixteen percent (N = 10) of the mothers were black, and the remainder of the mothers (N = 4, 7%) were Asian, Hispanic, and American Indian.

Educational Level. Most of the mothers (N = 49, 82%) had 12 years or less of education. The range of educational level was 9–17 years.

FAMILY PROBLEMS

Since the NPACE program was individualized and designed to address family needs and concerns, it was believed helpful to determine the most common problems encountered by these families (see Table 2). These designations were made by the nurse assigned to the family on the basis of her clinical judgment using specified criteria which are available from the authors on request. As shown in Table 2, 52% of the mothers lacked adequate information for optimal parenting. The majority of this group (27 of the 31) were first time mothers, so it was not surprising they lacked adequate parenting information. Forty-seven percent of the mothers also lacked adequate parenting skills, and the majority were first time mothers. The information and skills they lacked were fairly basic and ranged from cord care and diaper rashes to burping and feeding problems.

Another major problem with 52% of the NPACE families was financial, with either the partner unemployed or the family on welfare. The NPACE mothers were also concerned about their support system. Either they had an inadequate support system of reliable friends and family (N = 23, 38%), or they had no supportive partner (N = 28, 47%). Many of these mothers with no supportive partner actually had partners, but they were not emotionally supportive to the mother.

These problem areas are not unusual and perhaps would not be problems if the families faced only one at a time. However, many of the NPACE families experienced several of the problems simultaneously and were living in disorganized environments. There were 16 of these multi-problem* families in the NPACE program. The range and combination of problems with each family were staggering. One family had as many as 12 of the 23 problems. The father was an unemployed alcoholic who physi-

---

*Families living in disorganized environments, who were always in a crisis state and/or experiencing a lot of life change.

TABLE 2. Most Common Problems as Identified by
NPACE Nurse[a]

Problem Areas	Number	Percent
Mother Lacked Information	31	52
Financial or Unemployment	31	52
Mother Lacked Skill	28	47
No Supportive Partner	28	47
Baby's Physical Health	26	43
Inadequate Support for Mother	23	38
Depressed or Emotionally Upset Mother	17	28
Child Rearing (child abuse, neglect)	17	28
Mother's Physical Health	17	28
Multiproblems	16	27
Adolescent Mother	14	23
Mother-Infant Interaction	14	23
Mobility	13	22
Cesarean Births	11	18
Cultural Differences	10	17
Abused Mothers	9	15
Death or Grief	7	12
Alcohol or Drug Abuse	7	12
Mother without Transportation	7	12
Intellectually Slow Mothers	4	1
Premature	4	1
Other Problems with Partner, Other Children, Relatives, Housing	21	35

[a]Problem definitions can be obtained from the authors.
N = 60 families.

cally and emotionally abused the mother. The mother was an adolescent with her first baby. The baby had frequent illnesses, and the mother was depressed. The time and energy required to sort out and determine a focus with such a family were considerable. In the face of this family's crisis and disorganization, the NPACE program with its systematic assessment and individualized approach was extremely valuable in providing a framework for focus and organization.

THE SUPPORTIVE PROCESS

Since we found parent participation and cooperation critical in developing and carrying out a program of care and services to these families, much time and effort were expended in building relationships. In reviewing the cases, differences were found in the amount of progress made in establishing the relationships and the degree of satisfaction gained in working with the families. NPACE nurses found that an important aspect of their program was the establishment of a caring, trusting relationship with the parents. The nurses defined it as a caring relationship, because according to Mitchell and Loustau (1981), they assisted parents to grow toward whatever aspect of healthy functioning they could attain relative to their current state. The nurses did not attempt to change or cure the parents; rather they attempted through caring to maximize the parenting potential at the parents' current level of functioning.

FRAMEWORK

For the purpose of describing the NPACE program, the nurses utilized Brammer's (1973) helping relationship sequence since it incorporated many models, such as problem solving, skill development, life planning, and awareness, which have been found to be beneficial to parents during this transitional period. The goal of the helping relationship was to assist the parents to work toward independence and ultimately assume responsibility for their decisions.

The eight stages in Brammer's helping process include entry, clarification, structure, relationship, exploration, consolidation, planning, and termination. Two important points to remember about the helping relationship is: 1) the process may not progress sequentially, and differing amounts of time may be given to different stages; and 2) one's ease with terminating the relationship and/or the degree of satisfaction with the relationship are often directly related to a progression through all the stages, even if this is out of sequence. A definition of each stage of the helping process and how the NPACE nurses utilized the content are presented in Table 3.

ESTABLISHMENT

Relationship building differed for many of the families. The nurses identified three basic relationship progressions: ideal, difficult, and incomplete (see Figures 2, 3, and 4).

The first relationship illustrated in Figure 2 depicts the "normal" or "ideal" progression through the NPACE program. The norm was generally six to seven home visits. By the end of the first visit, the nurses had a firm commitment from the mother to participate in the program, with the relationship generally well established. There was little need to focus long on the mother or her needs since she was generally confident and competent as a mother and a person. By the fourth to fifth visit, she became actively involved in making decisions and setting goals regarding types of services she desired for follow up.

In contrast, mothers in the second type of relationship illustrated in Figure 3 experienced difficult progression through the stages of the

TABLE 3.   NPACE Adaptation of Helping Process with Supportive Nursing Measures

Stage[a]	Definition	NPACE Supportive Nursing Measures
1. Preparation and Entry	Prepare the parent, open the relationship, set the stage	Program explained to parent, i.e., what we had to offer and what benefits they could expect. Since parents were asked to select site for first visit and this was generally in the home, they were in control.
2. Clarification[b]	State problem, concern, and reasons for seeking help or giving services	We clarified why we were there and what their consent entailed. Discussed: 1) how visits would proceed, i.e., use of assessment, observation, flexibility in our approach, and length and frequency of visits; 2) role of the nurse, i.e., listening, observing, note taking, and providing feedback; and 3) our expectations of parent, i.e., sharing her observations, record keeping, goal setting, etc.
3. Structure[b]	Formulate the contract and structure	In verbal contract parent agreed to active participation by: 1) keeping scheduled appointments; 2) notifying if appointment needed to be rescheduled; 3) keeping records of infant's behavior, sleep, feeding; 4) reading suggested materials as interest and abilities allowed; 5) sharing

(continued)

TABLE 3.   NPACE Adaptation of Helping Process with
Supportive Nursing Measures (*continued*)

Stage[a]	Definition	NPACE Supportive Nursing Measures
		observations about baby; and 6) engaging in play and interacting with her child in mutually agreed upon activities, i.e., teaching.
4. Relationship[c]	Build the helping relationship	Goal is to increase depth of relationship and intensity of parent's commitment. Termination is a possibility. Relationship usually established by end of Stage 4, i.e., trust and openness are increased, and parent is committed and ready to work toward goals of program (stage where relationship deepens and trust is established).
5. Exploration	Explore problems, formulate goals, plan strategies, express feelings, learn skills	This working stage of the relationship involves assessment, intervention, data gathering, information exchange, joint problem solving, and mutual goal setting. Parent often has need to talk about self, problems, and possible plans, but is not ready to take next step, i.e., consolidation.
6. Consolidation	Explore alternatives, work through feelings, practice new skills	Decisions by parent to decide or act. Goals of this stage are to clarify feelings and pin down actions to take and new skills

**TABLE 3.   NPACE Adaptation of Helping Process with
Supportive Nursing Measures** (*continued*)

Stage[a]	Definition	NPACE Supportive Nursing Measures
		to practice. Flows from exploratory stage, blends into planning stage.
7. Planning	Develop plan of action, consolidate and generate new skills, behaviors, to continue self-directed activity	Time to evaluate progress, give feedback, encourage setting of new goals. Long-term goals established.
8. Termination	Evaluate outcomes and terminate relationship	This stage planned in advance and discussed several visits prior to last. Prepare for follow-up if needed and enlist mother's involvement in future needs, also anticipatory guidance for growth and development. Time for summary of progress and feedback to mother.

[a]From Brammer (1973).
[b]The first three stages take place on first visit so the mother knows what to expect and what is expected of her if the relationship is to continue.
[c]This stage may occur as early as the first visit, or it may never develop.

helping relationship. These mothers seemed to require much more time with the nurse, and they had a great need to talk about themselves, their problems, and possible plans for the future. They were not ready to take action, however, or to set concrete goals and follow through. Most of the time with these families was spent in the stages of relationship building and exploration in order to develop trust, explore their problems, and deal with the many crises that characterized their lifestyle (see Figure 3). These mothers characteristically withdrew, broke appointments, or became physically or emotionally ill. Termination was often problematic. Although the termination date was planned in advance, i.e., 3 months, many mothers were not at the point of terminating since it took as long to establish trust. It was frustrating for them as well as for the nurses to end the contact.

The third type of relationship, illustrated in Figure 4, depicted incomplete progression. This relationship was characterized by a fewer

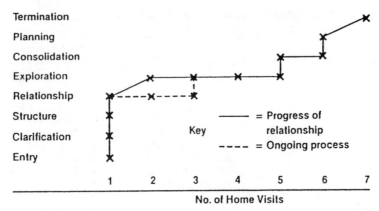

Figure 2.   Ideal progression through the stages of the helping relationship.

number of visits (two to five) and an unwillingness on the part of the mother to become involved in the program offerings. The commitment to participate in NPACE on the first home visit was rarely made. It was very difficult to see these mothers a second or third time. There was a great deal of resistance. A relationship was not established per se, although all the mothers agreed to remain in the study and were seen at 3 months by the evaluation team. Their reasons for not participating ranged from being disinterested, to not having the time, or simply not fully understanding what they had signed up for in the hospital. Figure 4 illustrates the abruptness or incompleteness of this type of helping relationship.

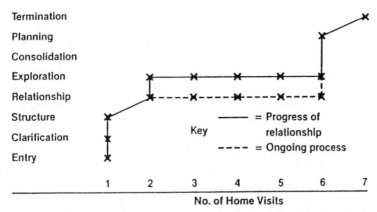

Figure 3.   Difficult progression through the stages of the helping relationship.

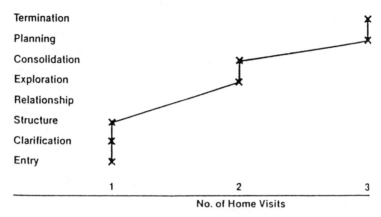

Figure 4.   Incomplete progression through the stages of helping relationship.

ACHIEVEMENT FACTORS

It was more difficult in some instances and in few cases impossible to provide support to the mothers. We had additional information about these families which we analyzed and reviewed to better understand this dilemma. By doing case reviews of the families, some further characteristics of the mothers were identified. In order to accomplish this case review, we chose the process of initially reviewing all cases the nurses felt they were successful with and subsequently those cases that were deemed failures.

The differences that emerged with these families had to do with the mothers' goal setting and decision making styles. There were three categories of mothers identified: involved, less involved, and uninvolved. The involved, interested mothers (N = 27) who entered into a mutual goal setting dialogue with the NPACE nurses had goals of their own, asked questions, and readily accepted the nurses' feedback and suggestions. Most of these mothers had a mature approach to problem solving and decision making, i.e., they sought solutions to their problems and were more independent in their actions. These mothers exhibited what some authors have called an internal locus of control; they were responsible for their own actions. The nurses were able to move through the stages of the helping relationship without difficulty, and these mothers exemplified the ideal progression model of the helping relationship.

The second category, mothers who were less involved (N = 27), were not as eager or enthusiastic as the involved mothers. They merely tolerated the program and became only partially involved in setting goals for themselves. Fifteen of the 27 in this category were members of multiproblem families and demonstrated few skills in problem solving and decision making. They often let things happen and were caught up in the decisions of others. They exhibited an external locus of control. These mothers took little or no responsibility for their own actions. Nurses found it difficult to make progress in moving through the helping relationship with these mothers, and the difficult progression model exemplifies these interactions.

The third category, uninvolved mothers (N = 6), consisted of those mothers who stayed in the program but were not interested in getting involved or participating. These mothers did not set goals, and their decision making was diffused, i.e., scattered with no direction, or nonexistent. Their problem solving abilities were either finalized, inflexible, or undetermined. These mothers exemplified the incomplete progression model of the helping relationship.

Table 4 lists the three categories of mother (involved, less involved, uninvolved) and the problems they most commonly encountered. The involved mothers had fewer problem areas to contend with; thus, they had more energy to become involved in the NPACE program. They had

**TABLE 4. NPACE Most Common Problems
by Category of Mother**

Problem Areas	Involved N = 27	Less Involved N = 27	Uninvolved[a] N = 6
Mother Lacked Information	66%	59%	33%
Financial or Unemployed	33	70	50
Mother Lacked Skill	52	59	17
No Supportive Partner	33	59	50
Baby's Physical Health	33	49	67
Inadequate Support	33	52	33
Depression or Emotional Upset	29	48	33
Child Rearing Problems	30	30	17
Mother's Physical Health	22	37	33
Multiproblems	7	48	17
Adolescents	15	26	33
Mother-Infant Interaction	4	44	17
Mobility	11	48	17
Cesarean Births	15	26	33
Cultural Differences	19	19	0
Abused Mothers	7	26	0
Death or Grief	15	15	0
Alcohol or Drug Use	7	26	17
Lack of Mobility	7	33	17
Intellectually Slow Mother	7	4	17
Premature Infant	0	11	17
Other Problems with Partner, Other Children, Relatives, Housing	26	37	33

[a]The uninvolved mothers reported less problems, but these results are believed to have been influenced by the difficulty assessing these mothers, rather than less problems.

few financial problems; therefore, they did not have to expend energy worrying about adequate food, heat, or housing. They could use their energy to seek out answers to their concerns and could become more involved in setting mutual goals with the program nurse. There was a high percentage of these mothers who lacked information (66%), and this was because they asked for information more often.

Most of the multiproblem mothers were categorized as less involved (see Table 4). These less involved mothers typically had many financial problems, no supportive partner, inadequate support systems, and were often depressed. The mothers and infants had more physical health problems, there were more interaction problems with the infant, and they were more mobile.

The lack of involvement by these multiproblem families was understandable. Since multiproblem mothers were so overwhelmed with all their problems, they had little energy to become involved with or show interest in outside sources, especially if they were depressed or had a physical health problem.

In the third category of mother, uninvolved, the nurses identified fewer problems, except for the baby's physical health, cesarean birth, intellectually slow mother, and premature birth (see Table 4). These mothers were characterized as not going beyond the third stage of the helping process (structure); therefore, the information exchange that would have allowed the nurses to identify additional problems was often missing. These mothers were not thoroughly assessed.

SUPPORTIVE MEASURES

To gain a greater understanding of the NPACE process and program, it was helpful to look at the goals of the mothers and the decision/making categories (involved, less involved, uninvolved) in relation to the nurses' supportive acts (see Table 5). Figure 5 shows each of the mothers' goals and the nurses' supportive acts as identified in a post hoc analysis by each of the NPACE nurses. There were some commonalities across all the mothers' goals, i.e., the nurses tended to devote the same amount of time to active listening, information exchange, validation, and information giving. This was to be expected since these acts were the major thrust of the NPACE program.

Since the analysis of supportive acts was done on the basis of chart review and recall by each nurse for her own case at the termination of the program, the percentage of occurrence can only be regarded as a selective perception of the aspects of support. With that as a limitation, it was interesting to see some difference between the categories of mothers. The nurses did more social sharing, self-disclosure, and mutual sharing with the involved mothers than with the other mothers. This fits expectations

TABLE 5.   NPACE Nursing Support

Nursing Support to Meet Mothers Goals	Nurses' Acts
1. Self-Disclosure	Provide input regarding personal experiences. Use of self as therapeutic entity.
2. Mutual Sharing	Easy give and take, generally on feeling level. Dialogue. Focus more on client.
3. Social Sharing	Interaction that emphasizes other family members, pets, sports/activities outside context of program goals, i.e., offering tea, coffee; showing house; conversing with grandmother; etc.
4. Active Listening	Responding to emotional message, reflection, clarification, restatement of ideas, etc.
5. Information Exchange	Back and forth exchange of information regarding infant, mother, family, or problems (problem solving). Nurse or client initiation, with client an active participant.
6. Sounding Board	Being there, taking in, listening, but not necessarily responding.
7. Validation	Praise, encouragement, positive reinforcement, feedback, or discouragement that supports current activities (common words = admired, reassured, etc.)
8. Information Giving	Program content, pamphlets, resources, anticipatory guidance, teaching, suggestions, advice, discussion, instructions, demonstration of Brazelton behaviors. Client is a passive receiver of information.
9. Actions	Demonstration of infant care skills, bringing or arranging resources (calling agencies), grocery shopping, watching sibs, running errands with mother, bringing reading materials, cutting nails, etc.
10. Baby or Mother Touch	Any nonverbal gesture that results in contact between nurse and person or infant.

since these mothers were more involved and interested in the program.

A look at the less involved mothers revealed that the nurses served more as sounding boards (see Figure 5). Since a majority of these mothers were from the multiproblem families, it was not surprising that they had a lot to "sound off" about to the nurses.

The mothers who were uninvolved, although few in number (N = 6), required a different set of supportive acts from the nurses (see Figure 5). With these mothers, the nurses touched the baby more and performed more actions such as errands or giving physical help. Their babies were more often sick, which required physical touch for examination and physical assessment. Additional effort was also required on the part of the nurses to get the mother more involved with her infant.

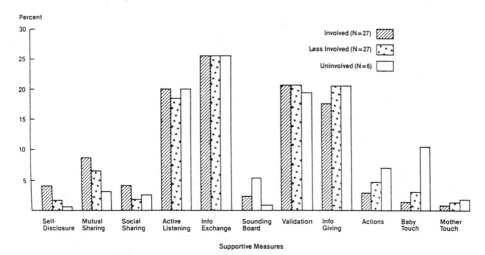

Figure 5.   Nurses' supportive acts by mother category.

One additional analysis was completed from the nurses' home visit recordings. The home visit recordings were analyzed by independently trained coders. The coders were graduate students in nursing, and the code had designations for the type, area, focus, basis, and topic of the nursing measure. There were 5 types of measures, 6 areas, 3 foci, and over 68 topics. Reliability for every tenth record was done; all were above 95% interrater agreement. Table 6 describes the types, areas, and basis, since these are the only categories concerned with this paper.

The analysis of the nurses' recordings revealed they spent significantly more time with the involved mothers in supporting their parenting and providing information on nutrition (see Table 7). The recordings also revealed that the nurses did significantly more specific assessments with these families. Because of the support and fewer problems, these mothers were available to complete the sequence of planned assessments. Consequently, the nurses utilized more assessments.

For less involved families, the nurses spent significantly more time with these mothers than with the uninvolved mothers, and more time was spent on the telephone with the mothers about work, school, support systems, and self-esteem (see Table 7). This was not surprising since the nurses felt the need to monitor these families more closely. As was seen in Table 4, these mothers lacked basic child care information and frequently they were without partners or supportive others. In addition, they and their babies had more physical health problems, the mothers were depressed more often, and they had more alcohol or drug problems.

The time spent with the uninvolved mothers was in actual monitoring of their physical problems and assisting them with resources. These

TABLE 6.   Nursing Activities Log Coding Guide

Each nurse's recording of the visit in the Visit Log is analyzed with respect to her stated activities. A nursing measure is defined as a recorded activity which pertains to a discrete type, area, basis, and topic. The definitions for each category follow.

Type

Monitoring is:
- collecting information
- keeping track of events
- making a diagnosis
- formulating problems
- identifying concerns
- subsumed in information, support, therapy, and planning

Information is:
- providing verbal, written, or behavioral guidance to a client
- role modeling, demonstration, discussion, showing
- mass media (pamphlets, books)

Support is:
- validating behaviors, reinforcing, praising, encouraging ongoing behavior
- listening
- giving resources, supplies (diapers, etc.)

Therapy is:
- providing methods for an identified problem, i.e., information, discussion, problem solving, prescription of medication or physical treatment regime

Planning is:
- a program action to achieve goal
- nurse gives information to client to plan so the client is the planner

BASIS

No specific assessment used

Specific assessment identified

Area

Physical refers to body structure or physiological function due to physical growth.

Nutrition is foodstuff or nutrient intake: type, amount, frequency, method, and pattern. Does not include interaction.

Parenting is any act of taking care of a child, e.g., interacting, mediating, stimulating, caretaking, or the process of parenting or caretaking. Includes the development of role of parent.

Developmental pertains to integration of biopsychosocial systems to level of behavior.

Resources/Environment are finances, housing, material resources.

Psychosocial (Intrapersonal) includes neighbors, friends.

---

mothers were from families least available to the nurses, so when the nurses did get into the homes, they used the physical parameters of assessment which seemed more acceptable to the families and were more comfortable for the nurses to use.

Another significant difference was the total time spent with the three categories of mothers (see Table 7). Based on a Kruskal-Wallis 1-way ANOVA, significantly less time was spent with the uninvolved mothers. It was interesting and enlightening that an equal amount of time was spent

TABLE 7.   Nurses' Contact with NPACE Families (Minutes)

Category of Mothers	Mean	SD
Involved	664.48	250.08
Less Involved	682.00	342.41
Uninvolved	335.66	115.19

with the involved and the less involved mothers. It was expected that more time would have been spent with the less involved because of the many problems encountered with these families.

VARIABLES

In attempting to further understand the factors contributing to these differences, an examination of the demographic characteristics yielded useful information. The two variables which showed significant differences among the groups were social status and social risk. Social risk included the presence of the following factors: husband/partner absent; maternal age less than 18; and mothers had no financially supportive person, no emotional help, no person to share concerns, negative feelings at birth, no phone, no contact person, and heavy use of alcohol during pregnancy. Kruskal-Wallis 1-way ANOVA showed the involved mothers had a significantly lower social risk score than the less involved mothers, who, in turn, had a significantly lower score than the uninvolved mothers.

The social status score (Hollingshead, 1975) was statistically significant in the direction expected. More of the involved mothers had the highest social status score, while mothers who were classified as uninvolved scored the lowest among the three categories.

RESULTS AND IMPLICATIONS

The purpose of this paper was to define our experience in supporting vulnerable families. Although all the families in the NPACE program were high risk, some benefited from the NPACE approach more than others. Ideally, the NPACE's individualized approach would be desirable for all high-risk families; but due to the time required and the usual public health nurse caseload, it would be highly impractical. While client outcomes are not the focus of this paper, the parent-infant outcome data suggest that the NPACE approach has the most positive influence on multiproblem families compared to the Nursing Support Infant Bio-Behavioral (NSIBB) and Nursing Standard Approach to Care (NSTAC) programs.

These multiproblem families were appropriate for the NPACE program for two reasons. First, since they were living in disorganized environments with daily crises, they required a lot of time and energy from the nurses attempting to reach them. The NPACE program design was not limited to a specific amount of time that could be spent with each family. Secondly, the families represented those most in need of services, i.e., these families were among the hardest to reach and the most difficult to provide with services. In reviewing the nurses' supportive acts, however, we found that the mothers from multiproblem families were more similar to the mothers categorized as involved than with the mothers in the less involved category who did not have multiple problems. The nurses' supportive measures for multiproblem families with the less involved mothers were similar to measures provided for involved mothers with fewer serious problems in relation to mutual sharing, active listening, information exchange, validation, and information giving. The involved mothers seemed to know they had problems, and they sought some help. To cite a cliche — support is only support when it's needed and sought.

We believe we could be more effective using the NPACE approach with high-risk families if contact would begin in early pregnancy. The first 3 months of life is a time of crisis and disorganization; therefore, the postpartum period is not the ideal time to begin nursing intervention. First of all, an effective working relationship requires the establishment of a trusting relationship. The timing to initiate such a relationship is critical to its success, and the point at which a mother is developing a relationship with her new infant is not the appropriate time to initiate a relationship with a nurse. This period is often referred to as a closed period for forming new relationships outside the family unit, and this concept led us directly to our current research in which we are studying relationship building during early pregnancy (Barnard, 1981 – 1987). Although we are still in the early stages, we have discovered pregnancy is an ideal time to begin intervention with multiproblem families. The pregnant women are interested and more psychologically available for a working relationship during this period.

Since our results show differences in the number of assessments accomplished with the three categories of mothers (involved, less involved, and uninvolved), we believe that a more structured approach over a longer time would prove more effective with the uninvolved families. One of the overall strategies of the current project is to continue our systematic approach and be more persistent, focused, and structured with the less involved mothers. Having a longer period of time to work with these mothers should enhance the development of the helping relationship. These changes may prove to be less threatening for those mothers who tend to become withdrawn or apathetic when faced with the task of forming a new relationship. We also will incorporate more information about infants' behavior and developmental changes during the first 3 months after birth in order to be sensitive to mothers' needs. Since a working relationship has already been established in the prenatal period with the mothers in our current project, more time can be spent on focused activities. During this time of crises and family reorganization, therefore, the family will not only have a relationship with a professional who can listen to their concerns, but they will also have someone to provide needed information and guidance in creating a more optimal environment for the newborn. Therefore, the current project with its initiation during the prenatal period, the additional time spent maintaining a relationship with the nurses, and its structured focus hopefully will allow these women to maintain a satisfactory relationship with the nurses. This experience should enable them to become more independent, confident, and competent in their parenting and social abilities.

SUMMARY

We have shared a review of the process of helping vulnerable families within the framework of testing a specific model of nursing intervention. The nursing care was offered during a transitional period for families, i.e., immediately following the birth of their infants.

The intent of the nursing care was to be supportive of the family, particularly of the mother. We found some families were difficult to support; these tended to be families who by our definitions of problems had more reasons why they could benefit from help. We also found that mothers who did not have clear goals or the ability to make decisions easily were difficult to involve as mutual participants in the helping process. These mothers came from families that tended to have higher social risk, lower social status, and less evidence of a supportive network. We have concluded that the critical elements to consider in supporting these families are when contact is established and the length of time supportive nursing measures are provided. We speculate it would be more productive to be involved with high social risk families who have low support in early pregnancy and continue the support until they begin to use a network of family, friends, and other professionals in a supportive, helping relationship. To obtain support requires individuals who actively seek the information and support they need to optimize their parenting role.

CRITIQUE

Sharron S. Humenick, R.N., Ph.D.

Kathryn Barnard, Charlene Snyder, and Anita Spietz have presented a partial report from a larger study of nursing interaction with high-risk families of newborns. They have documented what many nurses may have previously surmised, i.e., those families which appear to need the most help may be the hardest to serve.

NURSING SUPPORT

Another documented finding is that characteristics of the mother, such as her eagerness to engage in problem solving, are related to the nature of support given by the nurse. Involved mothers evoked from the nurse an increased amount of mutual sharing, active listening, information exchange, validation, and information giving. The other group who evoked these same increased nursing responses were the less involved mothers from multiproblem families (as opposed to less involved mothers from families with fewer problems).

A comparison of three nursing approaches—NPACE, NSIBB, and NSTAC—was not the major thrust of the current paper under review. However, it is encouraging to note that NPACE, a supportive approach based on systematic assessment, was described as producing the most positive outcome with high-risk families. This individualized approach, based on reinforcing strengths, is a positive approach as compared to a problem oriented deficit model.

The problems under study in this research project are most relevant. For years public health nurses have made home visits to families of newborn infants, especially to those with physical and social high-risk factors. There has been very little research available to guide the content, approach, or timing of such visits. Over the years little has been done to document the value or cost effectiveness of such nursing services. As a result, in many health departments newborn family home visiting is not the well-funded service it once was. In some areas of the country, public health nurses have even asked nursing educators why newborn home visiting is still taught to student nurses. It is clearly time to evaluate the methodology and document the value of nurses making home visits to families of newborns. Although the road to definitive answers is long, it is gratifying to note the inroads made through the present study.

Perhaps one of the most important questions raised by the reported findings is—How does a nurse provide support for hard-to-serve, high-risk parents? The report indicates that these mothers were of a lower social status and demonstrated less evidence of a supportive network in addition to being high risk. Clearly this study provides a picture of mothers needing more support than they are receiving, but not responding, or perhaps being unable to respond, well to nursing support offered.

The additional research which was described as in progress and based upon the investigation of establishing a trusting relationship with a nurse during pregnancy appears promising. This approach allows a longer time for relationship building and has several other potential advantages as well.

ADDITIONAL BENEFITS

It has been asserted that women move faster and further in a therapeutic relationship while pregnant. Thus, pregnancy may prove to be one of the most effective times for a nurse to establish a working relationship with young women who are characterized by a lack of support systems. If researchers should find that nurse-client relationships formed in pregnancy are especially productive, the common practice of casually reassigning a new nurse when the client relocates in a neighboring nursing district would be called into question. Continuity of care might receive more emphasis in planning nursing care.

Nuckolls and associates (1972) reported that in the presence of stress, pregnant women with a large amount of support were associated with a one-third decrease in the incidence of complications. Brown and Harris (1978) found in a study of 485 women that under conditions of high stress, women with support had a 25% less incidence of depression.

Thus, in providing supportive nursing acts for high-risk pregnant mothers, there is a potential to accomplish far more than establishing a relationship which will be useful in the postnatal period. If a combination of support and individualized education were to be offered at prenatal visits, there is a potential to decrease infant complications and/or depression in the mother. Either outcome might affect the number of subjects who eventually become doubly vulnerable, as were some of the subjects in the study at hand.

Furthermore, researchers have provided evidence that active participation in childbirth is associated with an increase in internal locus of control (Felton & Segelman, 1978) and instrumental personality attributes among women (Humenick & Bugen, 1981). If the prenatal nursing contacts include intervention which results in a more active, satisfying birth experience for the mothers, it is possible that prenatal nursing visits would influence mothers towards exhibiting attributes of internal control in the postnatal period. These mothers, therefore, would be more like the mothers of the current study who were classified as involved.

The hypothetical, potential benefits of supportive prenatal nursing acts are described in Figure 1. In addition to the need for research to further test the implied hypotheses, there is also a need to evaluate the content, timing, approach, and cost effectiveness of such prenatal visits.

Of interest in the current study is the use of relationship progression and case reviews to differentiate mothers into categories of involved, less involved, and uninvolved. In systems theory terminology, engaging a client in active collaborative interactions is termed systems entry. The fact that systems entry is not always readily negotiated has been previously described in the literature (Hall & Weaver, 1977). Although any type of health professional is likely to find variation in ease of obtaining client involvement, the problem appears especially pertinent in relation to home visits for newborns. When the client initiates health care ser-

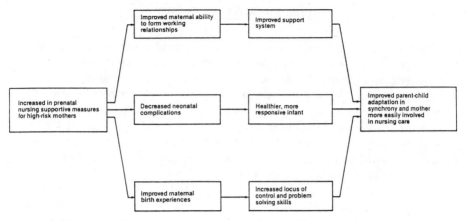

Figure 1. Hypothetical benefits of supportive nursing measures with high-risk prenatal women.

vices, she typically comes believing she has a situation which can benefit from interaction with the health care provider. In home visits for newborns, however, the service is often initiated by the nurse or a referring agency. It is no surprise, therefore, that it is difficult to involve some mothers, especially those with an apparent external locus of control and a poor support system.

MATERNAL INVOLVEMENT

In this study, the authors found a difference in the type of nursing activity based on the level of involvement of the mother. Since we have come to accept that the infant, in part, shapes the behavior of the caregiver, it is not difficult to accept that clients, in part, shape the behavior of the nurse. The surprise in this study was the finding that less involved mothers from multiproblem families evoked similar responses from the nurses as were evoked by the more involved mothers.

In explaining this finding, the authors suggest that being faced with multiple problems led the less involved mothers to know they needed help. While this explanation is possible, rival hypotheses also exist. Perhaps it was nursing factors which led the nurses to respond differently. For example, in multiproblem situations, it is probably exceedingly clear to the nurses why they need to be there. Thus, they may be motivated to exert extra effort even when clients lack motivation to become involved. It also might be worthwhile to hypothesize that most home visiting nurses have a tendency to be internal locus of control personality types. Perhaps nurses with an internal locus of control relate better to clients with an internal locus of control such as the involved mothers were surmised to be. Although the less involved mothers appeared to be external locus of control personality types, perhaps a certain percentage were internal locus of control types whose typical responses were masked by depression resulting from the multiple problems they faced. It would be conceivable that if a number of the less involved were basically internal locus of control types, some aspect of their behavior evoked nursing responses typically given to internally controlled clients.

Whatever the actual reason for different types of nursing responses to different types of clients, this finding provides very fertile ground for future research. For example, one might ask if the differences in nursing measures were actually appropriate given the client characteristics. The answer to such a question might help to formulate guidelines for influencing nurses to respond in appropriate ways, given certain types of clients. Measures such as locus of control on both mothers and nurses might be useful.

RESEARCH IMPLICATIONS

The description of levels of mother involvement during nursing home visits brings up yet another question — What are the cost/benefit ratios for visiting each type of mother? Maternal-child nurses, on the whole, do not like to put dollar values on services they see as benefiting humanity. It may be our lack of documentation of cost/benefits, however, that has led to a general decrease in the funding of this type of service. Such a question is, therefore, an important one to research.

The family that is hard to serve may show little short-term benefit, even with extensive nursing visits. The families described in this study were doubly vulnerable through high maternal risk, high infant risk, and additionally they had poor support systems and lack of involvement with the visiting nurse. They could be hypothesized as headed for further problems which will be exceedingly expensive to society in the long run. If they can eventually become involved in nursing care, there is the possibility of cost effectiveness even though the cost of the initial service is high. First of all, nursing researchers need to document whether or not nursing support has the potential to make a significant difference with such families; then, it would be possible to determine if philosophically, preventive supportive care should be offered. Likewise, it would be useful to obtain documentation of cost/benefit ratios for intervention with high-risk involved clients, as well as low-risk families. The ground work provided by this study would be very useful as the basis for some long-term cost/benefit studies.

The remaining aspect of this study upon which I wish to comment is the positive, supportive approach used with clients. When nurses are taught problem solving skills, problem oriented charting, and problem oriented nursing diagnoses, there is the potential to become problem oriented and to lose sight of maintaining a supportive balance. In addition to solving problems, nurses can and do support client strengths, assist clients to build stronger support systems, and in general help clients become adept at self-care. Several nursing research studies have documented the benefit of supporting clients' strengths in families with newborns (Barnard & Neal, 1977; Anderson, 1980; Poley, 1979). Yet, it is not atypical for some nurses to feel that they have no role in situations where they are not given a problem to solve. Studies such as the presentation are important to continue to build a strong theoretical basis for nursing services which provide a balance between a positive approach to support and a problem solving approach.

DISCUSSION

J. Bumbalo: I was struck by the fact that the process in this study started with these families with a systematic assessment, and I would put forth the proposition that it really did not just use an assessment but a very sophisticated level of nursing process all the way through. I would ask us to look at the fact that there is an interplay between the interpersonal process, the therapeutic process, and nursing process; they do indeed interact with each other and facilitate one to the other. I think where nurse researchers run into difficulty is they don't look at the interface between what they are asking in relation to the nursing process and what they are asking in relation to interpersonal factors. For example, at the point of assessment we want the most information; and we know from an interpersonal point of view that when we're in the orientation phase in the interpersonal relationship, we're going to have people least willing to share information. At the other end of the continuum — termination of the relationship and evaluation — nursing process fits in very nicely. Using good nursing process helps with both aspects of the relationship. What I've tried to look at with a lot of graduate students relative to their clinical practice is what's the interface between nursing process and interpersonal factors, and when do you back off from your nursing process to build on your interpersonal process to allow you to go back to your nursing process. I think the study that was just described to us is a superb example of this type of interface.

A. Spietz: I think that was our monumental task, and I think we've grappled with this for a long time in trying to separate the two processes and yet maintain the integrity that is there between them. That's enlightening for us too, but I think the difficulty is in trying to teach it.

J. Bumbalo: I have a comment that relates to trying to teach it. We teach students some things about how to apply the nursing process, but I wonder if we do not avoid teaching them how to use the interpersonal process ("Interpersonal Relationships," 1966). I've found one model that is especially helpful. McGrath's (1963) group in Utah talked about three parameters that influence relationships: attraction, influence, and attitudes. They built a model that says that you very specifically try to manipulate those things that you're trying to influence; for example, show the person what common bases you have. And that would be how you would work on attitudes. Some of the attraction factors are not known, but I think that is what Dr. Humenick was alluding to when she said that maybe the attraction is that the nurses and the less involved mothers were both examples of external locus of control type personalities and they were better able to build a relationship. I think, however, that we should do a more analytical analysis of why a particular nurse is able to work very well with a certain type of patient. Maybe we don't need to change nurses; maybe we do need to be very systematic about finding the basis to interact with a certain family.

J. Fawcett: I have two comments. First, some of this discussion refers to what sociologists call interpersonal attraction. This is a very difficult area to investigate, perhaps even more difficult than social support, due to many theoretical and empirical problems. Like other behavioral research, studies of interpersonal attraction do not yield definitive and concise explanations for the reasons why people are attracted to certain people, but not others. Second, I am concerned about the apparent separation of the nursing process and the interpersonal process in some of our discussion. I think that Carper's notion of types of knowledge needed for nursing practice combines the two processes in a meaningful way. She maintains that nursing practice ". . .depends on scientific knowledge of human behavior in health and illness, the esthetic perception of significant human experiences, a personal understanding of the unique individuality of the self and the capacity to make choices within concrete situations involving particular more judgments" (1978, p. 22). Nursing practice, then, is a combination of science, art, the therapeutic use of self, and ethics. The nursing process is a systematic manner of applying this knowledge. The interpersonal process is what transpires between client and nurse as the nursing process is applied.

J. Bumbalo: In my previous comments, I was obviously using the term nursing process to refer to the methodology of the practice of nursing, i.e., a problem solving approach involving assessment, intervention, and evaluation. I was referring to interpersonal process as a separate phenomenon. However, let me attempt to clarify my position. In the sense that nursing process forms the basis for one's contract with the patient or client and is the basis for nurse-patient interaction, it is definitely interpersonal and therapeutic in nature. Whether or not it is possible or appropriate to empirically differentiate between nursing process and interpersonal process is debatable; however, I have found it a valuable teaching strategy to have students analyze them theoretically as separate but concurrent processes.

D. Magyary: I notice that the study indicated more adolescents in the less involved group, and I thought of Dr. Mercer's comment about how hard it is to get them to participate in a study. Did you notice the nursing process taking on a different orientation when dealing with adolescents versus middle-aged women?

C. Snyder: I would say yes. Adolescents were much more difficult. As you can see, they did fill up that group. Often times, the teenagers were living with their mother or living in disorganized environments with or without boyfriends. The increased numbers of people, as well as the disorganization, made it difficult to focus.

D. Magyary: Did you find anything that linked them with the nursing process?

C. Snyder: I think it was just a sensitivity to where they were in their developmental process more than anything else.

P. Brandt: Perhaps we need to study a variety of treatment approaches to determine what enables adolescents to adapt to parenting. For example, the helping process may be more therapeutic with adolescents if peers are utilized rather than or in addition to professionals. Group sessions versus individual sessions could also be examined in relation to selected desired child or parenting outcomes.

K. Barnard: I'd like to speak toward alternative approaches. Our approach did not work with these less involved clients. I would like to indicate that possibly one approach to working with people who find it difficult to become involved in a relationship is a type of structuring which the NSIBB program did provide, in which it was not necessary for the mother or the nurse to get as involved in a therapeutic relationship. There were certain activities that the nurse provided for the mother and the rest of the family, both in terms of talking about and leaving little pamphlets about infant crying, keeping a sleep activity record, and so forth. The nurses who were involved in this program were absolutely frustrated because they had to keep this agenda and they felt that it was not meeting the needs of the families, etc. We also almost had a major office rift because we discourage people from talking to one another during the project since we're working on opposite teams and fear contamination. This rule had a sizable effect on office morale. We did carry out the project, but the nurses were constantly coming to me and saying "We've just got to do something different. We can't carry out this program. They have so many needs." I talked to them, but unless it was a case of murder, child abuse, or something like that, I tried to encourage them to maintain the program.

When we looked at the 3-month data, particularly for the multiproblem families, the infants in the multiproblem family group in the NSIBB program had the highest mental development. One of the things this suggests to me is that if you continue structuring for very disorganized, multiproblem families, the constant structuring and focusing allowed them to focus on the needs of those infants, maybe in a better way than all the therapeutic relationship building in the other program. However, when you looked at the 10-month outcomes, what was apparent in these multiproblem families was that the NSIBB kids had plummeted on the Bailey measurements while the NPACE infants had taken an upward shift. It was as if by focusing on the mothers, which was a predominant activity in the NPACE program, you energized them and they finally began to focus on the infants; whereas the mothers in the NSIBB were not energized, and when they lost the structure and focusing, their focus on the infant decreased.

I think there are alternatives, and it's very clear to me that the NSIBB program, although carried out with master level prepared nurses, could be modified and carried out by less trained individuals, e.g., neighborhood aides, etc. I think that we have to quickly move to begin to reconceptualize how we work with some of these multiproblem families, and I think a simpler model with less individualization might be the model to use.

B. Bishop: I wondered if you were able to look at the hard-to-reach teenagers. In my experience it is really tough to reach these teenagers. When you look at their histories, very often those youngsters, particularly if they were living in the home with their mothers, had been set up to have the baby. The baby was not their baby; it was for their mothers who could no longer have a baby. They could not take care of their baby as a mother because they were a vehicle for their mothers and their job was done. They have incubated a baby so that their mothers have a baby, and they're ready to return to school, etc.

Also, I have some reflections in relation to Dr. Barnard's comments about alternative approaches. I was a school nurse for pregnant teenagers, and maybe one of the approaches we need to look at much more is the school nurse in the high school. It's a beautiful way to monitor teenagers. They don't have to come see you; you're there, and they're there. You can keep track of them, and you can get reinforcement from the group. Other teenagers can recommend you if you work well with them, and after a while, more teenagers will come to see for themselves what the nurse is doing and the help she can offer to them. The most successful program that I know of as far as adolescents is the one in St. Paul where they put the maternal-infant care program right into the high school and the nurse was there all the time. What they found first is that the fertility rate went down for the entire population in that school since family planning was available. Second, for those teens that became mothers, they had no cases of abuse or neglect a year after the child was born and also teen mothers' fertility rate went down. In a school situation, one can cover a large population without one to one because of the grapevine and the results of teens interacting with each other to spread information. And it can affect everyone, not just the pregnant adolescents.

P. Brandt: By providing opportunities for peers to teach or support each other in parenting, we actually encourage the natural process of helping that occurs between adolescents on other topics. Peer teaching has been found to be important for the development of communication in young handicapped children and for facilitation of social competence in juvenile delinquents. There appears to be potential importance for adolescent parents also. For example, the adolescent mother I am presently seeing in the clinic demonstrates skills in contingently relating to her infant, and she is enthusiastic about sharing these skills with other teen mothers. She would be an excellent resource for a peer teaching program.

A. Spietz: That is one of the techniques we use when we distribute some of the books we want them to read. We ask them to review this particular book and let us know how it would work for them so that we could use it for other mothers in the program. They just love that because it is an esteem building type of exercise.

P. Brandt: I recently talked to a researcher in Ohio who had nurses train neighborhood/community people to develop skills in relationship building and infant care. The community people subsequently worked with new parents to develop parents' skills in infant care.

S. Humenick: There is a term that I really like which Hall and Weaver (1977) attribute to Smoyak. It is "professional hanging around," a tactic used when systems entry is not readily negotiated with the client system. Sometimes we need to give ourselves permission not to do anything that looks therapeutic, but rather just hang around in an effort to become part of the environment. Eventually, we may be seen as more acceptable and we may then be better able to negotiate a therapeutic relationship.

M. Curry: It seems that we need to put some of these approaches into operation with families whose infants fail to thrive, and perhaps use lay or community workers to do the relationship building. This approach may be much more cost effective than using nurses, and it may accomplish the same outcome. I would certainly agree that we need both second and third order change in how we define and operate our health care systems. I would also like to follow up on Dr. Norbeck's comments regarding the use of the research process as a clinical intervention. I have had a similar experience in my study of antepartum hospitalization (Curry, 1983), in which women completed both Sarason's Life Experience Survey (Sarason, 1978) and the NSSQ (Norbeck, Lindsay, & Carrieri, 1981). Many women have commented that they found completing the questionnaires helpful, both in terms of helping to pass the time and in helping them to gain a different perspective on their situation. Further, after delivery, most sample women described participating in the study as one of their most effective coping mechanisms. It is clear that we need to systematically document these effects and begin to describe both their positive and negative effects.

K. Pridham: I think this a very rich study in many ways. One way is in the language which this study develops to describe nursing and nursing actions. I wonder if you are developing a language with which to characterize the family strengths that you have identified. It seems to me that one of the things which has been lacking in the currently available nursing diagnosis classification system is a means of identifying strengths or competencies that one wants to enhance or support.

A. Spietz: I think we are. We have developed profiles for each family whereby we will divide up each assessment tool that we do use and cite the strengths that we find from that assessment. For example, having realistic developmental expectations for her infant at birth is a strength, i.e., knowing a newborn can see, hear, and is aware of surroundings, etc. A weakness, on the other hand, might be if she perceives that talking to the baby isn't important until 12 months of age. Our assessments can lead to identifying the strengths, as well as the weaknesses. I think that the problem many nurses have is in translating and intervening from the actual assessment. We find it very easy because it is a skill we have developed in doing the research during the past 10 years. For example, if you find a mother who scores low on sensitivity to cues, we interpret it immediately and give some kind of positive feedback. We initially started collecting data, then we began to slowly intervene and collect small bits of information, and now we're intervening totally.

C. Snyder: In addition, we share the assessments freely with the mothers. We do an assessment, tell them their strengths, and show them the areas they can work on if they are interested. It seems to build their self-esteem to focus on their strengths.

In this new project (Infant-Family Focus), one major focus has been to try to help them improve their social skills and help them survive in the community so to speak. We assess their social skills at the beginning, and then reassess them to look for any improvement. They also need community skills. Many of these mothers don't even know where the nearest bus stop is; and they don't know how to use the yellow pages, the telephone book, or the library. We get some dialogue going on this skill; and some will try to develop the skills, while others won't. We also try to get them involved in building their skills, not just around the pregnancy, but as a woman. We try to build self-esteem and nurture these mothers so that they, in turn, can nurture their baby. It's very exciting.

One of the tools that we use in the new project is Dr. Cranley's Fetal Attachment Scale (1981). We've started using the scale during the latter weeks of pregnancy; and at the same time, we've also incorporated some of Jessup's work of getting the mother to focus on her unborn baby (Carter-Jessup, 1981). We ask her to talk to her fetus and try to interact by massaging or rubbing her belly. She then keeps track of these activities, as well as the fetal movements, on a Nursing Child Assessment Sleep/Activity (NCASA) record. This simple record keeping has been very helpful in promoting and enhancing the acquaintance process.

B. Bishop: One of the things that is not included very much in the nursing literature is documenting how to identify and use strengths to build nursing plans. Most of the available information is too vague. We all know how to assess weaknesses better than strengths. I think that this kind of information is available in this study, and it is time to share some of this information with colleagues.

S. Feetham: You have indicated that nurses do not know how to use the instruments for obtaining a systematic assessment as reported in your research. It would be helpful to practitioners and nurse researchers for you to publish what you have gained in your intervention research through the use of systematic assessment.

K. Barnard: I'd like to go back to something Sharron Humenick mentioned, which I call the collapse of the public health nursing services in communities. These services are disappearing. We need to find ways to support their continuance, but there is a problem proving their effectiveness and also a significant burn out problem in public health nurses. They encounter on a daily basis really hard families to work with; the way they cope is not to contact these families, or to stop visiting after one or two visits. One of the things we've been thinking about is to provide a structure for the nurse to survive in these situations. For instance, we had the nurses complete a 9 point scale after each visit to determine their satisfaction with their performance on that contact. Our data suggested that public health nurses are very dissatisfied with what they can accomplish, but the use of the assessment does increase their satisfaction. The nurses in our study on Newborn Nursing Models that were the most satisfied with their performance were the nurses that were using the NSIBB program. The NSIBB was the most structured model where the nurses had definite objectives and specific interventions for each home visit. I think that out on the battlefield, it may be necessary to have some structuring and some guidelines. I'd like to encourage those of you who are involved to begin to turn some of your energies toward developing protocols that can be used in the field by nurses who really are dealing with some monumental societal problems in the families we serve. In many respects, these nurses are holding communities together.

G. Anderson: There seems to be a common problem being reported by almost everyone here these 2 days, and I have a suggestion that may help to build both the mothers' self-esteem and the nurses' satisfaction. The common problem is the crying of an unsootheable infant. There are ways to help some of these infants, and these measures could be very easily instituted. If these infants become more sootheable, I believe many other problems will take care of themselves. Social support will still be needed, but it will have a much better chance of being more effective. One approach is based on research by Jakobsson and Lindberg (1978, 1983) in Sweden. In a double blind crossover study, these investigators found that when mothers stopped ingesting cow's milk, cow's milk products such as cheese, and products containing cow's milk, colic disappeared in 35 of 66 breast-fed infants and reappeared on at least 2 challenges (cow's milk to mother's) in 23 of these 35 infants (Jakobsson & Lindberg, 1983). A second approach is something that I learned from Jack Paradise who told me that otitis media in young infants is very difficult to diagnose because both otitis media and crying cause a very red tympanic membrane.* Because infants are likely to cry during an ear examination, otitis media can be missed, and it can become a chronic problem and the cause of much crying in some infants. The third approach is that very simple chiropractic techniques may be needed, each for different problems that may have occurred during birth, e.g., as a result of forceps deliveries or with pressure that is sometimes placed on the neck in order to deliver the infant's shoulders. At present, the best reference on this material is by Frymann (1966). The techniques she described have been modified and extended by chiropractors, but they have not been described by them in the literature as yet, in part because the techniques are so easily taught and so effective that it did not seem necessary at first (M.D. Chance, personal communication, September 1982). However, background material is available now (Walther, 1981, 1983), three more volumes are planned, and the fifth one will specifically address the pathology of colic as viewed by chiropractors and the recommended procedures for treatment. Chiropractic treatment is not symptom-oriented, the processes and rationales make sense, the results are convincing, and this alternative seems worthy of our consideration.

S. Feetham: I think also the work Dr. Barnard is doing on infant massage identified some areas for soothing infants. Have you used that in teaching the parents?

K. Barnard: We did teach infant massage, and we found a variable response. Some mothers cannot use infant massage well, and it sends them and their baby into hysteria. It would be very interesting to follow those mother-infant pairs later. Other mothers find it a very useful technique, and among the mothers we originally taught during the first 3 postpartal weeks, about 75% of them were still doing it at 8 months.

Our infant massage program included some techniques from the literature which use face, arm, hand, body, and foot massage in a sequence for approximately 8 minutes that we taught mothers to do (Booth, Johnson-Crowley, & Barnard, 1983).

C. Snyder: I have had experience using these techniques, although I wasn't involved in Dr. Barnard's research on infant massage. The success of the technique really depends on the mother's personality. A very nervous, uptight mother simply cannot massage, and I also think you have to teach mothers some relaxation techniques. Instruct them to relax and

---

*Jack Paradise is a pediatrician in the Ambulatory Care Center, Children's Hospital of Pittsburgh.

tune into the baby. Then guide her; otherwise, these mothers overexcite the babies. You really have to be sensitive to the mother's personality. It's just like therapeutic touch. You really have to be sensitive to those energy fields.

K. Barnard: We teach mothers little games and exercises to play with their infants. I would say that the majority of them handle the games and exercises better than they do massage.

S. Feetham: One thing I've always been so impressed with is the strong clinical base in Dr. Barnard's work. Many nurse researchers come from a strong clinical base; yet we do not often acknowledge the strength of that base and overtly identify to others that this is the source of our research. When we use instruments from other disciplines and we feel uncomfortable about what is measured, it may be because the instruments are not consistent with our practice. We, as nurse researchers, need to recognize that there may be other ways to test the questions derived from our practice. A strength of so much of what has been presented and discussed during this conference is movement towards the recognition and development of research from the strengths of nursing practice.

REFERENCES

Anderson, D. J. (1980). Informing mothers about the behavioral characteristics of their infants: The effects on mother-infant interaction. Unpublished doctoral dissertation, The University of Texas, 1979. *Dissertation Abstracts International, 40,* 1119-B. (University Microfilms No. 79-200076)

Barnard, K. E. (1979). *Nursing child assessment satellite teaching manual.* Seattle: University of Washington.

Barnard, K. E. (1981–1987). *Clinical nursing models proposal.* (Grant No. MH36894). National Institute of Mental Health.

Barnard, K. E., & Eyres, S. J. (1977). *Results of the first twelve months of life.* Final report to the Division of Nursing, Bureau of Health Resources and Development, U.S. Public Health Service, Health Resources Administration, Department of Health, Education and Welfare on the Nursing Child Assessment Project. (No. 01700200142-9). Washington, DC: Government Printing Office.

Barnard, K. E., & Eyres, S. (Eds.). (1979, June). *Child health assessment, Part 2: The first year of life.* (DHEW Publication No. HRA 79-25). Hyattsville, MD: Division of Nursing.

Barnard, K. E., & Neal, M. V. (1977). Maternal-child nursing research: Review of past strategies for the future. *Nursing Research, 26,* 193–197.

Bowlby, J. (1977). The making and breaking of affectional bonds. *The British Journal of Psychiatry, 130,* 201–210.

Booth, C., Johnson-Crowley, N., & Barnard, K. E. (1983). *A program of massage and exercise for newborns: Description of program and results.* Unpublished manuscript, University of Washington, Seattle.

Brammer, L. M. (1973). *The helping relationship process and skills.* Englewood Cliffs, NJ: Prentice-Hall.

Broussard, E. R., & Hartner, M. S. S. (1976). Neonatal prediction of outcome at 10/11 years. *Child Psychiatry and Human Development, 7,* 85–93.

Brown, G. W., & Harris, T. (1978). *Social origins of depression.* London: Travestack.

Carey, W. B. (1972). Clinical applications of infant temperament measurement. *Journal of Pediatrics, 81*(4), 823–828.

Carper, B. A. (1978). Fundamental patterns of knowing in nursing. *Advances in Nursing Science, 1*(1), 13–23.

Carter-Jessup, L. (1981). Promoting maternal attachment through prenatal intervention. *MCN The American Journal of Maternal Child Nursing, 6,* 107–112.

Chance, M. D. (1982, September). Personal communication.

Cobb, S. (1976). Social support as a moderator of life stress. *Psychosomatic Medicine, 38,* 300–314.

Cranley, M. S. (1981). Development of a tool to measure maternal-fetal attachment. *Nursing Research, 30,* 281–284.

Curry, M. A. (in progress). *The effects of long-term antepartum hospitalization on maternal behavior and the family.* Funded by NIH Division of Nursing, No. ORS 1088C.

Dudley, D. L., & Welke, E. (1977). *How to survive being alive.* New York: Doubleday & Co.

Felton, G. S., & Segelman, F. B. (1978). Lamaze childbirth training and changes in belief about personal control. *Birth and Family Journal, 5,* 141–150.

Frymann, V. (1966). Relation of disturbances of the craniosacral mechanisms to symptomatology of the newborn: Study of 1250 infants. *Journal of the American Osteopathic Association, 65,* 1059–1075.

Hall, J. E., & Weaver, B. R. (1977). *Distributive nursing practice: A systems approach to community nursing.* New York: Lippincott.

Hollingshead, A. B. (1975). *Four factor index of social status.* New Haven, CT: Author.

Holmes, T. H., & Rahe, R. H. (1967). The social readjustment rating scale. *Journal of Psychosomatic Research, 11,* 213–218.

Humenick, S. S., & Bugen, L. A. (1981). Mastery: The key to birth satisfaction: A study. *Birth and Family Journal, 8,* 84–90.

Interpersonal Relationships: A review. (1966). *Regional Rehabilitation Research Institute Bulletin, 1.* Salt Lake City, University of Utah.

Jakobsson, I., & Lindberg, T. (1978). Cow's milk as a cause of infantile colic in breast-fed infants. *Lancet, 2,* 437.

Jakobsson, I., & Lindberg, T. (1983). Cow's milk proteins cause infantile colic in breast-fed infants: A double-blind crossover study. *Pediatrics, 71*(2), 268.

Lindner, K. (1982). *Life change, social support and cognitive problem-solving skills.* Unpublished doctoral dissertation, University of Washington.

McDonald, A. D. (1964). Intelligence in children of very low birth weight. *British Journal of Preventive and Social Medicine, 18,* 59–74.

McGrath, J. E. (1963). A descriptive model for the study of interpersonal relations in small groups. *Psychological Studies, 27,* 10–17.

Mitchell, P. H., & Loustau, A. (1981). *Concepts basic to nursing.* New York: McGraw-Hill.

Norbeck, J., Lindsay, A., & Carrieri, V. (1981). The development of an instrument to measure social support. *Nursing Research, 30,* 264–269.

Nuckolls, K. B., Cassel, J., & Kaplan, B. H. (1972). Psychosocial assets, life crisis, and the prognosis of pregnancy. *American Journal of Epidemiology, 95,* 431–441.

Paradise, J. L. (1966). Maternal and other factors in the etiology of infantile colic: Report of a prospective study of 146 infants. *Journal of the American Medical Association, 12*(1), 7.

Paradise, J. L. (1980). Otitis media in infants and children. *Pediatrics, 65,* 917.

Poley, B. A. (1979). Altering dyadic synchrony, maternal self-confidence, and maternal perception of the infant through a teaching-modeling intervention with primiparous mothers. Unpublished doctoral dissertation, The University of Texas, 1979. *Dissertation Abstracts International, 39,* 5313. (University Microfilms No. 79-11012)

Sarason, I., Johnson, J., & Siegel, J. (1978). Assessing the impact of life changes. Development of the life experiences survey. *Journal of Consulting and Clinical Psychology,* *46,* 932–946.

Walther, D. S. (1981). *Applied kinesiology, Vol. 1: Basic procedures and muscle testing.* Pueblo, CO: Systems DC. (275 W. Abriendo Ave., Pueblo, CO 81004).

Walther, D. S. (1983). *Applied kinesiology, Vol. 2: Head, neck, and jaw pain and dysfunction–the stomatognathic system.* Pueblo, CO: Systems DC.

Werner, E. E., Bierman, J. M., & French, F. E. (1971). *The children of Kauai. A longitudinal study from the prenatal period to age ten.* Honolulu: University of Hawaii Press.

Willerman, L., Broman, S. H., & Fiedler, M. (1970). Infant development, preschool IQ, and social class. *Child Development, 41,* 69–77.

COMMENTARY

The contents of this report exemplify family-related theory development. Here, attention was directed to the mothers of high-risk infants. Barnard, Snyder, and Spietz identify the assumptions upon which their work was based, implying that a family systems approach was used by virtue of their reference to the parent-infant system and their illustration of the interaction of mother, child, and environment in the Nursing Assessment Interactional Model. The assumptions guided development of the a middle-range theory and the methodology. The theory as is expressed in a hypothesis states that "if either partner in the parent-child interaction had nonoptimal characteristics, the chances for parent-child adaption, especially for synchrony, would be markedly decreased [particularly when] both the parents and the baby have nonoptimal characteristics." Methodologically, the assumptions influenced the selection of families. Additional direction for the work comes from social support theory, which was used as the basis for the nursing intervention, an eight-stage helping relationship or process.

Barnard and her colleagues have made a significant contribution to family-related theory development in nursing by identifying specific supportive acts performed by the nurses as they engage in the helping relationship with mothers and by beginning to identify maternal, infant, and social variables that influence the progression of the helping relationship. Humenick further advanced the theory development effort by discussing and diagraming the outcomes of a suggestion made by Barnard and her colleagues to begin nursing intervention during pregnancy.

JACQUELINE FAWCETT

10

Affiliating in Stepfather Families: Teachable Strategies Leading to Stepfather — Child Friendship[1]

PHILLIS NOERAGER STERN

When a man marries a mother, he becomes a stepfather. He does not gain the status of father surrogate, with all its implications for managing the children's upbringing in full partnership with the mother, however, until he is able to allay the doubts of mother and children that he is equal to this enormously important task. Analysis of interviews with 30 stepfather families indicate that one of the most troublesome areas of adjustment for these families lay in the problem of when, and under what circumstances, the stepfather may properly discipline his wife's children. Although family standards differ, I found that the stepfather who affiliates with his stepchild prior to, or in concert with disciplining, settles more easily into the male-adult-co-manager position in the household.

This paper discusses the process of affiliating, meaning to befriend, discovered in the analysis of data from a grounded theory study of stepfa-

Reprinted from *Western Journal of Nursing Research, 4*, 75–89, 1982.

ther families. Affiliating was found to consist of ten related strategies that stepfathers and children used to overcome friendship barriers. The ten strategies of affiliating discovered in this study can be taught to other stepfather families by nurses who work with these families.

BACKGROUND AND SELECTED REVIEW OF THE LITERATURE

When she remarries, a mother and her spouse may think that they will merge immediately into a happy integrated family, but as nurses and other professionals working with families know, this is rarely the case. Although considerable literature deals with conflicts within stepfamilies, it is scattered and the findings are sometimes contradictory. Most authors agree, however, that discipline poses a serious problem in stepfamilies. Literature selected for this review concentrates on four areas: a) significance of the problem; b) conflict over child-rearing, particularly disciplining of children; c) the stepfather's self-image as opposed to the self-image of the child; and d) integration in re-married families.

Significance

Over 15 million children under 18 live in stepfamilies in the United States (Roosevelt and Lofas 1976). This represents about 13 percent of the total population according to the Population Reference Bureau (1977). About one million children and half a million adults become members of stepfamilies each year (Visher and Visher 1979). In most cases, children live with a full-time stepfather rather than a stepmother, because in nine out of ten divorces the mother keeps the children. A recent study in San Diego, California (Bohannan 1975), showed that nine percent of the city's population was made up of stepfather families.

Discipline

Disputes over discipline have been recognized as problematic by a series of authors (Simon 1964; Mowatt 1972; Maddox 1975; Roosevelt and Lofas 1977; Visher and Visher 1979). Haley (1976) also discusses sequences of conflicts over discipline in stepfamilies. Messinger (1976:196) found that children rejected the stepparent in the parent role, and "often reacted with feelings of guilt, hostility, rebellion or withdrawal." Fast and Cain (1966:486) in a classic study found that stepfathers, particularly, suffered from role confusion in their interactions with their spouses' children, being asked to act as "parent, stepparent, and nonparent."

Self Image

Stepfathers view themselves less favorably than do stepchildren. In a study comparing stepfather families with intact families, Bohannan and Erickson (1978) found that stepfathers had a more negative image of themselves as fathers. These stepfathers saw themselves as contributing less to family discipline than their wives, and in contrast with the opinion of their wives and stepchildren, viewed their stepchildren as less happy than children from intact families. Bohannan and Erickson (1978) reported that the self-image of stepchildren was quite positive and that the mental health, school achievement, and self esteem of children in stepfamilies was equal to a similar group of children in intact families. This finding supports a secondary analysis of two public opinion surveys (Wilson, Zucher, McAdams and Curtis 1975). The analysis showed no difference in a comparison between adults from stepfather homes with those from intact homes.

Integration

Initially, stepfathered families consist of two separate dyadic relationships: a husband-spouse subsystem and a mother-child subsystem. The integration of these separate dyads into an integrated family unit is a complicated and sometimes unsuccessful process. The mother-child alliance must relax its tight bonds so that the stepfather can participate in managing the child (Stern 1977a, b). Maddox (1975:88) describes the stepfather as the "watched parent." She suggests that the behavior of the stepfather must be such that the mother and children can consider him suitable to the father-surrogate role.

Roosevelt and Lofas (1977) point out that stepfather and child lack a shared history on which to base their relationship. Therefore, when the child attempts to test the limits of the stepfather's patience, the stepfather's resulting anger may set off a disciplinary action more harsh than would be the case if the two had a history of love and familiarity to support their relationship. Generally the mother reacts swiftly in the defense of her child. As Roosevelt and Lofas (1977:83) write, "Through one means or another she may build her biological fences beyond which the stepfather is not welcome."

Family integration was the subject of Duberman's (1975) study of 88 reconstituted families. Duberman used spouse self-rating and observations to determine that 45 percent of the families were high in family integration, 34 percent moderate, and 21 percent low. Duberman's findings, however, conflict with an earlier study by Bowerman and Irish (1962) who concluded that step homes with teenagers were more likely than intact families to have stress, ambivalence, and low cohesiveness.

Macklin (1980:910) in reviewing a decade of stepfamily research writes of the need to compare "successful" with "unsuccessful" stepfamilies. The process of affiliating is seen as contributing to the success of the stepfather family situation since it provides a means for bringing together biologically-unrelated members in a way in which the newly-formed unit can function with cohesiveness and mutual support. The present study stands alone in its attempt to describe *processes* that contribute to integration (or success) in stepfather families.

METHODOLOGY

This paper presents selected findings from a study of stepfather families based on Grounded Theory Methodology (Glaser and Strauss 1967; Glaser 1978; Wilson 1977; Stern 1980). The grounded-theory approach to the identification of social processes has been found useful in a variety of contexts (e.g., Maxwell 1979; Stern, Tilden and Maxwell 1980; Corbin 1980; Bozett 1981). The purpose of this study was to determine processes involved in stepfather family integration, or success. The strategies used by stepfathers and children to establish affectional ties, collectively called affiliating, were discovered through the traditional matrix of Grounded Theory wherein several research processes occur simultaneously. "In other words, the investigator examines data as they arrive, and begins to code, categorize, conceptualize, and to write the first few thoughts concerning the research report almost from the beginning of the study" (Stern 1980:21). Although analysis and data collection proceed simultaneously, a division is made between sample and data collection on the one hand, and analysis and data collection on the other, in order to provide the paper with some organization and clarity.

Sample and Data Collection

The proposal for this study gained approval of the Committee on the Research of Human Subjects, University of California, San Francisco. Interview and observational data were collected from an opportunistic sample of 30 stepfather families in the San Francisco Bay area in 1975 and 1976. Subjects were referred to the investigator by other stepfamilies and by nurse colleagues. I spoke with 62 persons in 85 hours of intensive interviews, collecting data on 132 persons from present and former marriages. The original intent was to interview whole families as a unit; however, because of family resistance, this was possible in only eight cases. The remaining interviews were conducted as follows: five couples, 12 grown stepchildren living out of the home, four mothers only, one stepfather only, and one aunt to children in a stepfather home. Separate additional interviews were conducted with six stepfathers, ten mothers, and four stepchildren living in the home. The social class of the subjects ranged from blue collar to professional, with the majority in the middle range. Ethnic representation included 86 percent white, six percent black, and the remaining eight percent consisted of mixed American-Indian-Caucasian, and Mexican-American persons.

Protestants predominated with 52 percent; 20 percent were Catholic; 18 percent Jewish; three percent "other," and seven percent "none" for religious affiliation. Several families were of mixed religions. The majority of the children were born in California, while most parents came from elsewhere. The age of the 61 children at the time of the spouse union ranged from two to 19 years, with a fairly equal distribution of 31 percent pre-school, 38 percent school age, and 31 percent teenage.

Years of marriage at the time of the interview ranged from one-and-one-half years to 20 years. The mean fell roughly between three to five years.

Data Collection and Analysis

Affiliation, a theoretical construct, emerged from an analysis of the data. It consisted of ten strategies to be defined and discussed below. For the moment, let us note that these strategies were discovered by asking stepfathers, "what do you think your stepchild likes about you?" or "what did you do to get your stepchild to warm up to you?" The child was asked, "what do you like about your stepfather?" and "what things do you and your stepfather do together that you enjoy?" Mothers were similarly questioned.

Affiliating and its constituent strategies were of course dimensional, with positive and negative poles. The negative pole, non-affiliating, was in each instance determined by asking stepfathers, "what do you think your stepchild would like you to change about your behavior?" or "what things do you do that turns your stepchild off?" Stepchildren were asked, "what do you wish your stepfather wouldn't do?" or "what would you like to change about your stepfather?" And again mothers were questioned in the same areas. Children were asked similar questions about their own behavior.

Grounded Theory (Glaser and Strauss 1967) served as the basis for the analysis of data. Briefly described, it is a means of generating categories of social processes that do not depend upon *a priori* pigeonholes developed by the investigator but are instead "grounded" in the data themselves. Data in their simplest forms, statements by interviewees, were examined as they were collected until similarities were noticed, and were then coded together to form a number of different concepts. For instance, the interviews contained repetitive references to the process "teaching" stepchildren, and a category of "teaching" emerged. Similar process categories emerged from that data. For example, several stepfathers made references to "accepting kids the way they are." That data was labeled "accepting." These codes "are called substantive codes because they codify the substance of the data" (Stern 1980:21).

Next, substantive coded data which seemed to cluster together and relate, were formed into categories. Teaching emerged as a category of affiliating strategies. When more data were compared, categories of trusting, spending time, and liking were similarly discovered.

Concept formation and refinement consist of clustering categories under a higher-order category to form a theoretical construct, or core variable which explains the action or main problems in the situation under study, and how the interactants deal with these problems. The main problem experienced by the families in the present study in their efforts to become a "happy family," as some described it, resulted from negotiations regarding the disciplining of the mother's children: whether the stepfather should participate equally or not. In families which reached some consensus on this issue among all family members, the process of affiliation seemed to be operating between stepparent and child. Taken together the categories formed the theoretical construct of "affiliation" at the highest level of generality.

FINDINGS

The discovery of the following ten affiliating strategies is important because it is through their use that stepfathers and children in the present study managed to make friends with one another. While it may seem obvious that family members must act as friends in order to attain a state in which individual members become coordinate behaviorally and affectively into a harmonious unit, it was not obvious to some stepfather families.

Affiliating Contexts

About half of the stepfathers in this study concentrated on their disciplinarian role in the family at the expense of more companionate interactions. In these cases, the mother generally intervened, assuming the role of go-between, thus effectively separating children and stepfather affectionately and physically.

Affiliating allows the child to view the stepparent as a person of value; it reduces fear in, and gains the confidence of the child. Failure to befriend the child may cause the stepfather to be viewed as a person worse than valueless. The child has no faith in the nonaffiliating stepfather, and may be frightened by him. Mutual respect is essential if friendship is to evolve between stepfather and child. If either persistently belittles the other, the stepfather will not expend the energy necessary to win over a recalcitrant adversary, and the child will persevere in protective behavior against the intruder.

Affiliating is seen as additionally important in helping men who, like several in the present study, lack the skills necessary for making friends with a resentful child. These men didn't know how to begin the process. Many had never considered asking their stepchild what they liked or didn't like about them until the time of the present interviews, and many had never shared their reciprocal feelings with the stepchild.

Temporal Considerations

Less than half of all families interviewed established a state of integration or "happy family" existence. But no matter what the outcome, all families reported a period of disequilibrium following the marriage during which structural patterns were established. The disequilibrium proved to be temporally specific. Almost all families reported a period of between one-and-one-half to two years before "things settled down." Figure one represents a schematic model of temporal relationships and bi-polar, affiliating-nonaffiliating strategies.

Affiliating Strategies

Affiliating social processes are by their nature interactional. They involve strategies used by the child as well as the adult. Data from the present study indicate however, that it is generally necessary for the stepfather to initiate the process.

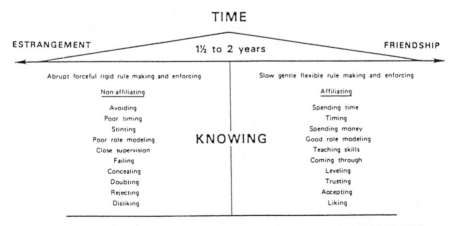

FRIENDSHIP-ESTRANGEMENT IN STEPFATHER-CHILD RELATIONSHIPS

Figure 1. Bi-polar AFFILIATING-NON-AFFILIATING dimensions. Affiliating points in the direction of stepfather-child friendship; non-affiliating points in the direction of stepfather-child estrangement. Temporal dimensions are illustrated at the top of the figure.

The strategies described separately here, relate closely with one another, and in some cases tend to overlap. Because they were presented to me as separate entities however, I have retained that distinctness.

SPENDING TIMES VS AVOIDING

Time spent is essential in forming friendly relationships with a stepchild: time to know, time to trust, time to consolidate values. Data from field notes indicate that spending time can be placed on both a quantity and quality continuum. One stepfather, Ed, who could be placed at the positive end of such a continuum, spent a great deal of time alone with his stepson Kent, teaching him a number of skills. Ed made it clear that he enjoyed the company of his stepson. Ed's temporal contributions were high quality and high quantity.

Floyd, a member of the least cohesive group in the study, rarely spoke to his stepchildren, and rarely spent time with them. Floyd *avoided* his stepchildren. Avoiding is the opposing property to spending time. Floyd, who avoided his stepchildren had a particularly distant relationship with his teenage stepdaughter. She described his presence in the in the home this way, "he comes home, usually late, goes to the TV in their bedroom, shuts the door, and that's it for the evening." Floyd's temporal contributions were low in quality and quantity.

TIMING VS POOR TIMING

Data from the present study indicate that a well-placed act of friendship makes a memorable impression on a stepchild, but an attempt to achieve a close relationship before the child is ready can meet with failure.

A part of affiliating is saying the right thing at the right time to bolster a child's self-esteem; in other words, good timing. Rose, 12, sometimes found her stepfather too strict. Rose was a little formal with her stepfather, Karl, when the interview began. During the course of the conversation Rose said that her best friend, whom Rose considered prettier than herself, now preferred another girl's company. Karl then compared Rose with her former friend. He said he thought Rose was "prettier, more tractable, sweeter; she is able to think better, and is more sophisticated." Karl's timing had been perfect. There was a visible change in Rose's attitude. She sat straighter, and gazed fondly at her stepfather during the remainder of the interview.

When stepfathers use poor timing, the responding rejection prevents some men from making another attempt at affiliation. However most stepfathers are willing to overlook initial rejection and report, "giving it another try." Emery's early attempts to be friends with Joey were disappointing. Emery used the same teaching approach on three-year-old Joey which had delighted his own children. Joey burst into tears. But, Emery was willing to keep trying. Experience is needed to learn proper timing in stepfamily relationships.

SPENDING MONEY VS STINTING

Children in the present study appreciated that good will may prompt a small introductory gift from a stepfather, but they also liked material gain for its own sake. A child who lives in a single-parent household has often had first-hand knowledge of financial matters. Children in this study were often told by their mothers that "things would be better" if she found a "new daddy." If the relationship between stepparent and child was a poor one, and there was no financial gain, children in this investigation found the condition unforgivable. They were bitter in their complaints about a stepfather guilty of stinting.

Teenagers have particular difficulty adjusting to a step-relationship, but Milo was that rare adolescent who liked his stepfather. Milo expressed delight over his appointments. Milo had private quarters and his own outside entrance. He had a stereo, color TV with electronic games, and a waterbed.

By contrast, Ruby was a grown woman when I talked with her, but she still resented the man her mother married when Ruby was 13. One of her chief complaints was the way her stepfather, Leonard, stinted when it came to spending money. Leonard took his own daughters to town to shop for clothes, but he never took Ruby and her sisters. Years later, Ruby still talked about the unfairness of it.

GOOD VS POOR ROLE MODELING

Like all strategies of affiliating discussed in this report, modeling is mutually beneficial: the child who models behavior after a stepfather flatters the model. When the child begins to pattern behavior after that of a stepfather, it works to win over the stepfather. Biological identification is absent in step-relationships; social identification becomes paramount. In the present study, every stepfather who recounted some way in which the stepchild was "just like me," beamed as he said it. This concept of modeling is supported in the literature as well as data from fieldnotes. Maxwell (1979) stresses the importance of role models. Lynn writes about the importance of the father in sex role development:

> Still other experts emphasize the importance of a masculine model in the home, not only for the boy's sex-role development, but for the girl's as well. We have seen that the father can influence the feminine development of his daughter and serve as a model of what a man is (Lynn 1974:255).

I had the opportunity of observing several pre-teen girls interact with both biological and stepfathers as masculine role models. All of these girls used the same familiar young-girl-talking-to-daddy gestures: they cocked their heads, looked side-long, and pouted a little.

The poor role model sets an example that repulses the child. Field-notes record these children stressing the differences between their biological and stepfathers — often in the presence of the stepfather, "You're not my father!"

The child who does not pattern behavior after the stepfather seems like a stranger. Typical is the comment of one man who said that he likes his ten-year-old stepson, but that he didn't get along well with the six-year-old, "He's not like us — he doesn't fit in so well."

TEACHING SKILLS VS CLOSE SUPERVISION

Teaching was found to be a conscious effort to impart knowledge. The process of affiliation often began by the stepparent teaching something to the child. Data reveal that the stepfather who teaches the child something useful feels like a "good guy." Children who learned new skills enjoyed a feeling of mastery. Children in this study reciprocated by teaching stepfathers family history and customs. They let the man "in on" family jokes, showed him where the canned goods go, explained where the scar came from, and interpreted the language of a younger sibling.

Close supervision emerged in this study as a non-affiliating activity that involved the stepfather following a child about to see if assigned chores were done properly. Such supervision was found to make clear to the child the inequality of its position in comparison with the supervising stepfather. Several children said, "He doesn't think I can do anything right — I hate that." Gouldner (1964), in his classic study of a new manager in a factory, makes the point that the factory workers resented close supervision, and that the outcome was less work done. If one considers the stepfather as a new manager in the home, and compares that position with Gouldner's view, it would seem to be true that close supervision leads to non-affiliating.

COMING THROUGH VS FAILING

The affiliating property of coming through has to do with reliability; the stepfather can be counted on during times of stress to "come through" for the child. Mothers in the present study saw "coming through," as they named it, as particulary important. It meant to them that they had support during a crisis period. For example, the mother of a teenager said of her spouse, "in times of trouble, Greg was great. When Arthur was arrested for having an open bottle in the car, Greg was on the phone to his lawyer immediately." On the other hand, stepfathers who failed their stepchildren during a crisis, were the object of extremely disparaging evaluations by the mothers in this study, "who needs him?" was the point of view.

Coming through emerged as a strategy acknowledged by stepchildren concerning their stepfather, but one that did not necessarily increase their affection for the man. Typical was Erica, now grown, who said, "As much as I used to hate him sometimes, he was always there to help you out of a jam if you needed it. And I *did* need it."

LEVELING VS CONCEALING

Leveling is speaking the truth about what one feels, thinks, and wants. Leveling emerged as essential to a close, friendly relationship between stepfather and child; it also appeared to be the solid ground upon which discipline can be based. One stepfather spent time playing with his wife's two children, showing them new skills of ball playing and hill climbing, but after a day's work on the farm, he was sometimes to tired for such sport. His wife reported:

> The kids got mad, you know, because he wouldn't play with them, but he just told them all he had to do around the farm, and that he was tired. The next morning they were up early wanting to help him with the milking.

Concealing emerged as the opposing process to leveling. Data demonstrated that the stepfather who was honest in what he said was considered to be reliable in other areas. The stepfather who concealed his feelings, however, created social distance between himself and the child, and could not be trusted. Eleanor's stepfather practiced evasiveness in the area of affection:

> It was clear to me that he preferred his own children, but he would never admit it. That caused me a lot of trouble in life: I would have gotten along a lot better if only he had been open about his preferences.

While Eleanor's stepfather "would never admit" how he felt, he cut off conversation with her about this important aspect of their relationship. She could not then tell him how *she* felt. The outcome was disintegrative social distance: there was an area of their lives which they could not discuss, the vital area of how they felt about each other.

TRUSTING VS DOUBTING

Trusting although closely related to the strategy of leveling is discussed separately here because adults in stepfather homes often expected children to trust the new member on sight. When questioned, they revealed that although they themselves recognized a temporal quality in their ability to trust another adult, they had not anticipated the same time lapse in children. They expressed surprise at the shyness and evasiveness of stepchildren. Stepfathers who were doubted for too long a time often stopped making overtures to their stepchildren.

Stepfathers, it was revealed, often doubt their stepchildren: the child's word, his or her ability to perform tasks, and in some cases, the child's basic honesty. For example, it took Justin a year and a half to realize that he could count on his stepson to complete assigned duties. "Suddenly" he said, "I realized, hey, I can really count on Garth."

ACCEPTING VS REJECTING

A major finding that emerged from the field data was that abrupt, intensified attempts by the stepfather to change a child's behavior lead to disintegration of their relationship, at least for a time. On the other hand stepfathers who accepted the total child, including the undesirable behavior were less inclined to attempt rapid, radical changes of behavior in the child. Typical of the man who accepts the child in its own right was the stepfather who found his "hyperactive" stepson a "challenge" but not "impossible." "Heck," he said, "you just have to accept kids for what they are, that's all."

Acceptance of a stepfather is an important strategy for children in promoting stepfather-child affiliation. Some children and stepfathers interacted in such a way that mutual rejection was the outcome. Zane found his stepson Ollie very different from his own children. According to Ollie's mother, "Zane tried, but having been rejected, doesn't try anymore."

LIKING VS DISLIKING

Liking emerged as either initial or terminal, and proved to be both a property and an outcome of affiliating. When liking is both initial and mutual between stepfather and child, the pull toward affiliation is stronger. Although very few stepfather-families practiced all the affiliating strategies listed above, where a majority of these strategies were in operation, stepfather and child reported "liking" one another.

Some stepfathers and children never learned to like one another. As mentioned in the section on spending money, teenagers are particularly troublesome in this regard. According to the data this stems from the fact that stepfathers often see teenagers as out of control, and needing a "firmer hand." For their part, teenagers who enter a developmental period where they attempt to take control of their lives become distressed at the appearance of a new manager in the home who attempts to enforce not only old rules, but a new set of rules as well. Amy, a teenager when her mother married Mac, reacted to her stepfather's new rules by crying out, "Well, and who are *you*?"

IMPLICATIONS FOR
NURSING INTERVENTION

Affiliating provides strategies for improving the relationship between stepfather and child. The strategies used successfully by stepfathers and children in the present study can be taught to other men taking on the surrogate-father role. These men are often advised to become friends with their stepchildren, but they are not told how to accomplish this feat. The present study provides pragmatic suggestions for making friends with a stepchild. Stepchildren too might learn these strategies. Nurses working with troubled families can supply concrete learning experiences useful to the stepfather, mother, and child in establishing their family roles.

Classes teaching affiliating strategies could serve as enhancers to integration in stepfather families. Such classes would provide avenues for health maintenance, and would be aimed at the family not yet in desperate straits. Families in the present study were asked specifically about the usefulness of a "group" for stepfather families. While they were generally resistant to the idea of a therapy group, a class, especially one taught through the public school system or along the lines of a preparation for childbirth class (in this case a preparation for stepfathering class), had more appeal. Nurses, particularly those working in primary care settings, public health, and practitioner roles, are in a position to provide classes to the stepfather family struggling to integrate, but from whose point of view a therapist is out of the question, because as they described it, the persons in the stepfather family are not "mentally ill."[3]

FURTHER STUDIES

Processes similar to those described above may occur in stepmother families. A future study focusing on affiliating strategies operating in stepmother families would reveal this information.

Although the qualitative study reported here separates the various strategies of affiliating into fairly discrete categories, some of the categories are closely related. A future study involving the construction of a psychometric scale with items representing the various strategies could be field tested and factor-analyzed. In this way, some of the categories might be found to collapse into a few salient factors. Such a scale when properly developed for validity and reliability might be a useful assessment tool for stepfamilies.

NOTES

[1]The manuscript was prepared while the author held the position of Assistant Professor, School of Nursing, University of California, San Francisco. The author wishes to thank Holly Skodol Wilson, Associate Dean for Academic Programs,

University of California, San Francisco for her helpful suggestions in the preparation of the manuscript. Robert J. Maxwell and Milton Stern served as editors for this paper. This study was supported in part by HEW — PHS — HSMA, Maternal-Child Services Pre-doctoral Traineeship, Project 935. Preparation of the manuscript was supported in part by Faculty Development Grant #2-405231-09501, University of California, San Francisco.
[2]An opportunistic sample is a sample of convenience.
[3]Since the completion of this study, classes using the strategies described here have been implemented through the Stepfamily Foundation of California, Inc.

REFERENCES

Bohannan, P. J. (1975) Stepfathers and the Mental Health of Their Children. NIMH Final report, La Jolla, California. Western Behavioral Sciences Institute.

Bohannan, P. J. and R. Erickson (1978) Stepping In. Psychology Today. January:53 – 59.

Bowerman, C. E. and D. P. Irish (1962) Some Relationships of Stepchildren to Their Parents. Marriage and Family Living. 24:113 – 121.

Bozett, F. W. (1981) Gay Fathers: Identify Conflict Resolution Through Integrative Sanctioning. Alternative Life Styles, 4:90 – 107.

Corbin, J. (1980) The Process of Management of a Pregnancy Combined with a Chronic Illness. Communicating Nursing Research — 13th Annual Conference of the Western Society for Research in Nursing of the Western Council on Higher Education for Nursing, Los Angeles, April 30.

Duberman, L. (1973) Step-kin Relationships. Journal of Marriage and the Family. 35:283 – 292.

Fast, I. and A. C. Cain (1966) The Stepparent Role: Potential for Disturbances in Family Functioning. American Journal of Orthopsychiatry. 36:485 – 491.

Glaser, B. G. and A. L. Strauss (1967) The Discovery of Grounded Theory: Strategies for Qualitative Research. Chicago: Aldine.

Glaser, B. G. (1978) Theoretical Sensitivity. Mill Valley, California: Sociology Press.

Gouldner, A. W. (1964) Patterns of Industrial Bureaucracy. New York: Free Press.

Haley, J. (1976) Problem Solving Therapy. San Francisco: Jossey-Bass.

Macklin, E. D. (1980) Nontraditional Family Forms: A Decade of Research. Journal of Marriage and the Family. 42:905 – 922.

Maddox, B. (1975) The Half-Parent. New York: M. Evans.

Lynn, David, B. (1974) The Father: His Role in Child Development. Monterey, California:Brooks/Cole.

Maxwell, E. K. (1979) Modeling Life: A Qualitative Analysis of the Dynamic Relationship Between Elderly Models and Their Proteges. San Francisco: University of California, unpublished doctoral dissertation.

Messinger, L. (1976) Remarriage Between Divorced People With Children From Previous Marriages: A Proposal for Preparation for Remarriage. Journal of Marriage and Family Counseling. 2:193 – 200.

Mowatt, M. H. (1972) Group Psychotherapy for Stepfathers and Their Wives. Psychotherapy: Theory, Research and Practice. Winter, 9:328 – 331.

Population Reference Bureau (1977) New York Times. November 27.

Roosevelt, R. and J. Lofas (1977) Living in Step. New York: Stein and Day.

Simon, A. W. (1964) Stepchild in the Family. New York: The Odyssey Press.

Stern, P. N. (1977a) Integrative Discipline in Stepfather Families (Doctoral dissertation, University of California San Francisco, 1976). Dissertation Abstracts International, University Microfilms No. 77-5276. b. 37.

1977b Stepfather Families: Integration Around Child Discipline. Paper presented to the

First Regional Congress of Social Psychiatry, Santa Barbara, California, September 7. Abstract available through the author

1980 Grounded Theory Methodology: Its Uses and Processes. Image. 12:20–23.

Stern, P. N.; Tildine, V. P. and E. K. Maxwell (1980) Culturally Induced Stress During Childbearing: The Pilipino-American Experience. Issues in the Health Care of Women. 2:129–143.

Visher, E. G. and J. S. Visher (1978) Major Areas of Difficulty for Stepparent Couples. International Journal of Family Counseling. 6:70–80.

1979 Stepfamilies: A Guide to Working with Stepparents and Stepchildren. New York: Brunner Mazel.

Wilson, H. S. (1977) Limiting Intrusion — Social Control of Outsiders in a Healing Community. Nursing Research. 26:103–110.

Wilson, K. L.; Zucher, L.; McAdams, D. C. and R. L. Curtis (1975) Stepfathers and Stepchildren: An Exploratory Analysis from Two National Surveys. Journal of Marriage and the Family. 37:526–536.

COMMENTARY

Stern's qualitative study makes an important contribution to family nursing theory development by expanding knowledge of stepfamilies. The family members of particular interest are the stepfather and the mother's children. Although Stern intended to interview whole families as units, she was able to realize her intent in only 8 of the 30 families included in the study because of "family resistance." Thus, the theory generated is appropriately classified as family-related.

Stern does not identify the underlying assumptions or conceptual model for her work. She does, however, note that the study was based on Grounded Theory Methodology. Proponents of Grounded Theory correctly claim that this research approach fosters non-theory-laden observations of phenomena that do not depend on *a priori* dimensions or categories or concepts. The aim of Grounded Theory, however, is as Stern points out, to identify social processes. And the focus on social processes implies certain assumptions about human life and behavior that reflect a particular conceptual perspective.

An outcome of Grounded Theory Methodology is generation of middle-range theories. As can be seen in the diagram, the middle-range theory discovered in this study is made up of the concept of affiliation and its categories. The categories encompass 10 strategies used by stepfathers and their stepchildren as they establish a relationship. Stern discovered that affiliation is a bi-polar concept with the dimensions of friendship or estrangement, and that each category also is bi-polar. She also discovered that the stepfather-child relationship required 1½ to 2 years to establish.

JACQUELINE FAWCETT

HEALTHY FAMILIES

11

The Family as a Unit of Analysis: Strategies for the Nurse Researcher

CATHERINE L. GILLISS

As interest in the family as a unit of health behavior and health service grows among nurses, nurse researchers are confronted with the complexities that impede family research. Despite the variety of approaches taken over the last 30 years, the literature on family research techniques repeatedly emphasizes the inadequacies of approaches and their lack of relatedness to a theoretical or conceptual framework.[1-3]

The appropriateness of research procedures in nursing is itself a controversial issue, and the study of the family is further complicated by difficulties of measuring the aggregate and its component parts. Examined here is the complexity of family evaluation through

- examination of the nature of the phenomenon;
- review and critique of the approaches that have been used to study the family; and
- identification of strategies appropriate to the nature of nursing research.

This work was supported in part by the Health Resources Administration, National Research Service Award 1F31-NU-05498-01, from the Division of Nursing.

Reprinted from *Advances in Nursing Science,* 5(3), 50–59, 1983.

NATURE OF THE FAMILY

The family has been described as a complex unit with unique attributes of its own but containing component parts that are significant as individual units, both independently and collectively. It is believed by many that the family is greater than (or different from) the sum of its parts. Consequently, there is lack of consensus about *what* should be evaluated and *how* selected methods might access the data that make the family unit more than the sum of its parts. Such concern is relatively new within nursing research; therefore, the development of thought in sociology and psychology serves as a basis for much of this discussion.

Literature

In an attempt to organize the measurable qualities of the family, numerous authors have proposed borrowing frameworks from other substantive areas to apply to family research. It has been suggested that the work of Argyris[4] on interpersonal competence might be useful in evaluating families. Cattell's[5] approach to the measurement of small group properties has also been used. It is based on

- population variables (measures of individuals within groups);
- structural variables (observed measures that illuminate processes and procedures); and
- true "syntality" (measures of the performance of the group as a whole).

Lazarsfeld and Menzel[6] suggest a parallel approach to the measurement of complex organizations. They propose that a *collective* (a unit comprised of individuals) has analytic, structural, and global properties. Its individual members have four types of properties:

1. absolute, which come from the individual and serve to describe him or her;
2. relational, which arise from information on the substantive relations between members;
3. comparative, which compare one member to another; and
4. contextual, which describe a member according to the qualities of his or her collective.

Straus[7] further develops the notion of analytical, structural, and global indicators as they relate to families. Analytical indicators are measures of characteristics of the individuals who comprise the family unit. In some cases these may be represented by summary scales or measures of central tendency (e.g., individual symptoms, age, religious interest, or alcohol consumption). Structural indicators are those that provide information about the relatedness of family members to one another and the interaction of the member individuals with one another. As described by

Straus, these are the most process-oriented of the indicators. They permit a view of function and interdependence. Self-reports and self-observation are appropriate techniques for studying these indicators. It is assumed that unit, dyadic, and triadic measures might be taken; the selection of one is dependent on the theoretical approach to the family and the research question. Finally, global indicators represent a category of static measures, somewhat apart from process. These are collective products that describe the unit, such as income, amount of money spent on health care, and socioeconomic status.

In view of these contributions, there is a need to constantly review which aspect of the family has been measured. Was it a collective property of individuals or a property of the unit? Most important, was it identified as such?

Theoretical Approach

It is the selection of a theoretical approach, or a philosophy about the family, that governs what is looked for and seen in the study of the family. A theoretical approach relevant to health care must permit viewing the dynamic individual, the dynamic unit, and their interrelatedness. The interaction approach, expanded through the use of systems theory, permits such a view of the dynamic family unit. In the terminology offered by Lazarsfeld and Menzel[6] and Straus[7] this combination of frameworks permits study of the analytical, structural, and global indicators.

The research questions developed for the study of the family are influenced by the theoretical framework used, as are the procedures of data collection. The striking diversity of approaches taken to family research is well summarized by Olson[8] and Lytton.[9] Some study mother–child interaction and describe it as family research, whereas others view the triadic unit in problem-solving activity and describe it as family research.

Hoffman and Lippitt[10] propose 11 causal-sequence schematic approaches for research relating family life to child behavior and development (see boxed material). Each of these approaches constitutes the focus of family research as it is collectively referred to in the literature.

The interaction framework has been used by early family researchers in psychiatry to focus on whether

- a family with abnormal members was different from other families;
- a family with one type of abnormal member was different from one with another type of abnormal member;
- one part of a family was different from another part; and
- a family changed into a different system following individual or family treatment.[1]

This framework has been used to focus on the character of individual

---

Approaches for Study of Family

1. Parental background
2. Current setting
3. Family composition
4. Relationship between parents
5. Character of the individuals who parent
6. Child-oriented parental attitudes
7. Overt parental behaviors
8. Child's orientation toward parents and siblings
9. Overt child behaviors toward other family members
10. Personal character of child
11. Behavior of child away from parents

---

members, the family structure (role fulfillment), patterns of interaction (including verbal and nonverbal communication), and the family as a working group.[1,3]

Although these family research foci are compatible with an interaction framework, the blending of principles from systems theory into that framework demands that the family unit assumes an essential focus in family research. The primary advantage of the recombination is the improved ability to relate individual to family behaviors and family to individual behaviors. This unit is fundamental to health care delivery and to the design of family research.

METHOD OF FAMILY STUDY

Critical overviews of family research methods are plentiful.[1-3,8,9] Each discussion presents much valuable information, and each is unique in its organization of methods. This analysis approaches the body of literature on research strategies from five methodological categories: (1) epidemiological, (2) self-report, (3) observational, (4) psychodiagnostic, and (5) treatment outcomes.

Despite differences that family researchers may have with respect to methodology, they agree on one issue. The selection of a method and related strategies is governed by the researcher's interest in maximizing the validity and reliability of the data. Variation appears as a function of beliefs about the factors that have the greatest impact on validity and reliability. Therefore, critique of these strategies will be focused accordingly.

Epidemiological Studies

Epidemiological studies of family generally provide analytical and global indicators of health. They have tended to use the individual members of a family as sources for data about other members and about the whole family as a collective. Health records, birth and death certificates, and hospital and clinic utilization rates have all provided data. Some investigators claim that their studies have yielded much valuable data; others are less enthusiastic. Muller et al[11] and Mechanic[12] identify the major failure of their studies as lack of reliability. Most often the strategies for data collection (records, telephone, interview, and health survey) involve only one heavily biased source. Although the health of all members may be the subject of inquiry, the mother is frequently the source of all the data. Schless and Mendels[13] have demonstrated that interviewing additional informants provides significantly more data.

Self-reports

As an approach to family study, self-report methods take several forms and are often used in combination with other methods. Health diaries have been used in an effort to access a wide range of everyday events. Roghmann and Haggerty[14] reported success with the technique because it provided them with specific details not accessible through retrospective interview. They suggest that the diary, or health calendar, is more reliable for everyday events than for serious family crises. This approach may reduce bias related to social desirability; however, the use of a singular informant for the entire family's symptoms and related health behavior represents an obvious threat to the construct in question. The *sum* of the family's health behavior appears to be more accurately reported by the sum of the family's individuals. Verbrugge[15] also points out the high costs to researcher and informant that are inherent in the diary strategy.

Other written approaches (questionnaires) have similar flaws. Lewis's Whole Family Questionnaire[16] and Moos's Family Environment Scale (FES)[17] are examples of widely used research instruments that conceptually emphasize the need for a *unit* measure and then seek data from each separate individual. Lewis makes little provision for summing or otherwise relating the scores, but the Moos FES allows calculation of a Family Incongruence score. Structured formats do, however, limit the respondent's ability to give the most accurate answer to the question asked. This is true of other written tools, such as those developed by Olson et al[18] and McCubbin and Patterson.[19]

Self-report, through the strategy of interviews, takes a variety of forms. An individual may provide personal data, perspectives on others, or perspectives on the family unit. A Rashoman technique, in which the perspectives of several individuals are compared and contrasted may be useful. Family units may be interviewed. Indepth interviews and family histories have been used successfully in conjunction with other strategies by numerous researchers.[20-27] The major threat associated with this technique is bias from both the informant and the coder. Mothers of schizophrenic children reveal their *own* reality when they provide a history of the child. The data are rich but must be recognized for their phenomeno-logical value. They tell the story of the informant. Too often they are generalized to the other members in a family. The threat to construct validity occurs when the data are interpreted as representing things that they do not actually represent. Coder bias is inherent because the re-searcher is constantly interpreting and reinterpreting the informant's data through a personal perceptual screen, most notably the investigator's feelings and thoughts about his or her own family.

Observation

Observation of families has taken several forms. Studies have used natu-ralistic settings and laboratory settings, and observers have been partici-pants and nonparticipants.

The naturalistic participant observers have provided extraordinarily rich data resulting in the development of frameworks for viewing families in various contexts. The method used by Hansen[20] and Henry[27] involved moving in (or spending approximately 10 hours a day) with a family for about 1 week. The observer joined in family events, accompanying others on shopping trips, visits to the doctor with children, and recreational trips. In-depth interviewing of all members continued throughout the week. Events and dialogue were recorded by the researcher.

Although Lewis[25] advocated the living-in method for providing ac-tion to structure and access to meanings, several threats to validity must be acknowledged. The distorting effects of observer presence were ad-dressed by Henry.[21] He believed that distortions were minimized because of the stability of family interaction patterns over time and the strain imposed by guarding against usual behaviors. Hansen[20] reported that after 3 days of being observed, the family relaxed, but she believed that each family tried to get along better than they would have if she were not there. The time and energy costs for this strategy are vast. Henry wrote that he had a high tolerance for living in and was generally able to control his angry reactions to family members. On the other hand, Hansen can-didly described the somatic symptoms she developed while she was living in.

Stack[26] and Howell[23] moved in. Their periods of data collection were a year and longer; the time was spent living in the communities and being involved in the daily lives of their informants. The intensity of their personal experiences may not have been of the same magnitude as for those who did not move in, but the ability to maintain objectivity over time must be questioned. The conflict between simultaneously being an insider and an outsider is recognized by anthropologists as a threat to first-rate field work.[28] The generalizability of these studies is limited; however, the studies are fundamental to theory building. From these qualitative works emerge the theoretical formulations that can later be confirmed through experimentation.

Researcher participation in a laboratory setting is uncommon; however, the work of Steinglass et al[29] falls into this category. In his work with alcoholics, he created some novel laboratory experiments. By conjointly hospitalizing couples and family members and permitting them to become intoxicated, he gained insight into the relationship between drinking behavior and family interaction. Watzlawick's Structured Family Interview[30] similarly allows for controlled observation of proverb interpretation and problem solving.

Other laboratory techniques have focused on nonparticipant observation in gaming or contrived situations and natural situations. Haley[31] pointed out that in contrast to experiments with individuals in which the interpersonal factor is *controlled*, family experiments seek to *measure* that interpersonal factor.

Among the more natural situations is the "plan something together" technique used by a variety of researchers.[30,32] Through a one-way mirror, family members are observed and evaluated for their patterns of interaction. Strodtbeck's revealed differences technique is a similar attempt to create a situation that requires the family to negotiate a resolution.[33]

Other laboratory techniques have been used to induce decision making, problem solving, and conflict resolution. Haley's Push Button Test[34] requires that a series of coalitions be formed with different family members. This highlights cooperation–competition themes in families. The Simulated Family Activity Measurement (M. Straus, I. Tallman, unpublished data, 1966) is a similar game that requires the family to *discover* the rules as they play.

These strategies need to be critiqued from two aspects — (1) the situation created and its approximation of a real-life situation and (2) the reliability of the coding or interpretation of the data.

The chief issue in relation to these efforts is whether they have any bearing on out-of-laboratory experience. Are they reliable indicators of real-life interaction? O'Rourke[35] demonstrated differences in similar tasks between performance at home and performance in the laboratory. Haley[31] echoed this finding when he cautioned that experimental behavior cannot be separated from the context in which it occurred. Zelditch,[36] however, has written that the purpose of experimentation is building and testing theory, which is abstract. He contends that experiments are relevant to theory and that theory is *applied* to natural settings. If one quantity resulted from an experiment and another from the natural setting, the role of theory would be to bridge the gap; the results need not be identical.

The second concern, the coding of data, is a major shortcoming that impacts on much of family research. It is a particular threat to reliability with respect to laboratory experiments. Bales' Interaction Process Analysis (IPA)[37] has been widely used with families. Waxler and Mishler[38] reported, however, that the IPA category system has actually been used in a variety of ways on various types of data. Pointing out that reliability coefficients were frequently not reported, they contended that this was secondary to low interrater reliability scores, which they acknowledged in their own research. Recent attempts to computerize the coding process may hold hope for the future. But the problem still remains: Someone must make an interpretation to rate the interaction.

Psychodiagnostics

Psychodiagnostic techniques have been used by researchers who are interested in the relatedness of personalities within the family.[22,25] Interpretation is again a concern. Projective techniques such as the Thematic Apperception Test and the Rorschach test permit a researcher to interpret data in isolation from a context. When used properly, they are interpreted by another investigator and serve as a check on the observations of the researcher.[39] Used without another technique, such as extensive interview, they make little contribution.

Family Therapy Outcomes

Finally, there are the outcomes of family therapy to evaluate. Although DeWitt[40] has indicated that conjoint family treatment is effective, treatment as a research strategy presents numerous threats to internal validity. Generally, there are no comparison groups available; there is little attempt made to adjust for extraneous variables. The threats presented by selection, history, or maturation are seldom considered. There is need for a family taxonomy that would aid researchers in beginning to make valid comparisons between and generalizations to families.

NURSING RESEARCH AND THE FAMILY

Nursing, as part of its involvement in promoting health, has become concerned with the impact of the health of individuals on the family unit and, conversely, the impact of the unit on the health of individuals. There is developing interest in the family as a context for individual health behavior and as a unit of health and illness.

When the family is treated as context to a research question, the collection of data may be validly undertaken with an individual client referent. In such cases, the client's perception of the family may be what is sought. This is exemplified by the work of Karlson,[41] who is attempting to relate the personal well-being and autonomy of adult children to the increasing dependency of their aging parents. The children are data sources in this study.

To a limited degree, family process can be studied by data provided by an individual family member. In ongoing work by Lobo,[42] the mother/ wife is asked to report the daily well-being of each family member and of the family unit. Using a multiple regression and correlation technique, Lobo is demonstrating which individual member's well-being was the greatest contributor to family well-being. This study has shown that questions can be asked about the family unit when access is limited to a single family member.

It is also possible to use the family unit as a source of data, yet learn little of the family's process. For several years, I have been concerned with the measurement of subjective stress in the family unit, using a minimum of two adult members from each family as data sources.[43] When the mean stress scores of individual family members were compared to a family unit score, which the family group reported, no differences were found. Dobbins[44] has essentially replicated this work with similar results. Yet the result of these studies is ambiguous. Is there no difference between the sum of individuals and the group? Or does the instrumentation fail to capture the aspect of the family that is greater than the sum of its parts? Observation of the family process for data collection activities might have clarified these findings.

Nursing research questions that address the family *unit* need to be conceptually, procedurally, and *analytically* appropriate to the aggregate. Data-analytic techniques must consider the highly correlated measures taken from family members; husbands and wives should not be treated as statistically independent samples. The researcher must carefully consider whether family data meet the assumptions of the selected techniques. Novel approaches to analysis should be encouraged.

Clinical nursing skills are an important resource to the nurse researcher studying the family. The nurse's level of skill development and knowledge about the family influences what can be observed or elicited. Observation of the family group is a complex skill. Attending to the global properties of the family group requires an ability to listen to the words spoken by family members, as well as an ability to simultaneously observe interactions. For example, the researcher who is invited to join the family for dinner not only listens to what is said but watches for the rules of the family as they are revealed. As the family tells its history and discusses its hopes, the researcher attends to the unit's definition of health and methods for achieving a level of health.

The nurse researcher who studies the family is subject to great bias in observations and interpretations. Therefore, some safeguard for that bias is necessary. This may be done through validation of findings with others through videotape or audiotape analysis. Alternately, multiple methods of data collection may be used to converge on similar findings; e.g., a clinical assessment of family functioning and a paper-and-pencil measure, such as FES by Moos[17] or Family Adaptability and Cohesion Evaluation Skill by Olson et al.[18]

Families are best studied over a period of time because the interesting questions are related to their health over time. More time series and longitudinal designs must be used to make interpretations regarding familial response to events.

Finally, these suggestions will result in a costly research undertaking. Therefore, it is recommended that family researchers explore creative methods for accessing samples and consolidating research with other activities. The point has been made that clinical practice skills are effectively used in data collection. Why, then, do we not conduct clinical experiments within our practices or while we are teaching practice skills to students? Perhaps, too, there are available subjects under the care of a nurse or physician colleague who might also serve as research collaborators.

• • •

Endless strategies have been developed for and used in family research studies. Despite the collection of creative strategies and the ever-increasing numbers of well-organized summaries of them, family research remains flawed. Attention must be paid to the logical consistencies among what is measured, about whom, from whom, and for what purpose. The theoretical framework must be congruent with the variables selected for study and the procedures used to source the data. Finally, techniques that are selected for data analysis must be reviewed for their theoretical consistency with family research.

REFERENCES

1. Haley J: Critical overview of the present status of family interaction research, in Framo J (ed): *Family Interaction*. New York, Springer, 1972.
2. Litman T, Venters M: Research on health care and the family: A methodological overview. *Soc Sci Med* 1979; 13A:379–385.
3. Riskin J, Faunce E: An evaluative review of family interaction research. *Fam Process* 1972; 11:365–456.
4. Argyris C: Explorations in interpersonal competence, I. *J Appl Behav Sci* 1965; 1:58–83.
5. Cattell R: New concepts for measuring leadership in terms of group syntality, in Cartwright D, Zander A (eds): *Group Dynamics*. Evanston, Ill, Row, Peterson & Co, 1953.
6. Lazarsfeld P, Menzel H: On the relation between individuals and collective properties, in Etzioni A (ed): *A Sociological Reader on Complex Organizations*. New York, Holt, Rinehart & Winston, 1969, pp 499–516.
7. Straus M: Measuring families, in Christensen H (ed): *Handbook of Marriage and the Family*. Chicago, Rand McNally, 1964, pp 335–402.
8. Olson D (ed): *Treating Relationships*. Iowa, Graphic Publishing, 1976.
9. Lytton H: Observation studies of parent-child interaction: A methodological review. *Child Dev* 1971; 42:651–684.
10. Hoffman L, Lippitt R: Measurement of family life variables, in Mussen (ed): *Handbook of Research Methods in Child Development*. New York, Wiley, 1960, pp 945–1014.

11. Muller C, Waybur A, Weinerman E: Methodology of a family health study. *Pub Health Rep* 1952; 67:1149.
12. Mechanic D: Influence of mothers on their children's health attitudes and behaviors. *Pediatrics* 1964; 33:445.
13. Schless A, Mendels J: The value of interviewing family and friends in assessing life stressors. *Arch Gen Psychiatry* 1978; 35:565–567.
14. Roghmann K, Haggerty R: The diary as a research instrument in the study of health and illness behavior. *Med Care* 1972; 10:143.
15. Verbrugge L: Health diaries. *Med Care* 1980; 18:73–95.
16. Lewis J: *How's Your Family?* New York, Brunner/ Mazel, 1979.
17. Moos R: *Family Environment Scale.* Palo Alto, Calif, Consulting Psychologists Press Inc, 1974.
18. Olson D, Bill R, Portner J: *FACES.* St Paul, University of Minnesota, 1978.
19. McCubbin H, Patterson J: *Systematic Assessment of Family Stress, Resources and Coping.* St Paul, University of Minnesota, 1981.
20. Hansen C: Living-in with normal families. *Fam Process* 1981; 20:53–75.
21. Henry J: My life with the families of psychotic children, in Handel G (ed): *The Psychological Interior of the Family.* Chicago, Aldine, 1967, pp 30–46.
22. Hess R, Handel G: *Family Worlds.* Chicago, University of Chicago Press, 1959.
23. Howell J: *Hard Living on Clay Street.* New York, Anchor Books, 1973.
24. Lewin E: Lesbianism and motherhood. *Human Organization* 1981; 40:614.
25. Lewis O: An anthropological approach to family studies. *Am J Sociol* 1950; 55:468–475.
26. Stack C: *All Our Kin.* New York, Harper, 1974.
27. Henry J: *Pathways to Madness.* New York, Vintage Books, 1973.
28. Ablon J: Field methods in working with middle class Americans: New issues of values, personality and reciprocity. *Human Organization* 1977; 36:69–72.
29. Steinglass P, Davis D, Berenson D: Observation of conjointly hospitalized alcoholic couples during sobriety and intoxication: Implications for theory and therapy. *J Fam Process* 1977; 16:116.
30. Watzlawick P: The structured family interview. *Fam Process* 1966; (2):256–271.
31. Haley J: Family experiments: A new type of experimentation. *Fam Process* 1962; 2:265–293.
32. Lewis J, Beavers W, Gossett J, et al: *No Single Thread: Psychological Health in Family Systems.* New York, Brunner/Mazel, 1976.
33. Strodtbeck F: Husband-wife interaction over revealed differences. *Amer Sociol Rev* 1951; 16:468–473.
34. Haley J: Experiment with abnormal families. *Arch Gen Psychiatry* 1967; 17:53–63.
35. O'Rourke J: Field and laboratory: A study of family groups in two experimental cultures. *Sociometry* 1963; 27:422–435.
36. Zelditch M: Can you really study an army in the laboratory? in Etzioni A (ed): *Complex Organizations.* New York, Holt, Rinehart, 1969, pp 528–539.
37. Bales R: *Interaction Process Analysis.* Reading, Mass, Addison-Wesley, 1950.
38. Waxler G, Mishler G: Scoring and reliability problems in Interaction Process Analysis: A methodological note. *Sociometry* 1966; 29:28–46.
39. Mench I, Henry J: Direct observation and psychological tests in anthropological field work. *Am J Anthropol* 1953; 55:461–480.
40. DeWitt K: The effectiveness of family therapy: A review of outcome research. *Arch Gen Psychiatry* 1978; 35:549–561.
41. Karlson S: A longitudinal study of social support, personal autonomy, and the well-being of adult family-member care-givers of aging parents. Read before the Fifth Annual Robert Wood Johnson Nurse Faculty Fellowship Symposium, Nashville, Tenn, April 1982.
42. Lobo M: Influence of mother on family health reports. Read before the 15th Annual Communication Nursing Research Conference, Denver, Colo, May 1982.
43. Gilliss C: The impact of event scale: Measuring subjective stress in families. Read before the Fourth Annual Robert Wood Johnson Nurse Faculty Fellowship Symposium, Nashville, Tenn, May 1981.
44. Dobbins E: Impact of event scale: Constructing a measure of subjective stress in families. Read before the Fifth Annual Robert Wood Johnson Nurse Faculty Fellowhip Symposium, Nashville, Tenn, April 1982.

COMMENTARY

Gilliss focuses on the family as a unit, both a unit of care/service and a single unit/variable of interest in research. The family unit is viewed as a system that is qualitatively different from the sum of its parts. Of interest, then, is the measurement of the whole rather than of the parts.

Gilliss offers alternatives and possibilities for the measurement of the family as a whole unit using various conceptual frameworks from disciplines other than nursing. She also identifies techniques that represent attempts to sample the whole family unit and the drawbacks of the techniques. Gilliss correctly points out that the congruence of the family "unit" measure with the overall study conceptualization and design is crucial.

Gilliss's paper represents a seminal effort that identifies methodological issues in the measurement of the family as a unit. As such, the paper has a secure place in the family theory development literature in nursing. Although the issues raised by Gilliss have not yet been resolved, the paper has facilitated ongoing discussion that is advancing family theory development in nursing.

ANN L. WHALL

12

Family Well-Being

SUSAN BLANCH MEISTER

The family, as a set of real human beings interacting with one another, transcends any model.

Abraham Kaplan

Conduct of Inquiry (New York: Chandler, 1964).

Family well-being is a construct that offers particular value and pertinence to nursing practice, theory, and research. Family well-being is a function of the fit between demands and resources, and dysfunctional fits are associated with decreased well-being and sometimes even violence. Currently, the empirical knowledge to define and measure family well-being is lacking. However, research in contributing disciplines substantiates the viability and importance of the concept. A representative subset of this research is presented in this chapter to describe "the family" as a convoy of relationships which is affected by the needs and abilities of its members, and contributes to defining and meeting both aggregate and individual needs. Results of extensive research in the well-being of individuals are also presented. The chapter closes with issues in family well-being which are pertinent to nursing care of violent families.

Reprinted from J. Campbell & J. Humphreys (Eds.), *Nursing care of victims of family violence* (pp. 53–73). Reston, VA: Reston Publishing Company, 1984.

209

THE CONCEPT OF FAMILY WELL-BEING

Family well-being is a hybrid concept. "Family" has been the subject of decades of research and theory building, while "well-being" has a shorter history in scientific study. Traditional frameworks for describing families have used significantly different definitions of and perspectives on the family. For example, the developmental framework defines the family as an aggregate and studies the developmental issues that confront that aggregate: establishing a home, negotiating school entry of the oldest child, managing the changes caused by the departure of the youngest child from the home. On the other hand, the structure-function framework emphasizes the organization of the family and studies the family functions that are achieved and ascribed: reproduction of the species, socialization of children, provision of adequate living environments. The roles framework emphasizes roles that are associated with each position in the family and describes how those roles are defined, enacted, and changed: establishment of spouse roles, enlargement of spouse role complexes to include parenting, and adjustments of parenting roles in response to development of the children. The interactionist framework focuses on the communication patterns within the family and describes short- and long-term effects of various patterns: effect of open communicative styles in young children and later impacts when those children are adolescents, effects of ritualized and rigid communicative styles in similar time periods. Systems frameworks emphasize systems within and beyond the family, and describe the mutual effects of those systems: family purchasing patterns and the larger economy, educational requirements and costs, and childbearing choices by families.

Each of these distinct frameworks in family studies offer unique information about families. However, the very nature of a framework requires assumptions about the subject. In this instance each family framework applies assumptions about the nature and composition of the family. These assumptions are valuable assets in scientific study, but those same assumptions may not apply to all families in our current society or violent families in particular. More to the point, the assumptions may define "family" in ways that are irrelevant, wrong, or too narrow for application to nursing practice with families. For example, how well does the developmental framework fit the family with adult children returning to the home? Can structure-function theory be applied to the voluntarily childless family? Does role theory apply to single parent families? Could the interactionist principles be applied to families with two employed parents who are working separate shifts? Would systems theory contribute to understanding the needs of the "reformulated" family with two previously divorced parents? Any one of these families might experience difficulties that result in contact with nursing; any one of these families might experience violence. Practice would be hindered by a scientific base that does not address the type of family in which the problems occur.

If the broad range of current family types is to be captured in the science that supports practice, then new family frameworks are necessary. These frameworks would be shallow if they did not incorporate the wisdom and findings of more traditional approaches, but more comprehensive and flexible concepts are needed as well.

"Well-being" is a comprehensive and flexible concept of a variable commodity that is larger in scope than "health." If you ask someone, "How do you feel about your life as a whole?" you are asking them to evaluate their degree of well-being. Because this concept emphasizes strengths and resources as well as problems and needs, it is congruent with the perspective of nursing.

Well-being has both objective and perceived dimensions, that is, comparative (objective) and subjective (perceived) indexes of current status. The two dimensions do not necessarily match. For example, an aging grandmother may simultaneously think that she is fortunate to be living in her family's home (objective sense of well-being), and feel that she has been cruelly stripped of a meaningful, productive adult role (perceived well-being). The concept of well-being can be applied to families as well. For example, consider a family that has a relatively stable economic status while also experiencing tremendous daily stress in meeting demands for heat, food, and other necessities. The objective well-being of this family is more positive than the perceived well-being.

Several characteristics of the interactions between the family and its members make family well-being especially relevant to the discussion of family violence. First, although the family comprises a most intense and enduring segment of each member's environment, the members also comprise vital components of the family's environment. The members affect the nature of demands on and resources for the family, and vice versa. Second, because both the family and its members experience ongoing development, they have concurrent changes in needs and abilities.

Ongoing development of the family member is a more familiar concept: the member grows and changes with help, and hindrance, from the family. This chapter emphasizes the family's perspective as well: a family faces old and new demands, and it sometimes finds new resources for meeting those demands. When the family does well in achieving resource/demand fit, then it has a greater capacity to contribute to the members — who are also juggling personal resources and demands. Similarly, members achieving functional degrees of fit have greater capacities to contribute to family-level resources.

If the family is not able to "fit" resources to demands, then the family is less able to contribute to the efforts of its members as they face individual requirements to "fit" resources and demands. Over time, members who are struggling to meet demands become less able to contribute to the family's processes of coping with demands. A wealth of data associates poor fit with illness, and these findings apply to families as well as to family members. It is the *dysfunctional fit of resources and demands* that bears directly upon family violence.

The victim of family violence is an especially acute example of recurrent cycles of poor fit. The breadth of content in this volume speaks to the complexity of the problems, and solutions, associated with such cycles. This chapter addresses family well-being as a basic component of those problems and solutions. Because there has been little direct study of family well-being, the discussion draws upon a range of theory and research in social networks, family functioning, social support, life span development, and person-environment fit. These concepts are central to understanding and responding to family violence, as it has already been established that violence and aggression have both social and environmental components — and the family produces an intimate relationship between those components.[1] The work reviewed here defines a context from which the concept of family well-being may be derived, and issues in disruption of family well-being may be defined. Most important, the work reviewed here comprises a baseline from which nursing may prepare to assist the victim of family violence.

FAMILY AS A CONVOY OF RELATIONSHIPS

The Convoy

Although there are differences, the constructs of family and social network have a number of commonalities. Social network is the more general construct, and refers to a constellation of cohesive and regularly activated bonds.[2] In other words, social networks are actually aggregates of social bonds. Family, therefore, is a specific form of social network and defined by particular types of bonds. A great deal of research has been designed to identify which bonds define the family network and the answer seems to be "it depends on who you ask." For example, a study of entire families demonstrated significant interindividual differences and intraindividual stability in perceived family networks.[3] Although the network of one subject was notably different from the network of another subject, each study subject was relatively consistent in defining his or her own network. One family in the study illustrates this pattern particularly well: the father consistently included his adult children and their spouses in his perceived network, the mother included the adult children and her daughters' husbands, and only the youngest adult child and his spouse included both parents in their networks. Given the importance and var-

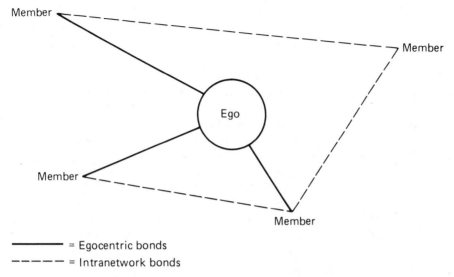

Figure 1.   Egocentric versus Intranetwork Bonds

iance of individual perception in defining family networks, this chapter examines the literature on the general construct of social network as the background against which an individual situation may be considered.

The issue here is egocentric social networks, where the social bonds all include "Ego," or the person defining the network (Figure 1). It may also be important to know which of the network members share bonds, but that level of network connectedness differs from the egocentric level and is not the focus of this chapter. Rather, the discussion focuses on the bonds that include the person and define a perceived, person-specific network.

Egocentric social networks are important because they are enduring, indigenous, and nonrandom. The network accompanies the person throughout the life span, and there are changes in the quantity, quality, and nature of individual bonds. R. L. Kahn and T. Antonucci noted this enduring quality of social networks and proposed the "convoy" as the construct for social networks viewed as part of life experience.[4] The network evolves around the person, and its particular nature is a reflection of that interaction. In other words, the egocentric network is indigenous and person-specific. The membership of a particular network is certainly not random. For example, emotional bonds are a foundation of family networks and the perceived membership in affective networks varies sharply from what stereotypical and sanguinal traditions would predict: mothers are not always included; children are not equally close; and spouses are not always important in perceived affective networks.[5]

The family has been identified as a special case of social networks. A number of potent variables are associated with this special social network, the family. For example, the family develops a paradigm, or framework, of shared assumptions, constructs, fantasies, and expectations about the world. This paradigm provides a central organizing force for the family.[6] Stress disrupts the texture of family life and challenges the substance of the family paradigm. When families are dysfunctional in response to stress, the dysfunctional behavior does not reflect the full potential of the family; it simply constitutes the behaviors which are most available at that moment in time. Although dysfunctional behavior may be destructive or even violent, it is essential to recognize that there are likely to be other responses which the family can utilize with assistance.[7]

The family has a set of vulnerabilities which alter the effects of stress. Both family organization at the point of stress and the nature of the larger social environment have major impacts on the manner in which the stressor is perceived. More important, family organization and the environment may either threaten or support the family paradigm, which in turn has a major impact upon the types of responses available to the family.[8] This cycle of effects is apparent in violent families; violence stresses the family, and the family often responds to stress with violence.

Even a family with a well-developed organization and a helpful environment is affected by change, and the effects of normative family life changes are especially pertinent to the convoy construct. As the years pass, each member experiences a unique trajectory of life span development and these changes present new issues to the family. Normative changes are associated with developmental patterns, and members' developmental milestones introduce gains and losses for the family. The birth of the first grandchild, the youngest child's school entry, the employment and apartment living of an adult child are each examples of normative changes that produce loss to the family. Precipitous loss of members has a major impact on the family, but even normative loss is a powerful variable in family stress.[9]

Society is also changing as the years pass. Social changes are pervasive and in recent years they have altered the ideology regarding families. B. Laslett describes the expectations of families as an overwhelming burden.[10] She emphasizes the psychological importance of the family as an attribute that gives the ability to alleviate, as well as cause, tremendous pain for members. She questions the degree to which families can realistically and effectively cope with this social ideology. For example, how can families faced with economic stress and uncertainty also muster the stability to provide a safe, secure environment? When the environment becomes so unsafe as to include violence, is the primary cause the family or the social ideology?

Of course, social changes are not perfectly organized and consistent. J. R. Miller identified coherence of issues as another factor in the effects of social changes.[11] Social issues with regard to women, work, dispersion of family members, and psychological propinquity are complex, and the degree to which they are coherent is the degree to which families may be expected to be able to cope effectively with them. Even social issues which are apparently quite general in nature eventually affect families in a profound manner. For example, Ann Wolbert Burgess demonstrated the potent reverberation of the recent American fuel and energy shortages across a wide range of day-to-day aspects of family survival and described the associated and subsequent stress perceived by the families.[12]

Effects of Members on the Convoy

Each member of the family is involved in a trajectory of life span development. This development changes the needs and abilities of the person. The changes echo through the family group, causing changes in family needs and abilities.[13] There is interaction between both of these types of changes and the mutual abilities of families and members to contribute to each other.

Life span development changes do not necessarily occur smoothly or in an organized fashion. There is ample opportunity for changes to cause both conflict and concordance among the members of the family. It is also clear that life change events do not have uniform meanings or effects across individuals.[14]

Attachment is central to the familial bonds that endure throughout these life span changes. John Bowlby defines attachment as a strong disposition to seek proximity to and contact with the attachment figure and to do so especially in situations involving emergencies, fear, anxiety, or threat.[15] Attachment is a persisting attribute and provides a strong, pervasive sense of security. Bowlby also emphasizes that although the behaviors associated with attachment change over the life span, the relationship continues to offer a secure base for testing and exploring the environment.

D. Heard suggests that the degree to which attachment relationships are adaptive is the degree to which the members of the family will gain confidence and the ability to cope from their familial bonds.[16] Roles have an effect in this process. Each member holds a number of roles within the family and as those roles are evolved and adjusted, the aggregate nature of the family is affected.[17] For example, parenting is a major role shift which affects the majority of adults. Maternal role characteristics and experiences are significantly different from those associated with the paternal role.[18] C. Jones demonstrated that expectations of the role change, readiness for the parenting experience, and match of temperaments between father and infant were central to explaining success in paternal role transition.[19] These findings describe one process of adjusting the "fit" between person and environment.

Unusual events are equally viable factors in the effects of members upon their families. In the instance of hospitalization, the crisis of one member reverberates through the entire family system. K. A. Knafl reported that when a sibling is hospitalized, parental expectations of non-hospitalized siblings and their roles in adjustment were related to the preexisting family structure.[20] J. R. Bloom found the same type of pattern in the case of adjustment to breast cancer, during which the amount of contact with significant others and type of family cohesiveness were both predictive of coping.[21] A significant amount of variance in self-concept was explained by the coping variables, and so this study serves as an illustration of the relationship between family and member characteristics.

M. L. Velasco de Parra demonstrated the processual aspects of family changes in a study of renal transplant patients and their families.[22] Following the transplant, the families reflected major shifts in alliances and relational hierarchies. These results emphasize the cyclic, interrelated effects of change in one member and resultant changes in the family.

The composition of the family changes over time, in relation to life span development patterns. The composition also changes with respect to social patterns of behavior, and the interaction of cohort and life span development changes is particularly evident in our society. One-half of recent marriages will end in divorce, one out of six women are unmarried at age thirty, there has been a rise in cohabitation, and one-third of today's young adults will eventually divorce and remarry.[23] To what degree will other social standards even permit, much less assist, people exhibiting these new behavior patterns? How could these new family forms "fit" their environments—and what nursing assistance will be most useful?

FAMILY CONTRIBUTIONS TO AGGREGATE AND INDIVIDUAL NEEDS

In theory, the family fulfills a number of functions that serve its own needs as well as those of its members. The family has been defined here as a convoy of relationships because of the importance of a life span view. This temporal dimension has several general implications for the outcomes of family functions. For example, family influences are different for each stage of development as well as each particular need or behavior of the members.[24] Therefore, time affects the relative impact of family functions for the individual because the importance of family influence varies across the life span. Erik Erikson's discussion of the eight ages of humans includes an example of the variability of family influence.[25] The generativity stage of later life requires a sense of guiding younger generations, while the identity stage of adolescence requires a sense of testing and establishing a unique self. Both stages can profit from, or be demolished by, family functions. It is equally important to note that the kinds of family functions that can contribute to each stage are different.

Time is also a factor in generational differences, which affect the outcomes of family functions. Parental influence on teens, stability of housing and energy sources, composition of the family, courtship and marriage mores, security and employment, and childrearing patterns each change over generations or cohort groups and carry real impact on the functioning of families.[26] Ethnicity is most certainly a viable factor which overlays the effects of member and cohort changes across time.

Family Functions

The primary outcome of family functions is to maximize coping and motivation. Members, at least potentially, gain psychological equilibrium as a result of family functioning, and that equilibrium is critical to engaging in effective coping responses.[27] The issue at hand is how does the family accomplish this formidable task? What are the mechanisms available to the family in terms of achieving this facilitation of successful coping by its members?

Research in family functioning measures the range of differences in family functions, but that research faces a number of conceptual and methodological problems. These problems are rooted in the fact that although one may interview every family member and strive to conceptualize all the information at the family level, the actual family is more than the sum of its parts.

Carolyn Sara Roberts and Suzanne L. Feetham measured two aspects of members' assessments of family functioning: what kind of family functioning each member perceived, and, what kind of functioning they believed "should be."[28] These assessments were applied to twenty-one examples of family functions, derived from three clusters of relationships (relationships between family and the broader social context, family and intrafamily systems, family and individual members). With a third question regarding how important each function seemed to the members, the researchers obtained a full measure of perceived family functioning. Their definition of family functioning provides the link between the perceptions of members and the aggregate family: family functioning includes the activities and relationships among and between persons and the environment which in combination enable the family to maintain itself as an open system. The Feetham Family Functioning Survey, both valid and reliable, provides a measure of discrepancy between expected and perceived family functioning. Reviewing degrees of discrepancy on each family function would provide a systematic method for identifying priorities for intervention. Functions with high discrepancies between expected and perceived are likely to be ones in which the family is limited in ability to contribute to either member or aggregate needs.

Perception has another, more basic, effect on outcomes of family functioning. The perceived nature of a relationship is associated with family contributions to the member. For example, Susan B. Meister found that an affective bond is not necessarily sufficient for providing assistance.[29] The 252 young adults in her study identified 4,544 network members. Network members were first classified in terms of affective, instrumental, and helping bonds, and then matched with the type of assistance offered over a four-month period of life change adjustment. Over one-third of the network members were reported as having an affective bond with the subject, yet offering *no* assistance during the adjustment period. This finding is important here because it highlights the errors which could result if affective family relationships were identified and then simply assumed to be functional or supportive.

Social Support

Much of what the family contributes to members can also be called social support. Defining social support has puzzled researchers for years, but we may estimate the definition as the provision of direct *aid*, expression of *affect*, and/or the *affirmation* of agreement or valuation of thoughts, feelings, or actions. Each of these forms of support describe what the family, or some of its members, might contribute to another member in need.

A review of the support literature confirms the existence and health effects of support. The theoretical value of social support lies in its dynamic effects within people's lives and its contribution to adjustment and well-being. Although researchers have employed a wide range of definitions of support, they have also had consistent success in showing effects of various forms of support. Most research has also used the more general construct of social network, rather than family, as the source of social support. Including this research in a discussion of family requires only two assumptions: (1) that the family is not wholly divorced from the egocentric social network, and (2) that holding a familial form of membership in the social network does not necessarily preclude the ability to offer social support. N. J. Pender and Susan B. Meister have demonstrated that these assumptions are defensible.[30]

Kahn and Antonucci propose a typology which is purposefully constructed for concordance with their concept of the convoy.[31] Recognizing that social support is important throughout the life span, they also note that the appropriate form and amount of support vary with age. Their typology is defined with an interest in exploring age, cohort, and individual differences in social support. Nursing and health care require the same kind of information and that concordance makes Kahn and Antonucci's typology particularly useful here (see Table 1).

The existence and viability of affective support has been demon-

TABLE 1.   Summary of Kahn and Antonucci's Typology

Form of Social Support	Definition
Affect	The expression of liking, admiring, respecting, loving Ego
Affirmation	The expression of agreement of acknowledgment of the appropriateness or rightness of Ego's acts or statements
Aid	The provision of direct assistance, things, money, information, time, entitlement to Ego

strated in several contexts: adjustment to job loss, prognosis and complication outcomes of pregnancy, hospitalization, and maintenance of mental health therapy.[32] In each instance, emotional support was associated with or predictive of an aspect of well-being.

Information and aid forms of support have also been empirically verified. J. S. House demonstrated their relationships to well-being in a series of work stress studies and B. H. Gottlieb produced them via a content analysis.[33] The combination of emotional informational support has also been tested. L. D. Egbert et al. Compared the recovery period of two groups of surgical patients. The experimental group received optimistic, enthusiastic, and reinforced preoperative teaching, and that group required less postoperative medication and length of hospitalization than did the control group.[34]

Affirmation has been demonstrated as a function of postpartum support groups. These volunteer groups were developed by the women who joined them and those women identified three principal elements of group support: an increased belief in their ability to parent, increased self-esteem and coping ability, and recognition of their postpartum feelings as normative.[35] These results suggest that affirmation may contain aspects of the other forms of support, that is, a statement of admiration is technically an expression of affect, but it contributes to increased self-esteem, which is associated with affirmation.

The arenas of work and home have been the context for many support studies. These two focuses of daily life involve many forms of support, induce and may meet needs for support, as well as define degrees of access to potential supporters.[36] Each arena includes some unique sources of support, but family members appear in each as well. The studies also demonstrated that some forms of support are situation (such as work or home) or relationship specific.

Family members are embedded in each of these studies of social support. The consistency of these results implicates familial bonds as support resources and emphasizes the specificity of relationships as a factor in support. For example, support which was sought out in relation to a particular concern was the most predictive of a sense of well-being at life change.[37] Patricia A. Brandt and Clarann Weinert, and B. L. Wilcox also found support to be associated with well-being; a sense of worth and social integration in the first study, psychological symptoms in the second.[38]

These findings are congruent with the basic elements of support. Support can buffer some stress effects, it can provide ongoing contributions to well-being, but it is neither a general panacea nor a completely independent factor in outcomes. There is disagreement about theoretical and methodological definitions of support mechanisms.[39] The majority of research demonstrates a modest and reliable association between social support and well-being, and the strength of that association mirrors the degree of stress in the person's situation.[40] Studies and theories of intra-family abuse often emphasize lack of social networks among abusers, suggesting a particular vulnerability to stress in the instance of limited sources of social support.

Utilization and Help-Seeking

The simple existence of network sources of support does not assure that the support is actually received. In some instances, supporters spontaneously offer assistance, but support is most often effective when it is sought out.[41] The family may contribute to members either by making them more able to seek support or by making its own support more accessible.

The majority of adults who experience a problem will initially seek some form of help from their social network, but perception of the network is a critical factor in this process.[42] For example, some people are "nonutilizers," that is, they attempt to manage problems in an independent fashion. Nonutilizers are not a homogeneous group. Awareness that help is available permits some nonutilizers to handle problems independently because they perceive their networks as effective backup, while other nonutilizers choose that route because they view their networks as insufficient, unpredictable, or inaccessible.[43] Therefore, how the family is perceived is a potent precursor to how it is (or is not) utilized by a member.

The network also has an effect on utilization of other resources, such as the health care system. B. A. Hamburg and M. Killilea describe the egocentric network as including both a lay referral system and a lay treatment network.[44] The network is needed during stress because a stressful event constitutes a situation with anxiety, impaired informational processes, and needs for new or expanded assistance. The indigenous, enduring network affects both the nature of these stress components and the options available to resolve them.

J. McKinlay found that utilization of routine prenatal services was strongly related to the types of network differentiation.[45] The pregnant women described their networks in two ways: either as a relatively homogenous group or as a group with clear subsets. The women who were utilizing prenatal services also reported networks in which they clearly distinguished between friends and relatives. Nonutilizing women made less of an intranetwork discrimination and were more likely to seek advice and opinions from their social network than from the health care system. This pattern of network perceptions affecting access to other resources is of great importance to health care providers. Patients are part of their enduring environment; thus, the effects of that environment upon episodic utilization of health services are pertinent to both theory and practice.

Not all studies have reported these types of extranetwork effects. For example, F. D. Wolinsky found no significant relationships between physical symptoms, subjective psychological well-being, social role, and utilization of health services.[46] It is important to note that the variables were coded as 0 (no) or 1 (yes) dichotomies. When symptoms, stress, and health care utilization are measured over time and coded in a more substantive manner, utilization *is* sensitive to daily, short-term family processes.[47]

When the issue is whether or not to see a doctor, the perceptions of *both* the person with a symptom and the network are viable, interactive variables. E. Berkanovic and C. Telesky studied two groups of people with symptoms: those who thought a physician contact was important and those who did not.[48] In the first group, when the network members did not endorse seeing a physician, only 68 percent actually had a physician contact. In the second group, when most of the network members thought it was important to see a physician, 33 percent of the subjects actually contacted a physician. In this study, network opinion played an important but not independent role in seeking health care. These results are noted here as evidence of the active role of the person. Opinions and actions of network, or family, members impact upon the person's choices, but they do not dictate final outcomes.

L. McCallister and C. S. Fischer have also demonstrated the importance of perceived social bonds as discriminators in networks.[49] Their subjects first defined a "probable exchange network"; they used a set of assistance functions to identify the set of individuals who were likely to provide each function. Many functions were suggested, including helping out during illness, responding to emergencies, loaning money. Subjects then identified any people who were "important to keep in touch with," and most subjects added names to their networks. At least one-half of the total network membership was *only* elicited by the importance criterion (51 percent in the first study, 62 percent in the second). This result illustrates that networks must be viewed across all relevant components. Failure to tap an important subset of the network will result in failure to identify all network members. More important, some levels of connection between members and subject will be missed. This issue of accuracy in range is one of the most difficult to address, as well as one of the major sources of measurement error.[50]

Accuracy in range is further complicated when networks are viewed across the life span. The attachment literature stands as powerful evidence of intraindividual life span changes in both particular bonds and the general nature of desired bonds.[51] For example, the women interviewed by S. G. Candy, L. G. Troll, and S. G. Levy represented a cross section of the adult life span, and particular functions of friends varied with the age of the woman.[52] There is clearly a temporal dimension to social bonds and this dimension requires recognition in research, theory, and practice.

FAMILY WELL-BEING: DEFINITIONS AND ISSUES

Person-Environment Fit

J. R. P. French, W. Rodgers, and S. Cobb developed the construct of person-environment fit and set it into the context of adjustment or adaptation.[53] Person-environment fit is a function of four factors:

E (objective):   The objective amount of environmental supplies that are available.

P (objective):   The objective amount of supplies that are necessary to meet current demands.

E (subjective):   The subjective amount of environmental supplies that are available.

P (subjective):   The subjective amount of supplies that are necessary to meet current demands.

The degree of balance between demand and supply defines the degree of "fit." French, Rodgers, and Cobb included both subjective and objective factors in their construct, and they emphasized that overall fit predicts outcome variables such as coping and strain. Because person-environment fit is a multidimensional construct, coping and strain are related to a number of demand/supply balances. French, Rodgers, and Cobb used the balance of relationships and privacy as an illustration: if one demand requires an increase in interpersonal contacts, then the supply of privacy must decrease. For example, when an infant is born, the family must strike a new balance of contact and privacy.

French, Rodgers, and Cobb drew attention to the multiplicity of demand/supply balance and suggested that the relative importance of each balance was critical to the overall degree of fit. In the affiliation and privacy example, if the person placed minimal importance on privacy, then the loss of a supply of privacy would have little impact on overall fit. On the other hand, if loss of privacy was important, then such a loss would define a new and unmet demand. Unmet demands decrease overall fit, and French, Rodgers, and Cobb cite such deprivations as part of the complex of motivations which precipitate the need for adjustment and adaptation. The magnitude, relative importance, immediacy, and duration of deprivations affect the type of responses people make in terms of achieving overall adjustments.

The objective and subjective components of overall fit are not necessarily related. In fact, French, Rodgers, and Cobb presented two primary mechanisms of adjustment: actually altering the discrepant fit, and, altering perceptions of the fit. These mechanisms include both useful and problematic coping strategies, although they differ in terms of objective or subjective emphasis.

Person-environment fit offers a comprehensive and specific description of human adjustment, coping, and strain. How might that description be quantified to obtain estimates of the relationships between fit, coping, and strain? The answer is far from complete, but measures of overall well-being and factors which predict it address a significant portion of the question.

Perceived Well-Being

F. M. Andrews et al. developed a measure of global perceived well-being and a set of specific perceived well-being measures.[54] The global well-being measure was the subject of extensive study. F. M. Andrews and S. B. Withey investigated sixty-eight global measures and demonstrated the importance of measures which tap general evaluations of life as a whole within a current time frame.[55] The measures which asked a subject to evaluate current well-being, using the full range of current experience, also clustered together regardless of wording or measurement scale. Andrews's "Life no. 3" is one of these measures and asks subjects how they feel about their "life as a whole."

This global measure was included in a test of the affective and cognitive components of global well-being measures.[56] It captured a fairly even representation of affective and cognitive dimensions and achieved a high degree of validity.

Specific perceived well-being measures request evaluations of particular domains of life. For example, subjects evaluate feelings about how much they are accomplishing in life (using a seven-point scale, "terrible" to "delighted"). Eleven such items, all measuring interactions between life domains and subjects' values were found to cluster into three dimensions.[57] Content, relationships, and psychological immediacy split the items into statistically and theoretically substantive groups.

Andrews and Withey pursued a larger test involving the prediction of global well-being from the specific well-being items.[58] Beginning with 123 items, they determined that a small subset formed a linear, additive, and highly predictive combination. Four major life domain indexes occur within that predictive subset: family index, efficacy index, fun index, and money index. These four life domain indexes account for 70 percent of the variance in global well-being.

Meister used perceived well-being as the outcome variable in a study of perceived social support and networks.[59] The results have particular meaning to nursing because support and network variables accounted for more variance in the efficacy life domain than in the global well-being measure. The subscale of efficacy asks the subjects in estimate how they feel about: themselves, what they are accomplishing in life, and how they handle problems. These results emphasize the focal effects of support and selected network members on the precise individual characteristic of greatest importance to nursing; the basis for self-care. J. S. Norbeck, also a nurse, has similarly underscored the importance of social support to nursing theory and practice, and there has been a recent increase in nursing research in this arena.[60]

We have now come full circle. The discussion began with the interactive nature of family and family members, worked through an overview of the convoy and member's life span development, examined social support as a function of families, and set those parameters into the larger theory of person-environment fit, as evidenced by perceived well-being. We now note that the family makes a direct contribution to well-being, and the next step is to recall that the well-being of the family determines its ability to make such a contribution.

The Promise of the Construct of Family Well-Being

Previous research has demonstrated the utility of well-being as a construct which can quantify the more general idea of person-environment fit. Because "fit" is a multivariate function of subjective and objective components of the person and the environment, it would be nearly impossible to measure each factor which contributes to "fit." Rather, research designs are planned to incorporate some of the most salient factors, and well-being is used as a measure which taps a large segment of the degree of "fit" achieved by an individual. This approach has been fruitful in terms of individuals, and this chapter has been developed to posit the promise of using the same approach in terms of families.

Family well-being, as a substantive indicator of family-environment fit, would answer a number of questions that are crucial to nursing practice with families in general. It is presented here because of its potential role in developing nursing responses to family violence.

Practice hinges upon the identification of not only the problems, demands, and needs of the person, but also the available resources, strengths, and options. Family well-being is an indicator of the types of help and hindrance that are forthcoming for the person. As such, family well-being is a major factor in the adaptive capabilities of the person and constitutes a pressing issue in nursing assessments.

The practice setting and role of the nurse will affect the interventions which are developed from the assessment data. In most instances, interventions will focus on the person and use knowledge of the family's well-being as a guideline. Some nurses will be in positions to develop family-based interventions as well, and family well-being measures will be of particular value to them.

Nursing research can intensify the practice value of family well-being measures. We need two particular types of information. First, what are the interactive effects of family and member well-being in an enduring context? These effects may well vary in terms of normative and nonnormative changes, and both types of change are viable factors in nursing practice. Second, what are the predictors of family-environment and person-environment fits? The relative predictive powers of the context, time, and developmental stage are not known, but they will define the relative priorities of the context, time, and developmental stage in nursing practice with families.

LINKS BETWEEN THE CONSTRUCT OF FAMILY WELL-BEING AND VIOLENCE

There are three links between family well-being and family violence which are particularly pertinent and promising to nursing: the *role of deprivation*, the contextual *meaning of change*, and *potential strategies* for intervention in social networks. Each of these links is based upon current knowledge of an aspect of family well-being and may explain major factors in family violence.

French, Rodgers, and Cobb identified deprivation as a powerful source of motivation to adjust person-environment fit.[61] Some deprivations are predictable aspects of the family life cycle, and nursing research has examined the effects of instituting, expanding, and contracting the family.[62] Those studies emphasized the range of individual differences which result from attempts to adjust to change. Failed or torturous attempts at adjustment, whether to normative or unusual episodes of poor "fit," may well contribute to family violence. Because deprivation is at the root of attempts to adapt, particular deprivations may predict adaptive failures among certain people. If so, those deprivations could serve as cardinal warning signs of the potential for family violence.

The predictive value of the deprivations would be associated with specific characteristics of individuals, which brings us to the second link between family well-being and violence. Change is always an active factor in human experience, but some changes are more threatening than others. D. A. Hamburg, G. V. Coelho, and J. E. Adams emphasized individual differences in perceived threats and identified the importance of coherence between skills acquired from earlier socialization and skills demanded by the current environment.[63] In other words, if the environment is relatively stable, then the adaptive skills learned early in life are likely to be useful during later years as well. Is violence associated with lack of coherence? L. Rubin painted a disturbingly grim picture of the struggles and slim hopes of working-class families today, and much of her data defines precisely the lack of coherence described by Coelho, Hamburg, and Adams.[64] The potency of coherence between skills and demands also reflects the enduring role of the family, as early socializer and later environment, in creating situations which can result in adaptive or violent outcomes.

Intervention strategies are the third link between family well-being and violence. The family, as a social network, is the seat of attachments that promotes or inhibits mastery of life experience.[65] Families can, and indeed must, change over time. The nature of this change defines both family well-being and the degree to which the family can contribute to its members. Intervention to promote positive changes is possible. L. C. Ford, A. L. Whall, S. R. Miller, and P. Winstead-Frye have each developed a framework for nursing interventions with families, and each addresses several aspects of health-promoting interventions.[66] Hamburg and Killilea have similarly emphasized the need to develop interventions which build upon inherent resources, such as the family.[67] They also raise a pivotal issue: which *member*-focused interventions are best accomplished by the family, and which are most effectively instituted by health care professionals? This issue takes on particular urgency when it is applied to violent families. The strengths and inherent resources of these families are essentially undefined in extant research and theory.

The issue of splitting contributions to member well-being between two potential resources presents the second step in developing the construct of family well-being. Once we can estimate such well-being, we are able to identify pathways to effective facilitation of the family as well as the parameters of a nursing role with the members. When the enduring family network has achieved a healthy level of well-being, that network is often a wise source of intervention for the members. The nursing role must expand significantly in the instance of decreased or fragile family well-being, which is the focus of the remainder of this volume.

The profession of nursing can respond to these needy families by continuing basic and applied research, while voicing political and professional endorsements of multiple, diverse supports for families. Each nurse can respond by continuing to seek fuller knowledge of these families and stretching to develop a more complete perspective on how to best meet their needs.

SUMMARY

Although traditional family frameworks have produced a broad and useful body of knowledge, nursing requires a more comprehensive and flexible conceptualization of families. Family forms are more widely variant in our society, and practice is hindered by a scientific base that does not address the type of family in which health problems happen to occur. Well-being is a concept with great promise for nursing theory, research, and practice with families.

Well-being is of particular value because it is an index of family-environment, or person-environment, fit. The degree of fit between supplies and demands affects both the family and its members. When the family does well in achieving fit, then it has a greater capacity to contribute to the members—who are also juggling personal resources and demands. The same principle determines the degree to which members are able to contribute to the family. Dysfunctional fit of resources and demands (decreased family well-being and member well-being) bears directly upon family violence.

The family is a specific form of social network (convoy) and its membership is a function of the bonds perceived by the members. Across the life span, developmental experiences affect both the members and the family. These changes result in both conflict and concordance within the family. Members are faced with normative and nonnormative personal changes, and their roles and well-being are affected. Social mores affect life span patterns, including familial ones. Each member-based change affects other members of the family as well as the aggregate nature of the convoy.

Family functions best serve the members when they contribute to the psychological equilibrium essential to coping. Family assistance may take the form of social support, which is not a general panacea, but rather relates to well-being in a number of situation specific and person specific manners. While the nature of family functioning and support also affects member utilization of other resources, neither family nor member effects are necessarily independent predictors of outcomes.

Practice hinges upon the identification of not only the problems, demands, and needs of the person, but the available resources, strengths, and options as well. Family well-being is an indicator of the types of help and hindrance that are forthcoming for the person. As such, family well-being is a major factor in the adaptive capabilities of the person, and it presents a pressing issue in nursing assessments of families in general, as well as nursing responses to family violence.

Research findings, the practice setting, and role of the nurse will affect the interventions which are developed from the assessment data. In most instances, interventions focus on the person and would use knowledge of the family well-being as a guideline. Some nurses will be in positions to develop family-based interventions as well, and family well-being measures would be of particular value to them.

Nursing research can intensify the practice value of family well-being measures. The degree of family well-being is a factor in determining pathways to effective facilitation of the family as well as the members. The family with a healthy level of well-being is often a potent source of intervention for the members, while decreased family well-being may indicate a greater need for nursing intervention. The vulnerabilities and needs of these fragile families are all the more compelling when viewed in light of the strength embedded in healthier levels of family well-being.

REFERENCES

1. D. A. Hamburg and M. B. Trudeau, "Behavioral Aspects of Aggression: An Overview," in *Biobehavioral Aspects of Aggression,* ed. D. A. Hamburg and M. B. Trudeau (New York: Alan R. Liss, 1981).
2. N. Friedkin, "A Test of Structural Features of Granovetter's Strength of Weak Ties Theory," *Social Networks* 2, (1980): 411–422.
3. S. B. Meister, "Measurement of Perceived Affective Networks Defined by Whole Families: Reliability and Validity" (unpublished research report, University of Michigan, 1980).
4. R. L. Kahn, and T. Antonucci, "Convoys over the Life Course: Attachment, Roles, and Social Support," in *Life-span: Development and Behavior,* ed. P. B. Baltes and O. Brim, vol. 3 (Boston: Lexington Press, 1980).
5. Meister, "Measurement of Perceived Affective Networks."
6. D. Reiss, *The Family's Construction of Reality* (Cambridge: Harvard University Press, 1981). M. E. Oliveri and D. Reiss "A Theory Based Empirical Classification of Family Problem-Solving Behavior," *Family Process* 20 (1981): 409–18.
7. S. Minuchin and H. C. Fishman, *Family Therapy Techniques* (Cambridge: Harvard University Press, 1981).
8. D. Reiss, *Family's Construction of Reality.*
9. M. P. Andrews, M. M. Bubolz, and B. Paolucci, "An Ecological Approach to the Study of the Family, *Marriage and Family Review* 3 (1980): 29–49. E. M. Duvall, *Marriage and Family Development,* 5th ed. (Philadelphia: J. B. Lippincott, 1977), R. B. Taylor, R. L. Michielutte, and A. Herndon. "Family Life Events: A Study of 198 Families" *Family Practice Research Journal* 1 (1981): 68–74.
10. B. Laslett, "The Significance of Family Membership," in *Changing Images of the Family,* ed. V. Tufte and B. Myerhoff (New Haven: Yale University Press, 1979).
11. J. R. Miller, "Family Support of the Elderly," *Family and Community Health* 3(1981): 39–49.
12. A. W. Burgess, "Energy Related Stress and Families' Coping Response." (paper presented at the annual meeting of the American Academy of Nursing, 1980).
13. E. M. Duvall, *Marriage and Family Development;* D. P. Hymovich and R. W. Chamberlain, *Child and Family Development: Implications for Primary Health Care* (New York: McGraw-Hill, 1980).
14. A. H. MacFarlane, G. R. Norman, D. L. Streiner, R. Roy, and D. J. Scott, "A Longitudinal

Study of the Influence of the Psychological Environment on Health Status: A Preliminary Report," *Journal of Health and Social Behavior* 21 (1980): 124–33.

15. J. Bowlby, "Attachment and Loss: Retrospect and Prospect," *American Journal of Orthopsychiatry*, 52, (1982): 664–78.

16. D. Heard, "Family Systems and the Attachment Dynamic," *Journal of Family Therapy* (1982): 99–116.

17. P. Robischon and D. Scott, "Role Theory and its Application in Family Nursing," in *Family-Centered Nursing: A Sociological Framework*, ed. A. Reinhardt and M. Quinn (St. Louis: Mosby, 1973).

18. W. K. Wilson and L. Cronenwett, "Nursing Care for the Emerging Family: Promoting Paternal Behavior," *Research in Nursing and Health* 4 (1981): 201–211. Bowlby, "Attachment and Loss."

19. C. Jones, "Father To Infant Attachment: Effects of Early Contact and Characteristics of the Infant," *Research in Nursing and Health* 4 (March 1981): 183–192.

20. K. A. Knafl, "Parent's View of the Response of Siblings to a Pediatric Hospitalization." *Research in Nursing and Health* 5 (1982): 13–20.

21. J. R. Bloom, "Social Support, Accommodation to Stress, and Adjustment to Breast Cancer," *Social Science and Medicine* 16 (1982): 1329–38.

22. M. L. Velasco de Parra, "Changes in Family structure after a Renal Transplant," *Family Process* 21 (1982): 195–202.

23. A. J. Cherlin, *Marriage, Divorce, Remarriage* (Cambridge: Harvard University Press, 1981).

24. B. Hamburg and A. J. Solnit, "Workshop on Family and Social Environment," in *Adolescent Behavior and Health: A Conference Summary* (Institute of Medicine, National Academy of Sciences, Washington D.C., 1978).

25. E. H. Erikson, *Childhood and Society,* 2d ed. (New York: W. W. Norton, 1963).

26. U. S. Congress, *Editorial Research Reports on the Changing American Family* (Washington, D.C.: Congressional Quarterly, 1979).

27. D. Mechanic "Social Structure and Personal Adaptation: Some Neglected Dimensions," in *Coping and Adaptation*, ed. G. V. Coelho, D. A. Hamburg, and J. E. Adams (New York: Basic Books, 1974).

28. C. Roberts and S. L. Feetham, "Assessing Family Functioning Across Three Areas of Relationships," *Nursing Research* 31 (1982) 231–35.

29. S. B. Meister, "Perceived Social Support Subnetworks and Well-Being at Life Change (Ph.D. diss., University of Michigan, 1982).

30. N. J. Pender, *Health Promotion in Nursing Practice* (Norwalk, Conn.: Appleton-Century-Crofts, 1982), Meister, "Perceived Social Support Subnetworks."

31. Kahn and Antonucci, "Convoys over the Life Course."

32. S. Cobb, "Social Support as a Moderator of Life Stress," *Psychosomatic Medicine* 38 (1976) 300–314; S. Gore, "The Influence of Social Support in Ameliorating the Consequences of Job Loss" (Ph.D. diss. University of Pennsylvania, 1973); G. deAraujo et al., "Life Change, Coping Ability and Chronic Intensive Asthma," *Journal of Psychosomatic Medicine* 17 (1973): 359–63.; F. Baekland and L. Lundwell "Dropping out of Treatment: A Critical Review," *Psychological Bulletin*, 82 (1975): 738–83; S. Cobb "Social Support and Health through the Life Course," in *Aging from Birth to Death: Interdisciplinary Perspectives*, ed. M. W. Riley (Washington D.C.: American Association for the Advancement of Science, 1979).

33. J. S. House, *Work Stress and Social Support* (Reading, Mass.: Addison-Wesley, 1981); B. H. Gottlieb, "The Development and Application of a Classification Scheme of Informal Helping Behaviors," *Canadian Journal of Science* 10, (1978): 105–115.

34. L. D. Egbert, G. E. Battit, C. E. Welch, and M. K. Bartlett, "Reduction of Post-Operative Pain by Encouragement and Instruction of Patients," *New England Journal of Medicine* 270 (1964): 825–27.

35. L. R. Cronenwett, "Elements and Outcomes of a Postpartum Support Group Program," *Research in Nursing and Health* 3 (1980): 33–41.

36. E. Bott, *Family and Social Networks*, 2d ed. (New York: Free Press, 1971); House, *Work Stress and Social Support;* R. L. Kahn, "Aging and Social Support," in Riley, *Aging from Birth to Death;* Kahn and Antonucci, "Convoys over the Life Course;" F. E. Katz, "Occupational Contact Networks," *Social Forces* 37 (1958): 52–55; B. Raphael, "Preventive Intervention with the Recently Bereaved," *Archives of General Psy-*

chiatry, 34, (December 1977) 1450–1454; R. C. Stephens, "Aging, Social Support Systems and Social Policy," *Journal of Gerontological Social Work* 1 (1978): 33–45.

37. Meister, "Perceived Social Support Subnetworks."

38. P. A. Brandt, and C. Weinert, "The PRQ—a Social Support Measure," *Nursing Research* 30 (1981): 277–80; B. L. Wilcox, "Social Support, Life Stress, and Psychological Adjustment: A Test of the Buffering Hypothesis," *American Journal of Community Psychology* 9, (1981): 371–85.

39. J. M. LaRocco, J. S. House, and J. R. P. French "Social Support, Occupational Stress, and Health," *Journal of Health and Social Behavior* 21 (1980): 202–18; C. Schaefer, "Sharing up the 'Buffer' of Social Support," *Journal of Health and Social Behavior* 23 (1982): 96–98; J. S. House, J. M. LaRocco, and J. R. P. French "Response to Schaefer," *Journal of Health and Social Behavior* 23 (1982): 98–101; P. A. Thoits, "Conceptual, Methodological, and Theoretical Problems in Studying Social Support as a Buffer against Life Stress," *Journal of Health and Social Behavior* 23 (1982): 145–59.

40. K. B. Nuckolls, J. Cassel, and B. H. Kaplan, "Psychosocial Assets, Life Crisis, and the Prognosis of Pregnancy," *American Journal of Epidemiology* 95 (1972): 431–41; R. J. Turner, "Social Support as a Contingency in Psychological Well-Being," Journal of Health and Social Behavior 22 (1981): 357–67; Meister, "Perceived Social Support Subnetworks."

41. Meister, "Perceived Social Support Subnetworks."

42. N. Gourash, "Help-Seeking: A Review of the Literature," *American Journal of Community Psychology* 6 (1978): 413–23.

43. B. B. Brown, "Social and Psychological Correlates of Help-Seeking Behavior among Urban Adults," *American Journal of Community Psychology* 6 (1978): 425–39.

44. B. A. Hamburg and M. Killilea, "Relation of Social Support, Stress, Illness, and Use of Health Services," in *Healthy People: The Surgeon General's Report on Health Promotion and Disease Prevention: Background Papers,* Department of Health, Education, and Welfare Public Health Service publication no. 79-55071A; Institute of Medicine, National Academy of Sciences, 1979.

45. J. McKinlay, "Social Networks, Lay Consultants, and Help-Seeking Behavior," *Social Forces* 51 (1973): 275–92.

46. F. D. Wolinsky, "Assessing the Effects of the Physical, Psychological, and Social Dimensions of Health on the Use of Health Services" *Sociological Quarterly* 23 (1982): 191–206.

47. S. L. Gortmaker, J. Eckenrode, and S. Gore, "Stress and the Utilization of Health Services: A Time Series and Cross-Sectional Analysis," *Journal of Health and Social Behavior* 23 (1982): 25–38.

48. E. Berkanovic and C. Telesky, "Social Networks, Beliefs, and the Decision to Seek Medical Care: An Analysis of Congruent and Incongruent Patterns," *Medical Care* 20 (1982): 1018–26.

49. L. McCallister and C. S. Fischer, *Studying Egocentric Networks by Mass Survey,* Working Paper no. 284 (Berkeley: Institute of Urban and Regional Development, University of California, 1978a); L. McCallister and C. S. Fischer, "A Procedure for Surveying Personal Networks," *Sociological Methods and Research* 7 (1978b): 131–48.

50. P. W. Holland and S. Leinhardt, "A Method for Detecting Structure in Sociometric Data," *American Journal of Sociology* 70 (1970): 492–513.

51. Kahn and Antonucci, "Convoys over the Life Course."

52. S. G. Candy, L. G. Troll, and S. G. Levy, "A Developmental Exploration of Friendship Functions in Women," *Psychology of Women Quarterly* 5 (Spring 1981): 456–472.

53. J. R. P. French, W. Rodgers, and S. Cobb, "Adjustment as Person-Environment Fit," in *Coping and Adaption,* ed. G. V. Coelho and D. A. Hamburg (New York: Basic Books, 1974).

54. F. M. Andrews and R. C. Messenger, *Multivariate Nominal Scale Analysis* (Ann Arbor: Institute for Social Research, 1973); F. M. Andrews and S. B. Withey, "Developing Measures of Perceived Life Quality: Results from Several National Surveys," *Social Indicators Research* 1 (1974): 1–26; F. M. Andrews and S. B. Withey, *Social Indicators of Well-Being* (New York: Plenum Press, 1976); F. M. Andrews and A. C. McKennell, *Measures of Self-Reported Well-Being: Their Affective, Cognitive, and Other Components* (Ann Arbor: Institute for Social Research, 1978); F. M. Andrews, and R. F.

Inglehart, "The Structure of Subjective Well-being in Nine Western Societies," *Social Indicators Research* 6 (1979): 73–90.

55. Andrews and Withey, "Developing Measures."
56. Andrews and McKennell, *Measures of Self-Reported Well-being.*
57. Andrews and Inglehart, "Structure of Subjective Well-being."
58. Andrews and Withey, "Developing Measures."
59. Meister, "Perceived Social Support Subnetworks."
60. J. S. Norbeck "Social Support: A Model for Clinical Research and Application," *Advances in Nursing Science* 3 (1981): 43–60; J. S. Norbeck, A. M. Lindsay, and V. L. Carrieri, "The Development of an Instrument to Measure Social Support," *Nursing Research* 30 (1981): 264–69.
61. French, Rodgers, and Cobb, "Adjustment as Person-Environment Fit."
62. K. A. Knafl and H. K. Grace, *Families across the Lifecycle: Studies for Nursing* (Boston: Little, Brown. 1978).
63. D. A. Hamburg, G. V. Coelho, and J. E. Adams, "Coping and Adaptation: Steps towards a Synthesis of Biological and Social Perspectives," in Coelho, Hamburg, and Adams, *Coping and Adaptation.*
64. L. Rubin, *Worlds of Pain* (New York: Basic Books, 1976).
65. "Changes in Human Societies, Families, Social Support, and Health," in *Health and Behavior: Frontiers of Research in the Biobehavioral Sciences,* ed. David A. Hamburg, Glenn R. Elliott, and Delores L. Parron (Washington, D.C.: National Academy Press, 1982).
66. L. C. Ford, "The Development of Family Nursing," in *Family Health Care,* ed. D. P. Hyovich and M. U. Bernard, vol. 2, 2d. ed. (New York: McGraw-Hill, 1979); *A. L. Whall, "Family Systems Theory: Relationship to Nursing Conceptual Models," in Nursing Models and Their Psychiatric Mental Health Applications, ed. J. J. Fitzpatrick, A. L. Whall, R. L. Johnston, and J. A. Floyd (Bowie, Md.: Prentice-Hall, 1982); S. R. Miller and P. Winstead-Frye, Family Systems Theory in Nursing Practice* (Reston, Va: Reston Publishing Co., 1982).
67. Hamburg and Killilea, "Relation of Social Support, Stress, Illness, and Use of Health Services."

COMMENTARY

This paper presents an excellent review of family frameworks from the disciplines of sociology and psychology and the implications of these perspectives for nursing practice. The review is informative and should facilitate reformulation of theory so that it reflects a nursing perspective.

The family is regarded as a unit, and questions regarding how and why an individual acts with violence are asked within the context of the family unit approach. More specifically, Meister discusses family violence from the vantage point of existing frameworks of the family, including those addressing family well-being, family convoy, and social support.

Meister has made a significant contribution to family nursing theory development by generating a potentially testable theory of family violence that is congruent with selected family frameworks from various disciplines, including nursing. The theory, therefore, offers several options for scholars interested in family violence.

Meister's theory development effort serves as a model for family theory development in various interest areas. The challenge stemming from this and other similar efforts is selection or development of empirical indicators and research designs that are congruent with the theoretical approach.

ANN L. WHALL

13

Family Social Support: Toward a Conceptual Model

CATHERINE F. KANE

Nursing clinical assessment and empirical investigations of the social support resources available to families are hampered by the lack of theoretical bases regarding the family social support process. This article presents a preliminary conceptual model of family social support in the interest of stimulating discussion and further development. Assumptions of the model are presented, family characteristics and interaction processes are identified, and propositional statements are derived from the model. The model proposes that social support is not an outcome or a resource but a process of interaction through which the family develops versatility and resourcefulness in identifying and using resources available in its environment. The conceptual model presents family social support as a process of relationships between the family and its social environment.

Social support of the family unit is an important dimension in the realm of nursing practice and theory development, as early discharge pressures increase the demand for home nursing services. In addition, the family is assuming more of the burden of care for family members with acute and chronic health conditions. The family is thought of as existing within a web of relatives, friends, neighbors, and community services ready to

Reprinted from *Advances in Nursing Science, 10*(2), 18–25, 1988.

provide needed assistance. However, empirical assessment of this "support system" is hampered by the lack of a conceptual framework amenable to evaluating the supports available to a family as a unit as opposed to a family as a set of individuals.

The literature presents numerous theoretical constructs with which to examine the relationship between social support for individuals and various abilities of the individual to cope with adversity.[1-7] There is very little theoretical conceptualization or empirical investigation of the family social support system because the concepts relating to individual social support are not directly applicable to theory construction in family social support. The purpose of this article is to describe a conceptual model[8] of family social support derived through an inventory of causes and effects.[9] This process involves identifying assumptions regarding family social support, providing a working definition, and identifying the factors related to family social support. These factors were selected from literature reviews[1-7] regarding social support for individuals, focusing particularly on literature concerned with mental health. The process of constructing a conceptual model of family social support will provide the pretheoretical bases for constructing a theoretical model amenable to empirical testing.

ASSUMPTIONS

The initial step in this concept analysis was to identify the assumptions regarding the conceptual model. Three assumptions were acknowledged: (1) the family is a system; (2) social support is a social process; and (3) social support is positive and helpful. The associated rationale for each assumption follows.

The first assumption of the family as a system advocates the perspective that the family engages in a process of interaction within itself and between itself and the environment. This also implies that there is a flow of energy in terms of information, goods and services, and emotions within the family and between the family and its social network. This family systems perspective is espoused by numerous theorists.[10-14] From a systems perspective the family and its environment are considered to be mutually dependent. The foci are the human relationships and interactions in which this interdependence is actualized. This distinguishes social support from other interdependent physical realms such as atmosphere, plants, and animals.

The second assumption regarding social support as a social process follows from defining the family as a system. Thus family social support is a process reflecting a pattern of interaction over time between the family and its social system. This assumption is in keeping with systems concepts and emphasizes family social support as a process rather than a sum of resources available in times of crisis. Thus family social support is considered to be a process of social relationships through which resources may or may not be accessed.

The third assumption regarding social support as positive and helpful must be recognized in order to address the perspective[15-18] that social support analysis must include negative and hostile relationships in the sphere of social support. In asserting that social support is positive and helpful, the connotation of encouragement and nurturance inherent in the meaning of support is emphasized. No doubt negative interactions happen in a social network. However, negative interactions cannot be considered congruent with support; thus it seems more accurate to conceive of them as stressors rather than as "negative supports." Thus family social support is conceptualized here as positive, nurturing, and encouraging.

The assumptions regarding family social support as a concept are that the family is a system interdependent with other human systems and that it is a process that is positive and not stressful. These assumptions provide the basis for a working definition of a family social support as an ongoing pattern of social relationships between the family and its social environment that reflects interdependence.

INVENTORY OF CAUSES

In presenting the causes of social support, it is necessary to employ a holistic view of the family to maintain a systems perspective and to view the phenomenon in its entirety. The box, "Family Characteristics," provides an inventory of various antecedents of family social support identified in the literature.[1-7] It is premature to discount any factor, whether conceptual or empirical, in attempting to delineate a model of family social support. However, this inventory is not exhaustive. The effort has been made to select the most salient antecedents presumed to be involved in family social support, given the stated assumptions. The factors

---

Family Characteristics

- Number of ties in the social network
- Variety of relationships in the social network
- Economic status of the family and social network
- Flexibility of family structure
- Commonalities between the family and its social network
- Positive perception of the family by its social network
- Availability of the social network
- History of relationships
- Developmental epoch of the family

having the most empirical support are social network variables, such as the number of network ties, the variety of relationships, and the impact of socioeconomic status.

Family Characteristics

Family characteristics describe the background from which interaction emerges. The characteristics of the social network, such as size, variety, and history, interact with the family structure in terms of the family's compatibility with its social network to provide the ground for social interaction. Likewise, the stability of the family is perceived in terms of how long it has lived in a certain locale to form relationships and in terms of other characteristics, such as the age of family members.

A family's ability to garner resources from a network of relationships is enhanced by long-term relationships, commonalities families have with their networks, and the family's level of esteem within the community. These factors exert influences on one another and ultimately on the family's ability to command or draw upon the resources available. However, social support is not the social network, nor is it esteem, stability, or family structure. These factors are preconditions to the emergence of family social support. As defined, family social support is a pattern of social interaction characterized by interdependence in social relationships. Such a pattern is not the flow of goods and services between the family and its neighbors. Social support is not the lending of a lawn mower. It is the *why* of the lending. Social support arises for a family out of its long-term relationships with its extended family, neighbors, co-workers, and community.

Interactional Characteristics

The box, "Interactional Characteristics," presents the interactional characteristics proposed as the processes involved in family social support. These characteristics have been identified in the literature as important dimensions of social support and appear more akin to process dimensions of social support than characteristics of families and their social networks. The five interactional characteristics tap the dynamics of the social support construct. There is mutual interdependence in support relationships characterized by reciprocal helping relationships. This helping occurs through system interaction. It would seem that the more interaction there is between the family and its network, the more opportunities for mutual helping interactions occur. Likewise, the quantity and quality of the communication between the family and its network would seem to tap two dimensions. First, the amount of communication would seem to be encouraged by frequency of interaction. Second, the quality of communication would seem to indicate the effectiveness of advice and feedback that a family would receive from its network.

Interactional Characteristics
- Reciprocal helping relationships
- Frequency of interaction between family and social network
- Quantity and quality of communication
- Intimacy of relationships
- Trust within relationships

The last two interactional characteristics are intimacy and trust. These characteristics arise frequently in the support literature and are the dimensions of social relationships that clearly indicate supportive relationships. Intimacy reflects the level of sharing that a relationship reaches, such that a deep level of intimacy reflects personal and private information being shared relatively easily within the relationship. A superficial relationship indicates a shallow level of intimacy.

The interactional characteristics address the process dimension of family social support. They are shaped by the characteristics of the family but cannot be considered characteristics of the family. Rather, they are characteristics of the social support relationship. Since both the family and interactional characteristics are numerous and in some ways overlap, they were grouped within broader factors to better represent a conceptual model of the factors and consequently the process of family social support. The following model of social support was drawn from the inventories of causes as presented.

FAMILY SOCIAL SUPPORT: A MODEL

Fig 1 presents a conceptual model of family social support that includes family characteristics and interactional factors. Family characteristics are the ground from which interactional factors emerge. The crux of family social support lies within the interactional realm. The first interaction factor is reciprocity. Initially presented by Cobb,[19] reciprocity is the notion that an individual is involved in a network of mutual obligation. This belonging is demonstrated by behaviors in which an individual shares resources with others and is able to ask for and receive help from others. Reciprocity has since stood the test of time as an important dimension of social support for individuals and is compatible with family social support as a systemic process. Family involvement in a network of mutual obligations connotes interactions being initiated by the family, as well as its network, for mutual benefit.

In addition to reciprocity, the quality and quantity of communication between the family and its network is involved in social support. Caplan[20] emphasized the importance of significant others providing cognitive guidance to help an individual improve his or her handling of a

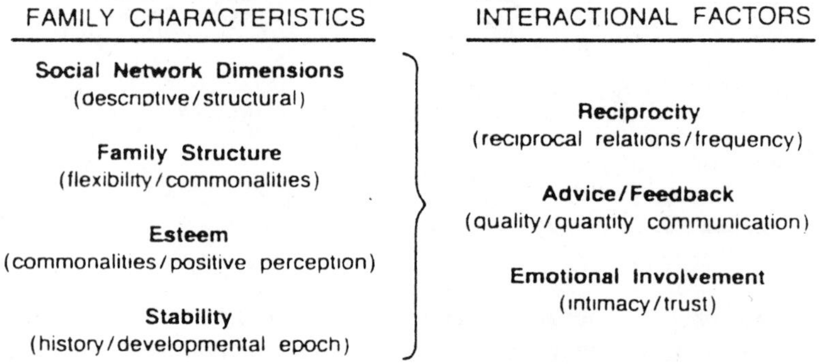

FAMILY CHARACTERISTICS   INTERACTIONAL FACTORS

Social Network Dimensions
(descriptive / structural)
                                            Reciprocity
                                    (reciprocal relations / frequency)
Family Structure
(flexibility / commonalities)
                                            Advice / Feedback
                                    (quality / quantity communication)
Esteem
(commonalities / positive perception)
                                            Emotional Involvement
                                    (intimacy / trust)
Stability
(history / developmental epoch)

Figure 1.   Conceptual model of family social support.

situation. The concept of cognitive guidance has also survived as an important dimension of social support for individuals. Within the proposed model the concept of advice and feedback is similar to cognitive guidance but is not considered a type of social support. Advice and feedback are conceived of as inherent qualities of social support such that a family is involved in sharing perceptions of itself with others and likewise of receiving evaluations from others as to how the family is perceived. The family explores options in handling crises and in fulfilling tasks. The family receives feedback from its network as to how well it is functioning and meeting its needs or the needs of the social network in which it is embedded. Again, the emphasis is that this feedback is an interactional factor of social support. It is not what results from social support or a type of social support.

Last, the concept of emotional involvement is presented as an interactional factor of family social support. Emotional involvement is proposed as the locus of the affect of the interactions between the family and its social network. It connotes positive emotional bonds between the family and others, such as love, caring, warmth, and compassion, but does not go beyond tolerance to a negative realm such as hatred, anxiety, or fear. The emotional dimension of family social support is at least positive, given the stated assumptions. Thus it is proposed that family social support involves a component of family feeling or positive orientation toward its social environment.

The three interactional dimensions of family social support are reciprocity, advice and feedback, and emotional involvement. These are the interactional components of a model of family social support that are influenced by those family characteristics presented in the inventory. The model posits family social support as characteristics of the family (social network, family structure, esteem, and stability) influencing interactional dimensions (reciprocity, advice and feedback, emotional involvement) of family social support within the family's social environment.

Propositions Regarding Family Social Support

- The larger the family's social network the greater the opportunity for reciprocity, advice and feedback, and emotional involvement.
- The more flexible the family structure the more reciprocity, advice and feedback, and emotional involvement.
- The more esteem the family has within its social network the more reciprocity, advice and feedback, and emotional involvement.
- The more stable the family the more substantial the reciprocity, advice and feedback, and emotional involvement.
- The more reciprocity occurring, the greater the family social support.
- The more advice and feedback occurring the more family social support.
- The more emotional involvement the more family social support.

The seven propositions regarding family social support (see box) show positive correlations between family characteristics, interactional factors, and family social support. These concepts represent the process of family social support. Once operationalized, they lead to hypotheses that can direct empirical tests of the model or parts of the model.

CONSEQUENCES OF FAMILY SOCIAL SUPPORT

This model emphasizes that family social support is a process that occurs over the life span. Thus, the various consequences depend on the particular needs and life stage of the family. Many outcomes of social support have been posited in the literature;[1,3,21] some of them have been considered to be social support, such as tangible assistance or resources in the form of goods and services, information, or protection from the effects of stress. In the proposed model the health and resources or help do not comprise social support. They are the outcomes of social support that become available to the family as it engages in the processes of reciprocity, advice and feedback, and emotional involvement.

Newman[22] conceives family health as fluctuating patterns of energy exchanges that may produce an increased range and quality of responses of family members to each other and to the world outside the family. Through this process the versatility and informational capacity of the family is enhanced. Newman's conceptualization of family health is a logical global consequence of family social support. Specifically, family social support is conceptualized as enabling the family to function with versatility and resourcefulness. For example, if the family social support is strong, i.e., characterized by the three dimensions, then the family becomes versatile and resourceful in its functioning and is exposed to a greater variety of goods and services, leading to the experience of health.

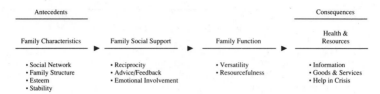

Figure 2.   Conceptual model of family social support: Antecedents and consequences.

Family social support makes resources available at the appropriate time for continued growth and development of its members and promotes the responsiveness of the social network of the family in times of crisis. Fig 2 incorporates the consequences of the interaction factors in a full model of family social support.

If the family fails to engage in reciprocal relationships or refuses to engage in the process of receiving feedback, it diminishes its family social support capacity and limits the resources available by restricting versatility and resourcefulness. Resources become available through the medium of social support; resources are not the medium. In this model health can be an outcome of social support flowing from the family's ability to function with versatility and resourcefulness.

• • •

This conceptualization of family social support begins the process of defining those dimensions of social support that can be identified for the family as a unit. Once conceptualized, these dimensions can be examined within the context of empirical research and clinical practice. The practitioner can assess the family in terms of reciprocity, advice and feedback, and emotional involvement. If the family process is lacking in one or more of these areas, strategies for strengthening the family process can be instituted. Family practitioners may be required to provide appropriate resources to the family in the interim. In addition, even though the family social support process is adequate, the family's social milieu may be incapable or lacking in the requisite resources. When the process of family social support results in insufficient resources for successful coping, it becomes the responsibility of family service providers to assist with appropriate services.

This preliminary conceptual model of family social support identifies the construct of family social support as a process of relationships between the family and its social environment. The model proposes that social support is not an outcome or a resource, but is a process of interaction through which the family develops versatility and resourcefulness and consequently achieves health.

REFERENCES

1. Turner R. J., Frankel B. G., Levin D. M.: Social support: Conceptualization, measurement, and implications for mental health. *Res Commun Ment Health* 1983;3:67–111.
2. Berrera B. Jr, Ainlay S. L.: The structure of social support: A conceptual and empirical analysis. *J Commun Psychol* 1983;11:133–143.
3. Leavy R. L.: Social support and psychological disorder: A review. *J Commun Psychol* 1983;11:3–21.
4. Israel B. A.: Social networks and health status: Linking theory, research, and practice. *Patient Counsel Health Educ* 1983;4:65–79.
5. Greenblatt M., Becerra R. M., Serafetinides E. A.: Social networks and mental health: An overview. *Am J Psychiatry* 1982;139:977–984.
6. Thoits P. A.: Social support and psychological well-being: Theoretical possibilities, in Sarason I. G., Sarason B. R. (eds): *Social Support: Theory, Research, and Applications.* Dordrecht, Holland, Martinus Nijhoff, 1985, pp 50–72.
7. Cohen S., Syme S. L. (eds): *Social Support and Health.* Orlando, Fla, Academic Press, 1985.
8. Fawcett J.: The "what" of theory development, in *Theory Development: What, Why, and How?* New York, National League for Nursing, pp 17–33.
9. Blalock H. M. Jr: *Theory Construction: From Verbal to Mathematical Formulations.* Englewood Cliffs, NJ, Prentice-Hall, 1969.
10. Broderick C., Smith J.: The general systems approach to the family, in Burr W. R., Hill R., Nye F. I., et al (eds): *Contemporary Theories about the Family.* New York, Free Press, 1979, vol 2, pp 112–129.
11. Miller J. R.: The family as a system, in Miller J. R., Janosik E. H. (eds): *Family Focused Care.* New York, McGraw-Hill, 1980.
12. Miller S. R., Winstead-Frye P.: *Family Systems Theory in Nursing Practice.* Reston, Va, Reston Publishing, 1982.
13. Swanson A. R., Hurley P. M.: Family systems: Values and value conflicts. *J Psychosoc Nurs Ment Health Serv* 1983;21:24–30.
14. Whall A. L.: Family system theory: Relationship to nursing conceptual models, in Fitzpatrick J. J. (ed): *Nursing Models and Their Psychiatric Mental Health Applications.* Bowie, Md, Robert J. Brady, 1982, pp 69–95.
15. Hammer M.: Social supports, social networks and schizophrenia. *Schizophrenia Bull* 1981;7:45–57.
16. Cohen C. I., Sokolovsky J.: Schizophrenia and social networks: Ex-patients in the inner city. *Schizophrenia Bull* 1978;4:546–560.
17. Wellman B.: Applying network analysis to the study of support, in Gottlieb B. H. (ed): *Social Networks and Social Support.* Beverly Hills, Calif, Sage, 1981, pp 171–200.
18. Tilden V. P.: Issues of conceptualization and measurement of social support in the construction of nursing theory. *Res Nurs Health* 1985;8:199–206.
19. Cobb S.: Social support as a moderator of life stress. *Psychosom Med* 1976;38:300–312.
20. Caplan G. (ed): *Support Systems and Community Mental Health.* New York, Behavioral Publications, 1974.
21. Heller K.: The effects of social support: Prevention and treatment implications, in Goldstein A. P., Kanfer F. H. (eds): *Maximizing Treatment Gains.* New York, Academic Press, 1979, pp 353–382.
22. Newman M. A.: Newman's health theory, in Clements I. W., Roberts P. B. (Eds): *Family Health: A Theoretical Approach to Nursing Care.* New York, Wiley, 1983, pp 161–175.

COMMENTARY

Kane has developed a formulation of family social support that is founded on three major assumptions dealing with the nature of the family and the nature and benefits of social support. These are true assumptions inasmuch as they are the "givens" from which further work proceeds.

The formulation encompasses an explicit definition of the concept of family social support and concepts gleaned from the literature that may be considered antecedents and consequences of family social support. The antecedents include several family and interactional characteristics that are grouped into categories, including the family characteristics of social network dimensions, family structure, esteem, and stability; as well as the interactional characteristics of reciprocity, advice/feedback, and emotional involvement. The consequences encompass the family function categories of versatility and resourcefulness, and the health and resources categories of information, goods and services, and help in crisis.

Kane has gone beyond identification of relevant concepts to specification of directional propositions linking the concepts. She also has included diagrams of the concepts and their connections. Note that in Figure 2 the categories previously labeled as interactional characteristics are under the heading "family social support."

The specificity of Kane's formulation and the strategy used for its development indicate that when the terminology used in this book is considered, it is more appropriately labeled a *theory* rather than a *conceptual model*. And inasmuch as the emphasis is on the family system, the formulation may be classified as family, rather than family-related, theory.

JACQUELINE FAWCETT

CHAPTER
14

Healthy Single Parent Families*

SHIRLEY M. H. HANSON

The purpose of this study was to investigate characteristics of healthy single parent families. The variables that were measured included socio-economic status, social support, communication, religiousness, problem solving, and the physical and mental health status of single parents and their children. The effects of the sex of custodial parents and the custody arrangements on health outcomes were also analyzed. A multimethod, multivariable approach was used. A total of 84 subjects participated in this study. Data collection included the completion of questionnaires and an interview in the home setting. Single parents and their children reported fairly high levels of both physical and mental health. Communication, social support, socio-economic status, religiousness and problem solving were also correlated with the mental and physical health of parents and children. Implications for practice and education are discussed and recommendations for future study are made.

*The author wishes to acknowledge Gretchen Dimico, Anne Mealey, and Jo Trilling at the Intercollegiate Center for Nursing Education in Spokane, Washington who participated throughout parts of this investigation. Also, Marion Sheafor, Elizabeth Byerly, Fred Bozett, Barry Coyne, and Julia Brown offered critical review of this manuscript. This study was partially funded by the American Nurses' Foundation and Washington State University.

Reprinted from *Family Relations, 35*, 125–132, 1986.

The American family has undergone rapid transition in the past 10 years resulting in new and different family structures. One common social phenomenon is the rapid increase in single parent families due to separation and divorce. While single parent families comprised only 11% of American families in 1970, this number nearly doubled to 25.7% by 1984. Reports indicated there were 8.5 million one parent families with children under 18 years of age in 1984 (U.S. Bureau of the Census, 1985). Correspondingly, nearly 12 million of 61 million children lived with single parents; approximately 88% of these children lived with mothers while 12% lived with fathers. Projections for the future indicate that the rising incidence of single parent households will continue. Seventy percent of children born in 1980 can expect to live with only one parent at some point before they reach age 18 (Hofferth, 1985).

Single parent families have received attention by family researchers since World War II. Much of this research has focused on the negative effects of father-absence on male children in single mother homes. These studies shared such common themes as tracing father-absence as a causative factor in juvenile delinquency, inadequate sex role identification, drug abuse, lowered school achievement, poor personal adjustment, and other forms of pathology (Bane, 1976; Biller, 1974; Brandwein, Brown & Fox, 1974; Hetherington, 1971; Kelly, 1980; Kelly & Wallerstein, 1976).

In recent years, the primarily negative approach to the study of single parent families has been criticized for a variety of reasons. For example, researchers have traditionally obtained their samples from clinical populations and have focused on problems to the neglect of strengths which exist in single parent families (Blechman, 1982; Herzog & Sudia, 1971; LeMasters, 1977; Ricci, 1981; Schlesinger, 1978). The present study incorporates the more recent concepts of family strengths and family wellness. Since not all single parent households experience multiple problems, nor are all children adversely affected by divorce. This positive framework focuses on the healthiness or strengths of the family unit rather than highlight its dysfunctional qualities.

The purpose of this research was to investigate the characteristics of healthy single parent families using dimensions previously identified in the research literature with healthy two-parent nuclear families. These characteristics included the parents' and the children's socio-economic status, social support systems, level of communication, and problem solving, degree of religiousness, and the physical and mental health of the dyad.

BACKGROUND

Several investigators have attempted to delineate characteristics and behaviors of healthy families. Otto (1973) was one of the first researchers to identify an area of study called family strengths. His original work delineated four important strengths of families: communication patterns, support systems, relationships, and crisis- or problem-solving ability. Stinnett and his colleagues also studied family strengths (Stinnett, Chester & DeFrain, 1979; Stinnett & DeFrain, 1981; Stinnett, DeFrain, King, Knaub & Rowe, 1981; Stinnett, Sanders, DeFrain & Parkhurst, 1982). They characterized healthy two parent families as those in which members express appreciation for each other, spend a good deal of quality time together, enjoy good communication, maintain a high degree of commitment to one another, share a religious orientation, and demonstrate the ability to handle crises positively. Pratt (1976) conducted research to delineate healthy families by examining various family structures. She concluded that the healthy or energized family was one in which: (1) all members were actively engaged in varied and regular interaction with each other; (2) the family had ties to the broader community through active participation of its members; (3) the family had a high degree of autonomy and a tendency to encourage individuality; and, (4) the family engaged in creative problem solving and active coping. Other theoreticians and investigators have also studied health and families. Lewis, Beavers, Gossett and Phillips (1979) identified nine dimensions of "healthy" families, Glasser and Glasser (1970) delineated five general criteria for the "adequate" family, Satir (1972) discussed patterns of vital and nurturing families, and Curran (1983) wrote about 15 common traits of healthy families.

Although the characteristics of healthy families varied throughout the literature according to conceptual or stylistic differences of authors, there were some similarities among the descriptors of healthy two parent families. Most of these similarities involved psychosocial dimensions, such as those cited above, but few researchers attempted to measure these dimensions or measure the actual physical and mental health of healthy families. Also no researcher has taken this model of healthy families and applied it to other types of family structure, such as the single parent family. Much of the prior work was exploratory with data obtained by interviewing families or professionals regarding what they perceived to be characteristics of the healthy family. Few investigations have actually *measured* families on the parameters identified for study here.

This investigator selected 5 variables commonly cited in the family literature as indicative of healthy families: good social support, higher socio-economic status, effective communication, degree of religiousness, and problem solving ability. She was not only interested in measuring these variables, but determining whether or not they were related to the actual physical and mental health of single parents and their children. The overall research question which guided this study was: Are there significant relationships among the socioeconomic status, social support, communication, problem solving, religiousness and the health of single parents and their children. Could these characteristics eventually be used to predict health outcomes in single parent families? Could these variables be used to guide intervention strategies of professionals who assist single parent families?

METHOD

Sampling Procedure

The subjects were recruited from a population of separated and divorced single parent families in the Pacific Northwest of the United States. A purposive nonrandomized sample was obtained through personal and professional contacts with a variety of community organizations and individuals. Families were also recruited through newspaper advertisement, and radio talk shows and television appearances. Families identified themselves as "healthy." Healthy families were defined as systems that were in a state of physical and mental well-being. Families were retained if the trained health care professionals also assessed the family as healthy. This system of selection was the same one used by Otto (1973), Stinnett, et al. (1982) and Pratt (1976).

Other criteria for inclusion were: (1) single parents who had lived only with their children for 6 months to 5 years; and, (2) single parents who had physical custody of at least one child between the ages of 12 and 18 years. In families where more than one child qualified for the study, the teenager closest to age 15 became the focal child. Upon initial contact, families were advised of the purposes, objectives, and procedures of the study. If both parent and child agreed to participate, an appointment was made and research questionnaires and consent forms were hand delivered or mailed. During the home visit several weeks later, the instruments were collected, checked for completion, and a parental interview took place. These interviews gave respondents an opportunity to ask questions and discuss their particular situation.

Summary Description of the Sample

There were 42 families who participated in this study, the parent and the focal child, for a total of 84 subjects. Twenty-two parents were fathers and 20 were mothers. The children's sample was comprised of 19 girls and 22 boys. Families were evenly divided regarding custody: 21 had joint custody and 21 had sole custody. Over 50% of the parents were Protestant but only 40% of the children claimed to be so. Approximately one-third of the sample never attended church whereas another one-third attended on a weekly basis. The mean age of parents was 41.6 years and the mean age for children was 14.1. Thirty-seven out of 42 parents (88%) had attended or completed college and/or some graduate school. Forty-one of the children were in junior high or high school; one was a high school graduate. The mean socioeconomic score was 49 (range 20–66); men had higher socioeconomic status than women. The mean income was approximately $18,000 whereas the pre-divorce income was about $22,000. Most of the parents were working full-time. Few of the children were employed, even part-time. Only 15 out of 42 (35%) single parents reported receiving child support from their former spouse and these recipients were single mothers. Nearly half of the sample consisted of two adolescent children and one parent in the home. The parents reported a mean of 14.3 years of marriage and 4 years since separation/divorce.

Instrumentation

A variety of instruments were employed to obtain an in depth measure of the multidimensionality of the single parent family unit. Parents and children alike completed all the pencil and paper instruments. Three of the 6 tools were developed by project personnel: Demographic Form, Interview Guide, and Family Health Inventory. Additionally, three standardized measurements were also adopted. Pilot testing and human subjects approval was completed. Below is a summary of the major variables studied and the instruments used to measure them.[1]

Variables	Instruments
1. Health	Family Health Inventory (FHI)
2. Social Support System	Personal Resource Questionnaire (PRQ)
3. Socioeconomic Status	Demographic Form (Hollingshead Four Factor Index)
4. Religiousness	Family Environment Scale (FES)
5. Communication	(Family Interaction Schedule (FIS)
6. Problem Solving	(Family Interaction Schedule (FIS)

The *Demographic Form* devised by the investigators was used to collect information such as birthdate, race, height, weight, religion, church attendance and activities, education, occupation, sources of income, past and current income, home ownership, custody arrangements, length of marriage, and time since separation or divorce.

The *Interview Guide* was developed to obtain information not readily obtainable through the other instruments. Parents only participated in the interviews. Examples of some of the questions asked included:

Have you or your children had professional counseling before, during or after divorce?

Have you joined any informal or formal support groups?

---

[1]To conserve space, the psychometric features of the Family Environment Scale, Personal Resource Questionnaire, and Family Interaction Schedule are not included in the narrative. Further information on these measurement tools can be obtained from the author or from the instrument developers, who are cited in the list of references.

What was the response of your children, extended family, and friends to the divorce?

What was your major support system during the divorce?

What are the informal and legal custody and visitation arrangements?

What effect do the custodial arrangements have on the children, former spouse, and yourself?

Additional questions were asked concerning the family's religiousness, the sexual behavior of the parents, and aspect of family functioning. The interview served as an important means to gather impressions about the family and their home environment. These data will be reported in a subsequent paper.

The *Family Health Inventory* (FHI) solicited information about the parents' and children's physical and mental health. Appropriate psychometric work (reliability, stability, and validity) was completed. The questions assessed dietary, sleeping, exercise and recreation patterns, drug and smoking habits, self-care practices, preventive health care measures, dental health, medical history, health services received, history of illness and accidents, and other items important to measure the physical and mental well being of the family members. Separate scores were obtained for physical health and mental health. Physical and mental health scores were also combined to achieve an overall health score.

The *Family Environment Scale* (FES) is a widely used standardized instrument originally developed to assess different dimensions of the home environment as perceived by family members themselves (Moos & Moos, 1976, 1981). Although subjects completed the entire instrument, only the Moral Religious Subscale was computed to measure the religiousness variable.

The *Personal Resource Questionnaire* (PRQ) is an instrument designed to measure the multidimensional characteristics of social support (Brandt & Weinert, 1981). Scores obtained from the Likert Scale in part two of this tool were used to quantify the amount of social support parents and children reported receiving from their networks.

The *Family Interaction Schedule* (FIS) is an instrument developed to measure communication and problem solving in families (Straus, 1965, 1968). The level of parent/child communication was derived from scores from one subscale of this instrument. Scores for dyadical problem solving were obtained from another subscale in the FIS.

FINDINGS

Parents and children reported their perception of their own physical and mental health on 5 discrete scales on the *Family Health Inventory* (poor, fair, good, very good, excellent). The parents perceived their overall health to be fair to excellent; the modal rating was very good. The majority of the parents rated their physical health either very good or excellent ($n = 28$) and their mental health the same ($n = 27$). The children of single parents perceived their overall health from poor to excellent. Children rated their physical health as good ($n = 11$), very good ($n = 13$), and excellent ($n = 15$). They also rated their mental health from good to excellent ($n = 37$). More children than parents scored lower on their perceptions of their overall health.

Socio Economic Status and Health

The score for socioeconomic status (SES) was derived using Hollingshead Four Factor Index (1975). As noted in Table 1, the mean SES score was 49.2 and the range was 22–66. Significance was set at .05. There was a significant negative correlation ($-.361$) between the children's scores on SES and their physical health. The higher the family's SES, the worse the physical health of children. Upon further analysis there was evidence that single fathers enjoyed a statistically significant higher level of socio-

TABLE 1. Parents' and Children's Scores on Measures of Family Strengths

Variables	M	SD	Obtained Ranges	Possible Ranges
Overall Health (FHI)				
Parents	120.3	9.1	100–134	51–164
Children	121.6	10.4	92–151	51–164
Physical Health (FHI)				
Parents	75.1	5.5	62–87	33–105
Children	76.6	7.7	60–99	33–105
Mental Health (FHI)				
Parents	43.4	5.7	29–54	18–59
Children	53.3	6.0	30–54	18–59
Social Support (PRQ)				
Parents	138.7	20.6	84–174	25–175
Children	130.0	15.0	97–158	25–175
Socio-Economic Status (Hollingshead)				
Parents	49.2	13.5	20–66	8–66
Children	49.2	13.5	20–66	8–66
Communication (FIS)				
Parents	79.7	16.1	51–111	0–140
Children	85.5	20.7	45–139	0–140
Religiousness (FES)				
Parents	4.7	2.4	0–9	0–9
Children	4.3	2.3	1–9	0–9
Problem Solving (FIS)				
Parents	52.0	19.7	18–104	0–140
Children	41.0	18.8	11–102	0–140

TABLE 2. Correlations between Parents' Major Variables

	Overall Health	Physical Health	Mental Health	Socio-Economic Status	Social Support	Communication	Problem Solving	Religiousness FES
Overall Health	1.0							
Physical Health	.800***	1.0						
Mental Health	.813***	.300*	1.0					
Socio-Economic Status	-.222	-.150	.206	1.0				
Social Support	.231	.011	.356**	.099	1.0			
Communication	.236	.013	.362**	.195	.216	1.0		
Problem Solving	-.031	.052	-.1	.161	-.105	-.119	1.0	
Religiousness FES	-.125	-.134	-.069	-.209	.04	.204	-.254	1.0

*p < .05; **p < .01; ***p < .001.

economic status than single mothers but the children living with single fathers had a lower physical health score.

Social Support and Health

Social support as measured by the *Personal Resource Questionnaire* resulted in a mean of 138.7 (range 84 – 174) for parents and a mean of 130 for children (range 97 – 158). There was no significant relation between parents and children on social support ($p = .153$). Parents enjoyed a wider network of social support than children. There was a significant correlation between parent's mental health and social support (.356) and between children's overall health and social support (.298). The greater the social support the higher the level of overall health.

Communication and Health

The mean communication score on the *Family Interaction Schedule* was 79.7 (range 51 – 111) for parents and 85.5 (range 45 – 139) for children. The relationship between parents and children's communication was significant ($r = .428$, $p = .002$). Children rated their communication higher than their parents. There was a significant correlation between parent's communication and mental health (.362) and between children's communication and their overall health (.382) and mental health (.369). The higher the quality of communication, the better the health, particularly mental health.

Problem Solving and Health

The score for problem solving was obtained from selected portions of the *Family Interaction Schedule*. Both parents and children were asked to report how fairly decisions were made around the household. Discrepancy scores between the dyad were then computed. The lower the discrepancy, the higher the problem solving between the pair. Parents reported more discrepancy between them and their children, therefore, children perceived better parent/child problem solving than did parents. There was a significant relationship between parents and children on problem solving ($r = .428$, $p = .002$). There were no significant correlations between the level of problem solving and the health status of each member of the pair.

Religiousness and Health

Religiousness was measured using the moral/religious subscale on the *Family Environment Scale*. Parents obtained a mean of 4.7 (range 0 – 9) and children 4.3 (range 1 – 9) hence parents reported a somewhat higher

TABLE 3. Correlations between Children's Major Variables

	Overall Health	Physical Health	Mental Health	Socio-Economic Status	Social Support	Communication	Problem Solving	Religiousness FES
Overall Health	1.0							
Physical Health	.804***	1.0						
Mental Health	.670***	.096	1.0					
Socio-Economic Status	-.222	-.361**	.079	1.0				
Social Support	.298*	.229	.212	-.220	1.0			
Communication	.382**	.215	.369**	.057	.479***	1.0		
Problem Solving	.037	-.143	.241	.002	-.276*	.114	1.0	
Religiousness FES	.275*	.422**	-.075	.261*	.160	.287*	.070	1.0

*p < .05; **p < .01; ***p < .001.

TABLE 4. Correlations between Children and Parents on Major Variables

Children's Major Variables	Overall Health	Physical Health	Mental Health	Socio-Economic Status	Social Support	Communication	Problem Solving	Religiousness FES
Overall Health	.260*	.162	.256	-.222	.037	.442**	-.113	.071
Physical Health	.050	.061	.020	.361**	-.034	.313*	-.054	.189
Mental Health	.373**	.196	.403**	.079	.105	.348*	-.122	.356**
Socio-Economic Status	.222	.150	.206	1.0	.099	.195	.161	-.209
Social Support	-.029	-.124	.074	.220	.162	.246	-.274*	.091
Communication	.076	-.050	.169	.057	-.082	.428**	-.025	.044
Problem Solving	.205	.199	.133	.002	-.001	.058	.428**	-.224
Religiousness FES	-.011	.001	-.019	.261*	-.090	.227	.023	.631***

$p < .05$; $p < .01$; $p < .001$.

level of religiousness. The relationship between parents and children was significant ($r = .631$, $p = .0001$). There was a positive correlation between children's religiousness and their overall health (.275) and physical health (.422) but no such relationship existed for parents. The higher the level of religiousness in children, the higher their health status.

Additional Results: Correlations

Additional correlations of interest were computed between other major variables. There were significant correlations between parents' physical health and overall health (.800), mental health and overall health (.813), and mental health and physical health (.300), all of which demonstrates the high positive interrelationships between the mind and body. If a single parent feels psychologically good, they are more likely to enjoy good physical health as well.

There were also significant correlations between children's physical health and overall health (.804), mental health and overall health (.670), communication and social support (.479), problem solving and social support (.276), and religiousness with socioeconomic status (.261) and communication (.287). In general, the variables measuring children were more highly correlated with each other than were the same variables measuring the parents.

Finally, correlations were computed between children's and parent's scores on major variables. The following correlations were significant: overall health of children with parent's overall health (.260) and parent's communication (.442); children's physical health with parent's socioeconomic status (.361) and communication (.313); children's mental health with the parent's overall health (.373), mental health (.403), communication (.348) and religiousness (.356). Children's problem solving was significantly correlated with parent's problem solving (.428). Finally, children's religiousness was significantly correlated with parent's socioeconomic status (.261) and religiousness (.631).

DISCUSSION AND CONCLUSIONS

The purpose of this study was to investigate the characteristics of healthy single parent families and to begin to identify those characteristics which might be used to predict the physical and mental health outcomes of divorcing parents and their children. A summary of the findings and concluding remarks follow.

In general, the *physical and mental health status* of these single parents and their children appear to be good. There were high correlations between the physical and mental health of parents and children alike once again demonstrating the interrelatedness of mind and body. Good health in parents is associated with good health in children.

There are some differences in the *health* of parents and children according to *sex*. Children living with female parents reported higher overall health than children living with male parents. Boys in particular enjoyed higher levels of health than girls, especially in relation to mental health. Boys living with their mothers had the best overall health whereas girls living with their fathers had the least. In terms of the parents, single mothers had poorer overall health than fathers. These findings suggest that mother's health is lower than their children's health but father's health is higher than their children. Are mothers sacrificing their own health for their children, or was this a spurious finding? One cannot help but wonder about the historical role that females play in our society in maintaining health of their families and what influence this may have had on these results. Also, do women generally see themselves as less healthy than men?

The health of parents and children also varied according to the *custody* arrangement. Fathers with sole custody of boys reported the highest level of mental health and mothers with sole custody of boys reported the lowest mental health; joint custody parents were about equal. This finding suggests that fathers feel better than mothers about sole custody of male children and that joint custody arrangements contribute to the mental health of mothers.

REFERENCES

Blechman, E. (1982). Are children with one parent at psychological risk? A methodological review. *Journal of Marriage and the Family*, 44, 179–195.

Brandt, P. A., & Weinert, C. (1981). The PRQ-A social support system. *Nursing Research*, 30, 277–280.

Brandwein, R. A., Brown, C. A., & Fox, E. M. (1974). Women and children last: The social situation of divorced mothers and their families. *Journal of Marriage and the Family*, 36, 498–514.

Curran, D. (1983). *Traits of a healthy family*. Minneapolis: Winston Press.

Glasser, P., & Glasser, L. (1970). *Families in crisis*. New York: Harper & Row.

Herzog, E., & Sudia, C. E. (1971). *Boys in fatherless families*. Washington, DC: U.S. Government Printing Office.

Hetherington, E. M. (1971). The effects of father absence on child development. *Young Children*, 27, 233–248.

Hofferth, S. L. (1985). Updating children's life course. Journal of Marriage and the Family, 47(1), 93–115.

Hollingshead, A. B. (1975). *Four factor index of social status*. New Haven, CT: 1965 Yale Station.

Kelly, J. (1980). Myths and realities for children of divorce. *Educational Horizons*, 59, 34–39.

Kelly, J., & Wallerstein, J. (1976). The effects of parental divorce: Experiences of the child in early latency. *American Journal of Orthopsychiatry*, 46, 20–32.

LeMasters, E. E. (1977). *Parents in modern America*. Homewood, IL: The Dorsey Press.

Lewis, J. M., Beavers, W. R., Gossett, J. T., & Phillips, V. A. (1976). *No single thread: Psychological health in family systems*. New York: Brunner/Mazel, Inc.

Moos, R. H., & Moos, B. S. (1976). A typology of family social environments. *Family Process*, 15, 357–372.

Moos, R. H., & Moos, B. S. (1981). *Family environment scale manual*. Palo Alto, CA: Consulting Psychologists Press.

Otto, H. (1973). A framework for assessing family strengths. In A. Reinhardt & M. Quinn (Eds.) *Family-centered community nursing* (pp. 42–56). St. Louis: C. V. Mosby.

Pratt, L. (1976). *Family structure and effective health behavior. The energized family*. Boston: Houghton Mifflin Company.

Ricci, I. (1980). *Mom's house, dad's house: Making shared custody work*. New York: Macmillan.

Satir, V. (1972). *Peoplemaking*. Palo Alto, CA: Science and Behavior Books.

Schlesinger, B. (1978). *One-parent families: Perspectives and annotated bibliography*. Toronto: University of Toronto.

Stinnett, N., Chester, B., & DeFrain, J. (Eds.). (1979). *Building family strengths: Blueprints for action*. Lincoln, NE: University of Nebraska Press.

Stinnett, N., & DeFrain, J. (1981). Strong families: A national study. In N. Stinnett & J. DeFrain (Eds). *Family strengths 3: Roots of well-being* (pp. 33–43). Lincoln, NE: University of Nebraska Press.

Stinnett, N., DeFrain, J., King K., Knaub, P., & Rowe, G. (1981). *Family strengths 3: Roots of well-being*. Lincoln, NE: University of Nebraska Press.

Stinnett, N., Sanders, G., DeFrain, J., & Parkhurst, A. (1982). A nationwide study of families who perceive themselves as strong. *Family Perspective*, 16(1).

Straus, M. (1965). Family interaction schedule manual. Durham, NH: University of New Hampshire.

Straus, M. A. (1968). Communication, creativity and problem solving ability of middle and working class families in three societies. *American Journal of Sociology*, 73, 417–430.

U.S. Bureau of the Census. (1985). *Household and family characteristics: March 1984* (Current Population Reports, Series P-20, No. 371). Washington, DC: Government Printing Office.

COMMENTARY

The study reported by Hanson focuses on self-identified healthy single-parent families made up of mothers or fathers and a teenage child. Just one child in each family was considered in the study, even if the family included other children. Hanson's definition of healthy families indicates an interest in systems and considers health as having physical and mental dimensions. These components of the definition represent assumptions that provided a particular context for the middle-range theory development work. Indeed, Hanson points out that her study is guided by a "positive framework [that] focuses on healthiness or strengths of the family unit rather than highlight its dysfunctional qualities."

Data analytic techniques emphasized individual level data, with variable scores obtained from the parents and the children. Given the methodological deviation from the conceptual perspective of the family unit or system, the work must be considered family-related theory development.

The intent of the study was to determine the scope of middle-range theory about healthy families. As Hanson points out, previous work relied exclusively on data from healthy two-parent families: The findings of her research, then, contribute to our understanding of the single-parent family in juxtaposition to the two-parent family.

Findings of particular interest in this study are the differences in health of parents and children on the basis of gender and custody arrangement. The implications of these findings for future family nursing theory development are intriguing.

JACQUELINE FAWCETT

THE IMPACT OF ILLNESS ON THE FAMILY

CHAPTER

15

Misogyny and Homicide of Women

JACQUELYN CAMPBELL

Homicide is defined as the "willful (non-negligent) killing of one human being by another."[1(p237)] In 1971 homicide was the leading cause of death for black women from 15 to 34 years of age and the third highest cause of death for white women from 15 to 29 years of age.[2(pp8-11)] In 1973 statistics listed homicide as the second leading cause of death for all women from 15 to 24 years of age.[3(p195)] Homicide must therefore be regarded as a major health problem of women, a problem that needs further study.

It can be viewed as a disease of society — and it needs to be analyzed in that context so that the direction that primary prevention should take can be identified. Herjanic and Meyer state: "The development of meaningful preventive measures depends on repeated epidemiological investigations to determine the changes in pattern of crime."[1(p 196)] Homicide rates over time and associated demographical characteristics of the victim and perpetrator are appropriate objects of evaluation in order to discover patterns and trends. The study on which this article is based used the police files of murdered women in Dayton, Ohio, a midwestern city of approximately 200,000 individuals, to examine in detail the patterns of homicide of women.

These patterns must be studied in conjunction with an analysis of their roots to provide a comprehensive model on which to base preven-

Reprinted from *Advances in Nursing Science*, 3(2), 67–85, 1981.

tive measures. Highriter calls for nursing research studies to combine descriptive analysis of statistics with theory in order to advance community health nursing science.[4] Pilisak and Ober demonstrate the need to view violence in a public health perspective, to conduct "inquiry into the distribution of the malady within the total population and into the facts about the social system that correlate with this incidence."[5(p389)]

The missing element from most theories of violence is a thorough analysis of the role of misogyny (hatred of women). In 1977, of the 2,740 American female homicide victims, 2,447 of the perpetrators were men.[6(p9)] During the same year, of 8,565 men murdered, 1,780 of the offenders — only 21% — were women.[6(p9)] During the period January 1, 1968, through December 31, 1979, of a total of 873 homicides in Dayton, 192 of the victims were women. A total of 175 (91%) of the murderers of these women were male; 17 (9%) were female. In contrast, of the 681 men killed during that period, only 19% (127) of the perpetrators were women.

The predominance of men killing women over women killing men in both local and national statistics cannot be explained solely by attributing the male predilection for violence to a biological tendency toward aggression, because of the fact that cultures exist in which there is virtually no homicide or other violence.[7,8] The possibility that misogyny is operating when men kill women needs to be considered and explored by scholars. Sills called for nursing research that examines "the relationships of sexism, racism, poverty, and other forms of deprivation to . . . health care."[9(p206)] Consequently this article examines the underlying causes of homicides of women in Dayton.

THEORETICAL FRAMEWORK: THE PATRIARCHAL SOCIETY

Steinmetz and Straus assert that "any social pattern as widespread and enduring as violence must have fundamental and enduring causes."[10(p321)] It is necessary to look at these causes when examining the aspect of violence in homicide of women. Biological, psychological, and sociological factors all need to be analyzed as part of the roots of violence. Although misogyny integrates all of these aspects, it has been absent from most theories regarding violence. Misogyny is a theoretical framework that needs to be considered in relationship to homicide of women. Misogyny derives from the patriarchal social system, which is an integral part of the social forces that Steinmetz and Straus state need to be understood, "because most aspects of violence, like most aspects of other human behavior, are the product of social forces interacting with basic human potential."[10(p17)]

Patriarchy can be defined as "any kind of group organization in which males hold dominant power and determine what part females shall and shall not play, and in which capabilities assigned to women are relegated generally to the mystical and esthetic and excluded from the practical and political realms."[11(p79)] Patriarchy has been the primary social form in recorded history, but growing archeological and anthropological evidence indicates that more equitable or matriarchal forms dominated society before recorded history. Violence, in terms of people killing each other, was virtually unknown.[7,12] These early cultural remnants show female deities sharing in power and in policymaking, and natural divisions of labor that were complementary and equally important, based partially (but not entirely) on sex.[12,13]

Fear of Women

The roots of the patriarchal societal organization probably can be most logically traced to men's fear of women in primitive times because of the unexplained mystery of reproduction.[14] Thousands of legends from all around the world indicate some crisis occurring when leadership was "wrested from the women, either by force or seduction or both" between 7500 BC and 1250 BC.[15(p203)] Early recorded history shows the efforts of men to overcome their fear by establishing a religious basis for the subjugation of women and depreciation of the woman's role.[16] Early Greek patriarchal formulations are based on the concepts of subjugation of nature and the linking of male "essential selves with a transcendent principle beyond nature which is pictured as intellectual and male."[17(p13)] Men eagerly accepted this paradigm, and the "first oppressor-oppressed relation, the foundation of all other class and property relations," became entrenched.[17(p3)]

Patriarchal Nuclear Family

The patriarchal formation was spread through religion, war, written history, and economics. Each subsequent sociological and economic development further divided the sexes and subjugated the female. Today every avenue of power is almost entirely controlled by men.[18] The male image of aggression is reflected in class and discrimination systems and attempts at controlling nature, wars, the arms race, ecological pollution, and widespread violence. Misogyny is embedded in patriarchy and is a basic part of the violence against women and nature in American society.

Childrearing Patterns

The patriarchal social and economic system has resulted in childrearing patterns where the mother has primary responsibility, especially during the early years. The lack of early parenting by fathers results in identification with mothers by both sexes. By school age, however, the boys are identifying with male figures and are often being taught to disown and fear all the attributes learned previously that might be considered "feminine" within themselves and frequently overemphasize the "masculine" attributes.[19] This rejection and fear of "feminine" characteristics is also transferred to women in general as misogyny.[19,20]

The sociological conditioning of men and women that begins in the home and is continued by the patriarchal society's institutions further teaches and encourages the expression of misogyny. Boys are taught the "male"[21-23] roles of competitiveness, aggression, superiority over, and disdain for women. The school-aged boy is thought normal when he avoids girls and talks openly of hating them. The major mechanism being expressed here may be misogyny rather than repression of sexual longings, the traditional explanation. This hatred, conceived in the parenting arrangements and the male psyche and nurtured by socialization of males, is then repressed later by sexual necessity.

Literature, History, and the Media

Exposure to literature, history, and the media, conceived mainly by men, continues to reinforce misogyny and the sex role stereotypes.[18] Male historians have selectively interpreted facts to make the traditional roles seem like the natural order, have negated the accomplishments of women, and have diminished female historical works.[12,18,24] Women are systematically discouraged from all creative endeavors, and their literary and artistic works are often maligned by male critics.[11]

The media are replete with sexism in print and advertising.[25] Television's heroes are the perfect embodiment of the male image of aggression and virility complete with frequent acts of violence against women.[26] Exposure to violent television can result in increased expressions of aggression in free play and moral approval of aggressive solutions to problems, especially in boys.[27] These outgrowths of the patriarchal system contribute to misogyny and its violent expression.

Religion

The unconscious hatred of women is nurtured and legitimized by religion. The Christian tradition depicts women as sinful. Much religious training is done while children are young and impressionable and unable to distinguish between myth and history.

Psychoanalytic Theory

In modern society "psychoanalysis has become the chief tool, replacing patriarchal religion, for rationalizing and sanctifying the inferiority of women."[28(p137)] Psychoanalytic theory, starting with Freud, has strengthened misogyny by accepting the idea that women are naturally defective and postulating that any woman who rebels against a stereotyped role is mentally ill and needs to be cast out by society or "cured" by the patriarchal figure of the psychiatrist.[24] In the psychoanalytic tradition mothers are blamed for most psychiatric ills, and yet motherhood is the only acceptable role for women.[11] By basing female psychology on "penis envy," Freud and his followers bolster the idea that women are inferior and therefore worthy of contempt.[18] If little girls envy little boys, it is their eventual succession to the elevations of prestige and power that girls see occupied by men that is envied, not their biology.[28] Thus psychoanalytic theories and treatment have served men by legitimizing further the oppression of women and contributed to male hatred of the female sex.

MACHISMO

The most virulent effect of growing up as a male in patriarchal society is the form of the masculine ethic known as *machismo*. This concept has been written about from the perspectives of many different disciplines and has variously been called "compulsive masculinity" and "macho" in the literature.[29,30] The following definition of machismo has been derived from a review and synthesis of most of this literature: the male attitude and behavior arising from and supported by the patriarchal social structure, which exalts strength and power, demands competition with and superiority over other men, glorifies violence, emphasizes virility, despises gentleness and expressing any emotion except anger and rage, and rigidly defines women as property, sexual objects, and subject of male domination. Misogyny is inherent in machismo. This doctrine is prevalent in most males in most patriarchal societies.

An extensive review of the literature surrounding violence, especially homicide, has shown that although seldom used as the central causative factor in theories of violence, machismo or a similar concept links violence theories from anthropology, sociology, criminology, psychology, and feminist viewpoints. For instance, Paddock, an anthropologist, studied two small towns 10 miles apart in Mexico that had basically the same socioeconomic and cultural backgrounds. One was virtually free of homicide while the other had a high homicide rate. One of the major differences Paddock found was that "machismo was all but absent" in the nonviolent community.[31] Whiting, another anthropologist, has also linked macho values to high rates of homicide and warfare in primitive societies.[32] The sociological subculture of violence theory was based on evidence better explained by a "subculture of masculinity," according to two separate reviews of the empirical research.[33,34] At least four separate psychological and criminological studies of murderers have noted a strong machismo ethic in the majority of subjects even while looking primarily for other characteristics.[35-38] Both Toch and Toby, in their studies of violent men, have found extensive machismo.[39-40] Men writing with a feminist awareness of the problems of patriarchal conditioning of men see the widespread prevalence of the macho ethic and warn of its violent, selfish, and otherwise destructive and misogynous nature.[19,41,42]

An Impossible Model

Male self-esteem is based on the impossible model of invulnerability, perfect competence, fearlessness, virility, power, and always winning.[40] Oppression of women or other classes or races enhances the power of men. The extreme oppression insisted upon by those described as being macho is often enforced by violence and is associated with shakier self-esteem than that of the normal male.

Powerlessness and Violence

When males feel that they are becoming powerless, violence or the threat of violence often results.[39,43] Toby stated that "violence may be the most appropriate way to protect one's honor, to show courage or conceal fear, especially fear of revealing weakness."[39(p22)] In the lower social classes the male is more likely to turn to violence because he is more impotent economically and politically.[43] He is more likely to claim authority on the strength of sex rank alone because he is usually forced to share more economic power with women.[18] These factors are reflected in higher rates of homicide and violence among poor males and their increased acceptance and respect for extreme machismo. Although poor women are more powerless than poor men, they do not generally turn to violence. Therefore powerlessness cannot completely explain the differences between the rates of homicide and violence in the poor versus the middle class unless the concept of machismo is added.

EVIDENCE OF MISOGYNY: GYNOCIDE

Homicide of women can be viewed within the context of other violent practices directed against women. Men use various mechanisms to generate fear in women and thereby ensure the continuation of the patriarchy and their continued domination.[44] Homicide of women is only one such practice. Dworkin defines gynocide as "the systematic crippling and/or killing of women by men."[45(p16)] Practices of gynocide can be considered as evidence of general misogyny and can be traced throughout history. There are no examples of correspondingly serious and lethal victimizations of men by women.

Witchburning

Witchburning, the slaughter of women who did not conform to the stereotyped role of the subservient medieval woman, is the earliest well-documented form of gynocide in history. "Tens of thousands of female peasant lay healers and midwives were burned as witches" in Europe from the 1500s to the 1700s.[46(pxxi)]

Suttee

Another form of gynocide occurred during the same period in India. The practice of *suttee*, or the inclusion of the widow in the male's funeral pyre, was firmly based on the belief that the wife was responsible for her husband's death, if not in this life, then in her previous lives. The practice included the man's many wives and concubines. Because men tried to marry child brides and concubines were also included in suttee, the practice exterminated many thousands of women. The widows were often drugged or coerced. Even if not forced, the women realized that their alternatives were to either sell themselves into prostitution or throw themselves on the mercy of their husband's relatives for a life of servitude and starvation. Suttee still occasionally occurs today, and the Indian beliefs about the expendable nature of the female sex continue to persist. The modern gynocide in India consists in insisting that men eat before women so that females often go hungry, in the starving of undesirable female babies, and in the killing of wives and daughters for "public embarrassment," especially "habitual disobedience," and for having illegitimate babies.[24,47(pp155,156)]

Footbinding

Another historical pattern of female destruction is the Chinese practice of footbinding. No Chinese woman was considered attractive to males unless her feet were tiny stumps that had been stunted by years of excruciatingly painful binding during childhood. She may not have been killed, but she was, in effect, crippled. She was made into the ultimate example of total dependency on her husband or father, unable to move more than a few steps without assistance.[24]

Gynecology

The medical practice of gynecology was and is a form of gynocide in Western society. It started with the late nineteenth century procedures of clitoridectomy, oophrectomy, and hysterectomy, used to cure female masturbation, insanity, deviation from the "proper" female role, overactive sexual appetite, and rebellion against husband or father. Gynecological gynocide continued through the "theft of childbirth" from women so that the event became a ritual in which the woman was reduced to a semi-helpless state, strapped into a position anatomically detrimental to delivery of a child but convenient to the physician, who became the star of the birth process. It has continued in the loss of life and reproductive capacity and mutilation of women being caused by superfluous hysterectomies, the Dalkon shield, diethylstilbestrol (DES), unnecessarily mutilating breast cancer surgeries, the originally poorly tested birth-control pill, and the coercive sterilization of poor women — all at the hands of predominantly male physicians.[46] Today's gynocide and misogyny may be more subtle, but the damage still occurs.

Female Circumcision

Today, in other cultures, gynocidal practices occur that are even more horrifying. The most extreme example is the genital mutilation practiced in much of east, west, and central Africa and parts of the Middle East. It can take the form of removal of the tip of the clitoris or excision of all of the external genitalia except the labia majora. It may be accompanied by infibulation, which refers to closure of the wound, except for a small opening for urination and menstrual blood, by sewing with catgut or by using thorns. This is often done in villages, without anesthesia, with razor blades, although it is also performed by physicians in modern hospitals. Rough estimates indicate that 25 to 30 million young girls are victimized by this brutal practice every year, because men in these cultures require the procedure before they will marry a woman. It denies the woman even mild sexual pleasure and leaves her sexual activity completely under patriarchal control because the husband can have her opened and refibulated at will. These operations are practiced in areas where the status of women is lowest.[24,48]

These same cultures reinforce male dominance with other forms of violence against women. Wives can be killed with little negative sanction for failure to obey their husbands.[49] In the Islamic culture: If an Arab woman commits adultery, either her husband, her father, or even her brother will kill her, because she has brought disgrace upon both her husband's family and her own family. The killing of the woman is called "the honor debt." Her dead body will restore honor to the family name.[50(p100)]

In Algeria if a bride is not proved to be a virgin on the wedding night, she will be killed by her father or brothers.[51] A Saudi Arabian princess was executed (along with her lover) by her grandfather for committing adultery in 1977, although her husband had left her.[52] An anonymous prominent Saudi woman interviewed in respect to that case concluded that the princess was made into an example because she tried to publicly revolt against the prescribed, completely subjugated role of women in that culture.[52]

These violent practices against women keep them subordinate through instilling realistic fear. Cultures that positively sanction such gynocide have also been linked with high general rates of homicide.[53] Machismo, misogyny, and violence are apparently tolerated and even encouraged in such cultures.

Rape

Rape is an example of violence against women that is prevalent in all patriarchal cultures. Brownmiller has documented the history of rape as an expression of hatred toward women and "a conscious process of intimidation by which all men keep all women in a state of fear."[54(p5)] Studies of rape and rapists have concluded that it is a crime of violence rather than of passion and that machismo attitudes and ambivalence toward women are found in the majority of rapists.[55,56] Rape takes many forms, including incest, marital rape, and the sexual abuse of clients by male psychotherapists, none of which are prosecuted criminally except in rare cases.[54]

Wife Abuse

Wife abuse is another gynocidal practice that is just beginning to be documented and fully examined. The patriarchal system that defines women as property of their spouses allows wife beating as an extension of that philosophy. Martin, Davidson, and the Dobashes have delineated the history of wife abuse as a lawful privilege of the husband until the late 1800s and as an unofficially sanctioned practice today.[58-60] The basic hatred of women that underlies this violence is brought out in the attitude of most wife beaters — that is, that she deserved it.[61] Intent, sadistic mutilation, the importance of male dominance as the main causative issue, and machismo attitudes in abusers have been documented by abuse researchers.[60,62,63] Wife abusers are generally men who feel powerless in some way and need to physically dominate their wives.[58] They exemplify the shaky male self-esteem that needs to be reinforced by oppression of others and the male hatred of female characteristics.

HOMICIDE AS A GYNOCIDAL PRACTICE

Obsession with Purity

Daly has identified several characteristics of gynocidal practices that tend to obscure the horror and misogyny of the crimes and allow men to escape full culpability.[24(pp131-133)] There is an obsession with the purity of the victims with each of these practices.[24] Jealousy as a manifestation of the male need for sexual control of his property is a form of obsession with purity that often leads to wife abuse and murder of wives, girl-friends, and former wives.[64] Homicide of young, virginal white women was found to generate much more publicity than other murders of women in Dayton, with frequent mention made of details of the undress of the victims.[65,66] Conversely, when the victim was sexually experi-enced, mention of this appeared frequently in the police files, but the community expressed little interest in the case, and the media generated little demand for the arrest of the killer.[67]

Erasure of Responsibility

The second major characteristic is an "erasure of responsibility for the atrocities," which can take the form of blaming cultural tradition, as with the practices of African genital mutilation and Chinese footbinding, or perpetuating myths that surround the practice and subtly blame the victim.[24(p132),62] Myths about victims of rape wanting to be violated or being able to fend off their attackers if they tried hard enough make it seem as though women are to blame for the crime.[54] The myth of female masochism and the traditions and cultural norms of husbands' hitting wives make wife abusers seem less guilty.[62] Myths associated with homi-cide of women also include female masochism and the ideas that men who kill women are psychotic or drunk, which makes them somehow less responsible for their crimes. Actual psychiatric pathology in criminal populations is estimated at only 18%, and the rates of violence for those patients labeled "criminally insane" is "not remarkably different" from the normal population.[68] Alcohol may neurobiologically reduce some of the normal inhibitions against violence, but "drunken deportment is situationally variable and essentially a learned affair" and can provide an "excuse in advance" for violence.[69(pp114-116)]

The Problem with Research

The final linking characteristic of gynocidal practices is that so-called "objective" research into each of the practices has lessened their impact by failing to question "the basic cultural assumptions which make the atrocious ritual possible and plausible" such as misogyny and female oppression.[24(p131)] Such research also fails to link the practice with the other similar instances of violence against women and tends in various ways to excuse the men.

RAPE

For instance, Amir found a 19% rate of "victim precipitation" in his study of rapes in Philadelphia.[70(p250)] The concept of victim precipitation was originally defined as when the "victim is the first to use physical force, show and/or use a weapon or strike a blow."[71(p2)] However, Amir classified all women who had a "bad reputation," were known as promiscuous, admitted having sex before with the offender, were not a virgin if younger than 18 years old, or had been raped before and did not prosecute as having precipitated their abuse.[70(p267)] In this way he has absolved close to one fifth of the rapists that he studied. Moreover, he has furthered the myths that substantial numbers of rape victims invite this atrocity.

WIFE ABUSE

Most wife abuse literature has also obscured the fact that coercive control of their wives is the main purpose of abusive men.[60,62,72] History provides extensive precedent for wife beaters, and the institutions of patriarchal society implicitly support the abusers rather than the abused.[61] Recent research into violence in the family has led one of the authors to create another mechanism to excuse a gynocidal practice that is already beginning to be reflected in other wife abuse literature.[76] Steinmetz has concluded that husband abuse may be as prevalent and serious as wife abuse.[73] However, she has used data that blur the differences between using all forms of violence, predominantly minor, and the kind of repetitive, frequent, prolonged, minimally provoked, serious assault that can involve sexual mutilation and other forms of sadism that most experts define as actual wife abuse.[60,62,72] Although a few wives undoubtedly beat their husbands, and some couples are equally assaultive toward each other, this kind of beating is reserved almost exclusively for women.[72] When family violence is examined in depth, the evidence supports the contention of the Dobashes: "Violence in the family is not randomly distributed among family members, but is disproportionately directed at females."[60(p433)] Except for the feminists, the experts on wife abuse fail to stress the misogyny suggested by the facts.

Research on homicide of women has also failed to connect the crime with other gynocidal practices and has served to minimize the realities, thus lessening the culpability of men. The literature generally has paid scant attention to homicide of women.[74] Theories of violence have been based on research carried out mainly by men using male subjects. This obscures the sex differences in aggression.[75] Crimes committed by women constitute less than 16% of the total, and violent acts are an even lower proportion.[75] Warren states: "This low contribution to the crime rate of a part of the population constituting more than 50% of the total remains the most consistent, significant and unexplained fact in criminology."[75(p145)] Machismo and misogyny in males may at least partially explain this disparity.

Victim Precipitation

Homicide of women by men is also legitimized by an emphasis on the statistics that show wives killing husbands approximately as often as the opposite. When authors like Langley and Levy conclude, "When it comes to spouse killing, there is true equality between the sexes," they are making generalizations without looking closely at the data.[76(p6)] Curtis found in his national survey of 17 major cities that victim precipitation in homicide and assault was "considerably more likely" among "males of both races" than females.[77(p84)]

Yet Curtis negates the impact of these data when he refers to victim precipitation as follows: "Husbands, in particular, may give their wives a push. . . ," making the precipitation sound minor.[78(p58)] The analysis of the Dayton data used the original strict definition of victim precipitation, as do most studies of homicide. In Dayton victim precipitation was always actual, showing a weapon or striking a blow (punching or slapping), and usually the blows were repeated. None of the offenders, male or female, was provoked to murder by "a push." The overall precipitation rate was 7.7% (5) for female victims compared with 60.5% (26) of the male victims. For females and males in intimate relationships, the percentages were 7.1% (2) of women who were first to use force and were subsequently killed versus 79.3% (23) of the men. Table 1 illustrates this difference and also compares other circumstances surrounding the intrasex homicides between intimately related men and women (husband-wife, girlfriend-boyfriend, or estranged same) in Dayton, Ohio, from 1975 through 1979.

Comparing Histories of Abuse

The comparisons of history of abuse by the victim and perpetrator in the intimate relationship category shown in Table 1 are also significant. Male victims had beaten their spouse in the past in 23 (79.3%), of the cases. Female victims had been at least equally violent toward the spouse prior to the homicide in only two (7.1%) of these cases. Eighteen (64.3%) of the male killers had beaten the woman involved, but none of the cases concerning female killers indicated prior husband abuse. More indication of prior abuse stems from the records of police calls to the home for family violence within the past 2 years in more than half the cases.

Because the prevalence of prior husband abuse is so low, it seems likely that most of the calls were because of wife abuse, although some of them could have been for violence with other people in or outside of the family. Police records of violent crime and witness reports of previous acts of violence revealed that 67.9% of the men killing women and 58.6% of male victims had histories of violence, indicating that violent men resided in most of these homes.

TABLE 1. Homicides of Men and Women in Intimate Relationships in Dayton, Ohio (1975–1979)

	Males Killed by Females		Females Killed by Males	
	Number	*Percent*	*Number*	*Percent*
Victim	29	100	28	100
Intoxicated	15	51.7	4	14.3
History of violence	17	58.6	3	10.7
History of abuse of partner	23	79.3	2	7.1
Offender				
Intoxicated	9	31.0	10	35.7
History of violence	9	31.0	19	67.9
Used excessive violence	5	17.3	17	60.7
History of abuse	0	0	18	64.3
Relationship				
Husband-wife	22	75.9	12	42.9
Boyfriend-girlfriend	3	10.3	5	17.9
Estranged husband-wife or boyfriend-girlfriend	4	13.8	11	39.2
Reasons				
Victim precipitation	23	79.3	2	7.1
Male jealousy	10	34.5	18	64.3
Female jealousy	2	6.9	0	0
Male dominance	8	17.8	5	17.9
Psychosis in offender	4	13.8	5	17.9
Previous police calls to home for family violence	15	51.7	15	53.6

The police had visited 11 of the 57 homes for "family trouble," assault, or other violence more than 3 times, and the police were called to one home 13 times and to another 12 times for these incidents. These 11 extremely violent households had also been involved in numerous other police dispatches; one had been visited a total of 56 times by the police in the 2 years prior to the homicide. These families were obviously well known to the police. It seems reasonable to assume that a criminal justice system more effective against violent men, especially wife abusers, might have been able to prevent at least some of the homicides.

Intoxication and Machismo

Men, either as victims or perpetrators, were also far more likely to be intoxicated than the women involved. Rather than as an excuse for violence, intoxication is best viewed as partially an indication of machismo ethic in which "drunken violence is the last line of defense" of a threatened male's masculinity.[79(p28)] However, alcohol's contribution to violence in the lessening of inhibitions can also be seen in the female offenders.

Jealousy

Jealousy is apparent as a large portion of the reason given for homicide of wives or girlfriends by their husbands or lovers. When male jealousy is cited as a reason for wives' killing husbands, this was the precipitating factor that began the wife abuse incident that terminated in the abuser's death. Male jealousy is also cited as a frequent cause of wife beating and is actually most logically and parsimoniously viewed within the context of a husband's or boyfriend's effort to maintain control over "his woman."[60,62,64] Because women are considered the possession of men in patriarchy, real or imagined sexual infidelity is the gravest threat to male dominance. The wife abuse literature suggests that most of the female sexual infidelity is imagined and, even if not, should not be considered as justification for violence.[60,62]

An important aspect of the jealousy cases in Dayton were the eight female victims who had left or divorced the man or had threatened to do so. In all but one of these cases there was also a history of wife abuse. These data strongly support the idea that abused women are being realistic when they cite being afraid of retaliation as a reason for staying in an abusive relationship.[62] In wife abuse literature this reason has traditionally been given little credence; instead the myth of female masochism has often been used to explain battered wives' staying.[62(p15)] Other male dominance issues such as the woman's refusing to get more wine, refusing sex, or refusing to give the man money began the altercation that accounted for 22.8% of these killings. The concept that women should be subordinate to their men can be seen as a lethal premise for some men and women.

Excessive Violence

Four of the intimate male-female relationship killings of women had elements of particular cruelty and sadism, such as the man's handcuffing the woman before shooting her or his keeping the woman a prisoner for 6 months as he slowly beat her to death. In 17 (60.9%) cases the man used excessive violence (shooting or stabbing more than once or beating to death). In five of the same cases there was evidence of premeditation. It is theorized that a single shot or punch or stab can be delivered in a momentary loss of control during an argument, without there being an intent to kill, but that excessive violence indicates more determination on the part of the perpetrator that the victim die.[80(p506)] Excessive violence and sadism used against women seem to also indicate misogyny. In comparison, excessive violence was used by only 17.3% of the wives or girlfriends who killed, and sadism and premeditation by none.

SUMMARY OF DAYTON HOMICIDES

A close analysis of data on homicide between intimately related men and women in Dayton, Ohio, revealed that despite the rough parity in numbers of male and female victims, which parallels national figures, the circumstances surrounding the cases are very different according to sex. Previously violent, abusive, intoxicated men motivated by issues of male control of women are most likely to be involved both as victims and perpetrators. Similarly, a study conducted in Kansas City and Detroit found that in 66 of 90 family-conflict homicides, the male was defining the female as an object of personal property and acting on that basis.[81(p24)] In stark contrast, in the Dayton sample, only three women killed their boyfriend, husband, or estranged boyfriend or husband without a history of having been battered by that man if not responding to violent precipitation. This is not to say that the women solved the problem of abuse in a healthy manner or that they did not act with violence, but it does point out the element of desperation and self-defense in their crime and the misogyny of the men that they killed. Most previous research has failed to indicate the magnitude of these differences.

Wife abuse is a strong linking characteristic between homicide of women and other gynocidal practices. In the wider examination of all the homicide of women by men in Dayton from 1975 through 1979, other justification for the concept of homicide as gynocide is apparent. A total of nine women, or 30% of the females killed by nonrelated males, were raped or otherwise sexually abused, as well as murdered. This can be considered the most violent of rapes, the most misogynous of murders. Male dominance issues accounted for 10% of homicides of women killed by men of no relation, while the remaining largest cause was robbery (33.3%). However, in over half of the robbery cases, $30 or less was obtained. Elements of sadism, machismo, and misogyny could be detected in those incidents, as much as or more than a desire for money. Men used excessive violence in 70% of the murders of women by nonrelated males, and the victim precipitated her own death by force in only one case.

There were two matricides committed by men in Dayton during the years of the study. The extensive review of literature on homicide revealed no instances of this practice being committed by women. The percentage of homicides in both national and local statistics of any women killing each other is also consistently low. In Dayton only 1.4% of the homicides between 1968 and 1979 involved two females, and the rates of such killings did not vary significantly from year to year. The 63% proportion of men killing each other can be partially explained by the machismo ethic, while the 20.5% segment of the total homicides of men killing women needs to be seen as predominantly gynocide. The gynocidal practices of homicide of women, rape, wife abuse, and male psychotherapy and medicine all work together in this culture to remind women that they are vulnerable. In other cultures homicide of women and other gynocidal practices are used with less negative sanction than in ours and, consequently the misogyny is more overt and the oppression of the women much more complete.

Men do not sit down together and *plot* how to keep women oppressed. They usually do not consciously use gynocidal practices to maintain dominance. Many of the violent practices used against women are part of tradition and culture, but that men can insist on their wives' being infibulated, for example, indicates sadism, pleasure with the status quo of dominance, and misogyny. When a man murders a woman or beats her, he is often reacting to a perception of threat to that dominance. In those situations of stress, anxiety, and resulting rage he strikes out blindly. He is not consciously thinking about maintenance of the patriarchy, but the effect of maintaining subjugation of a particular woman still exists, and the lesson is learned by other women hearing about it. When men are prevented from demonstrating dominance in their occupations or in their economic status, they are likely to insist on it with women and react violently if they perceive less than total submission.

THE SIGNIFICANCE FOR NURSING

The population most at risk for homicide of women has been shown to be battered wives. A total of 27.7% of the female homicide victims in Dayton were abused women, the largest group. Their husbands are also in danger. As Walker states: "As we begin to see more battered women, we also realize the high probability that as the violence escalates, they will eventually be killed by or kill their men."[62(p53)] The second largest group of female victims of homicide in Dayton was rape victims. The majority of women killed in Dayton from 1975 through 1979 were murdered by men who had a history of violence and jealousy. Male dominance issues accounted for a significant proportion of their motives to kill. Fifty-nine percent of these men used excessive violence when they killed; the matricides and rape-murders also strongly suggest misogyny. To prevent homicide of women, work needs to be undertaken to change the nature of a society that produces batterers, rapists, and other violent men who subscribe to the machismo ethic.

A Preventive Role

The study of homicide is unusual in nursing, yet nursing centers on promoting life and health. Evidence from peaceful cultures shows that with the right conditions, entire societies can be mainly cooperative, life supporting, and completely nonviolent. Nurses need to work at discovering these conditions and creating them in terms of primary prevention. Every life is precious, and each time a life is taken by violence an unnecessary death has occurred. The conditions that allow and promote violence in our society can be considered as producing disease and death and therefore within the realm of nursing to correct. Nurses can work within many contexts to prevent homicide from occurring at the societal, community, and individual level.

Abolishing the Patriarchy

To combat violence the patriarchal societal structure must be abolished. This is, of course, a long-term goal, but more than half the world's population is female, and by joining together women can accomplish the task. Great progress has already been made. As Morgan says:

> We know that serious lasting change does not come overnight, or simply, or without enormous pain and diligent examination and tireless, undramatic, every-day-a-bit-more-one-step-at-a-time work. We know that such change seems to move in cycles . . . and we also know that those cycles are not merely going around in circles. They are rather, an upward spiral, so that each time we reevaluate a position or place we've been before, we do so from a new perspective.[14(p14)]

Nursing must work to foster the attitudes that support life.

Legislation

Specific measures already being considered by elected officials can be brought to the attention of the public, shaped into bills, and passed into laws by a concerted effort of nurses spearheading public campaigns. Laws to eliminate violence and sexism from television, mental health promotion appropriations, laws to strengthen prosecution of rapists, and wife-abuse protection measures — none of these will eradicate violence in and of itself, but taken together they will promote life and health.

Community Efforts

On the community level, nurses need to work to change parenting arrangements and work against using physical punishment (which research has linked to adult violence) in disciplining children at home and in schools. This can be accomplished by supporting and teaching childbirth education classes, parenting classes, and family-living classes in high school and by conducting public education programs to explain the importance of fathers taking an equal part in infant care and the detrimental effects of physical punishment.

Therapy for Abusers

Nurses can create and support wife-abuse shelters. Nurses are also a necessary addition to the staffs of such shelters to provide holistic health care to the women and children staying there. Nurses in emergency rooms, physicians' offices, community mental health centers, and health departments need to start diligently looking for and asking about abuse so that these women who are so gravely at risk of being killed can be identified. Once found, these women need to be helped with their multiple health problems, but, more important, intensively counseled by nurses as to the serious dangers involved with abuse and what can be done.

Marital counseling should be looked upon as a final alternative instead of the treatment of choice.[60] The abuser is the one who needs therapy, and the woman should be supported emotionally, financially, and legally in leaving him, at least until he receives therapy. He can be considered as having a serious, potentially lethal disease that can be transmitted to others. The carriers of such diseases are isolated and given treatment until they are well. The criminal justice system has the potential to at least isolate these men, although treatment in such settings is unlikely without massive reform. The treatment for violence, machismo, and misogyny is as yet unknown, although unlearning of patriarchal formulations and acceptance of feminine characteristics does seem possible with supportive therapy.[19] Nursing should support treatment centers for abusive men where they could receive such therapy after being committed there by law, so that the woman could stay in the home and be protected from further harm.

Women's Groups and Nurses

The basic unit for health promotion and prevention of homicide of females is the individual woman. A mutual teaching process between groups of women and nurses is needed to instruct women of the nature of their oppression and the strengths that they have and those they need to develop. Nurses can learn from the women more about the nature of the problems that they face and the different cultural prescriptions that tend to keep them subordinate and therefore potentially abused. Most important, these groups will support the bonding and mutual self-awareness and support process between women that are needed for unity and power and concerted action.

CONCLUSION

Perhaps this all seems removed from homicide, but the violence inherent in patriarchy supports the violence in individuals who kill. All people have the potential for violence. Everything that shapes the characteristics of females—biology, learning, identification with the mother figure, promotion of empathy, emphasis on nurturance, ability to express positive emotions, and societal prescriptions of nonaggression—helps make women generally nonviolent except when "backed up against the wall." The parenting arrangements, socialization forces, and patriarchal structures that foster the development of machismo, misogyny, and violence in men, which in turn lead to homicide of women and other gynocidal practices need to be changed.

REFERENCES

1. Herjanic M, Meyer D: Notes on epidemiology of homicide in an urban area. *Forensic Sci* 8:235–245, 1976.
2. Martin L: *Health Care of Women*. Philadelphia, JB Lippincott Co, 1978.
3. Kreps J: *Social Indicators*. Washington DC, US Government Printing Office, 1977.
4. Highriter M: The status of community health nursing. *Nurs Res* 26:183–191, 1977.
5. Pilisak M, Ober L: Torture and genocide as public health problems. *Am J Orthopsychiatry* 46:388–392, 1976.
6. Webster WH: *Uniform Crime Reports*. Washington DC, US Department of Justice, 1975, 1976, 1977, 1978.
7. Fromm E: *The Anatomy of Human Destruction*. New York, Fawcett Crest Books, 1973.
8. Montagu A (ed): *Learning Non-Aggression*. New York, Oxford University Press, 1978.
9. Sills G: Research in the field of psychiatric nursing 1952–1977. *Nurs Res* 26:201–206, 1977.

10. Steinmetz S, Straus M (eds): *Violence in the Family*. New York, Harper & Row, 1974.
11. Rich A: *On Lies, Secrets and Silence*. New York, WW Norton, 1979.
12. Leavitt R: *Peaceable Primates and Gentle People: Anthropological Approaches to Women's Studies*. New York, Harper & Row, 1975.
13. Cade T: On the issue of roles, in Cade T (ed): *The Black Woman*. New York, New American Library, 1970, pp 101–112.
14. Morgan R: *Going Too Far*. New York, Vintage Books, 1978.
15. Robinson P et al: A historical and clinical essay for black women in the cities, in Cade T (ed): *The Black Woman*. New York, New American Library, 1970, pp 198–210.
16. Daly M: *Beyond God the Father*. Boston, Beacon Press, 1973.
17. Ruether RR: *New Woman, New Earth*. New York, The Seabury Press, 1975.
18. Millett K: *Sexual Politics*. Garden City, New York, Doubleday and Co, 1970.
19. Goldberg H: *The New Male*. New York, William Morrow & Co, 1979.
20. Miller JB: *Toward a New Psychology of Women*. Boston, Beacon Press, 1976.
21. Chapman J, Gates M (eds): *The Victimization of Women*. Beverly Hills, Calif, Sage Publications, 1978.
22. Rickel A, Grant L: Sex role stereotypes in the mass media and schools: Five consistent themes. *Int J Wom Stud* 2:164–179, 1979.
23. Hartley R: Sex-role pressures and the socialization of the male child, in Pleck J, Sawyer J (eds): *Men and Masculinity*. Englewood Cliffs, NJ, Prentice-Hall, 1974, pp 7–12.
24. Daly M: *Gyn/Ecology*. Boston, Beacon Press, 1978.
25. Pingree S: A scale for sexism. *J Commun* 26:193–200, 1976.
26. Gerbner B et al: Cultural indicators: Violence profile #9. *J Commun* 28:196–207, 1978.
27. Thomas MH: Desensitization to portrayals of real-life aggression as a function of exposure to television violence. *J Pers Soc Psychol* 35:450–458, 1977.
28. Firestone S: *The Dialectic of Sex*. New York, William Morrow & Co, 1970.
29. Gibbons DC: *Delinquent Behavior*. Englewood Cliffs, NJ, Prentice-Hall, 1970.
30. Weimer JM: The mother, the macho and the state. *Intl J Wom Stud* 1:73–82, 1978.
31. Paddock J: Values in an antiviolent community. *Humanitas* 11:183–194, 1976.
32. Whiting B: Sex identity conflict and physical violence: A comparative study. *Am Anthropol* 67:123–140, December 1965.
33. Erlanger HS: The empirical status of the subculture of violence thesis. *Social Problems* 22:280–292, 1974.
34. Hepburn J: Subcultures, violence and the subculture of violence: An old rut or a new road? *Criminology* 9:87–98, 1971.
35. Bach-Y-Rita G: Episodic dyscontrol: A study of 130 violent patients. *Am J Psychiatry* 127:1473–1478, 1971.
36. Gillies H: Homicide in the west of Scotland. *Br J Psychol* 28:105–127, 1976.
37. Maletzky BM: The episodic dyscontrol syndrome. *Dis Nerv Syst* 34:178–185, 1973.
38. Ruotolo AK: Neurotic pride and homicide. *Am J Psychoanal* 35:1–18, 1975.
39. Toch H: *Violent Men*. Chicago, Aldine Publishing Co, 1969.
40. Toby J: Violence and the masculine ideal: Some qualitative data. *Ann Am Acad Pol Soc Sci* 364:19–28, 1966.
41. Fasteau M: *The Male Machine*. New York, McGraw-Hill, 1974.
42. Pleck JH, Sawyer J: *Men and Masculinity*. Englewood Cliffs, NJ, Prentice-Hall, 1974.
43. May R: *Power and Innocence*. New York, WW Norton, 1972.
44. Frankfort E: *Vaginal Politics*. New York, Bantam Books, 1972.
45. Dworkin A: *Our Blood*. New York, Harper & Row, 1974.
46. Dreifus C (ed): *Seizing Our Bodies*. New York, Vintage Books, 1977.
47. Driver E: Interaction and criminal homicide in India. *Social Forces* 60:153–158, 1971.
48. Hosken FP: Female circumcision in Africa. *Victimology: In J* 2:487–498, 1978.
49. Malik MOA, Salvi O: A profile of homicide in the Sudan. *Forensic Sci* 7:141–150, 1976.
50. Mallik SK, McCandless BR: A study of catharsis of aggression. *J Pers Soc Psychol* 4:591–596, 1966.
51. Russell DE, Van deVen N (eds): *Crimes Against Women*. Millbrae, Calif, Les Femmes, 1976.
52. Public Broadcasting System. Death of a princess. May 12, 1980.

53. Mushanga T: Wife victimization in east and central Africa. *Victimology: Int J* 2:479–485, 1978.
54. Brownmiller S: *Against Our Will*. New York, Bantam Books, 1975.
55. Cohen M et al: The psychology of rapists, in Chapeu D (ed): *Forcible Rape*. New York, Columbia Press, 1977.
56. Groth AN: Rape: Power, anger and sexuality. *Am J Psychiatry* 134:1239–1243, 1977.
57. Schram D: Rape, in Chapman J. Gates M (eds): *The Victimization of Women*. Beverly Hills, Calif, Sage Publications, 1978.
58. Martin D: *Battered Wives*. San Francisco, Glide Publications, 1976.
59. Davidson T: Wifebeating: A recurring phenomenon throughout history, in Roy M (ed): *Battered Women*. New York, Van Nostrand Co, 1977.
60. Dobash RE, Dobash R: *Violence Against Wives*. New York, The Free Press, 1979.
61. O'Brien JE: Violence in divorce-prone families. *J Marriage and Family* 33:692–698, 1971.
62. Walker L: *The Battered Woman*. New York, Harper & Row, 1979.
63. Stark E: Medicine and patriarchal violence: The social construction of a "private" event. *Int J Health Services* 9:461–493, 1979.
64. Renvoice J: *Web of Violence*. London, Routledge & Kegan Paul, 1978.
65. *Dayton Daily News*. September 10, 1977.
66. *Dayton Journal Herald*. September 10, 1977.
67. City of Dayton Department of Homicide Police Files.
68. Mesnikoff AM, Lauterbach CG: The association of violent dangerous behavior with psychiatric disorders: A review of the research literature. *J Psychiatry Law* 3:415–445, 1975.
69. Gelles R: Violence toward children in the United States. *Am J Orthopsychiatry* 48:580–592, 1978.
70. Amir M: *Patterns in Forcible Rape*. Chicago, University of Illinois Press, 1971.
71. Wolfgang M: Victim-precipitated criminal homicide. *J Criminal Law, Criminology Police Sci* 48:1–11, 1957.
72. Gayford JJ: The aetiology of repeated serious physical assaults by husbands on wives. *Med Sci Law* 19:19–24, 1979.
73. Steinmetz SK: The battered-husband syndrome. *Victimology: Int J* 2:499–509, 1977–1978.
74. Lercher M: Black women and homicide, in Rose H (ed): *Lethal Aspects of Urban Violence*. Lexington, Mass, Lexington Books, 1979.
75. Warren M: The female offender, in Toch H (ed): *Psychology of Crime*. New York, Holt Rinehart and Winston, 1979.
76. Langley R, Levy R: *Wife Beating: The Silent Crisis*. New York, EP Dutton, 1977.
77. Curtis L: *Criminal Violence*. Lexington, Mass, DC Heath and Co, 1975.
78. Curtis L: *Violence, Race and Culture*. Lexington, Mass, DC Heath and Co, 1975.
79. Tolson A: *The Limits of Masculinity*. New York, Harper & Row, 1977.
80. Voss H, Hepburn J: Patterns of criminal homicide in Chicago. *J Criminal Law, Criminology Police Sci* 59:499–508, 1968.
81. Gates M: Introduction, in Chapman J, Gates M (eds): *Victimization of Women*. Beverly Hills, Calif, Sage Publications, 1978.

COMMENTARY

Campbell's paper is a compelling account of homicide and misogyny that reports the results of her early theory development work. Misogyny — the hatred of women — is the organizing theoretical framework.

The framework does not encompass the family per se but, rather, a specific type of relationship between married or unmarried men and women who are considered families or not related. The paper was included in this book because of its implications for family theory development. The editors believe that misogyny and homicide of women represent such vital concerns for those who work with families that Campbell's work should be included.

Campbell has, therefore, made an indirect contribution to family nursing theory development by drawing attention to violence that may well have its roots in family illness. The results of Campbell's literature review represent middle-range theory that requires empirical testing. As with other nonempirical theory development efforts, the challenge will be to formulate research designs that accurately address the theoretical relationships. Given the impact of the subject matter on human lives and the role of nursing in areas such as prevention, therapy, and community programs, systematic examination is warranted.

ANN L. WHALL

CHAPTER
16

Closing the Gap Between Grand Theory and Mental Health Practice With Families.
Part 1: The Framework of Systemic Organization for Nursing of Families and Family Members

MARIE-LUISE FRIEDEMANN

This paper proposes a nursing framework for individuals and families that was inductively derived from existing knowledge and the author's personal experience. The framework is based on the premise that all things are organized as systems. Individuals, family systems, and the environment are interrelated and the congruence of patterns and rhythms between systems and subsystems signifies health. Nursing involves assisting individuals and families to reduce anxiety by weighing against each other the two major dimensions of system control and congruence or spirituality with the aim of maintaining a dynamic equilibrium.

Reprinted from *Archives of Psychiatric Nursing, 3*, 10–19, 1989.

The family focus in nursing practice has existed ever since Florence Nightingale wrote instructions for district nurses and home missioners in 1876 (Miller-Ham & Chamings, 1983). Recently, all nursing disciplines have adopted an increasingly holistic perspective that includes the family system and the community (Murphy, 1986). Even though nursing conceptual frameworks are focusing primarily on individual clients and the nurse-client relationship, significant progress has been made in broadening the accepted nursing metaparadigm to include family system concepts (Clements & Roberts, 1983; Fawcett, 1975, 1977); and in applying these concepts in family practice (Whall, 1981, 1986).

Nevertheless, there is still a gap between grand theory and practice models, between nursing of physical illness and psychosocial problems, and between practice that encompasses various focal systems such as the personal, the interpersonal, and the social systems (King, 1981). The following two articles propose (a) a conceptual framework that integrates the concepts of family and family health and guides the thinking of all nurses involved with families, and (b) a practice model based on this broad conceptual framework. The suggested practice model is especially useful for family mental health nurse specialists and nurse family therapists.

The framework of systemic organization, originated at Wayne State University, presents a view of the world relative to nursing and suggests a way to perceive the nature of individuals and families as well as their basic processes of functioning within the environment. During a recent presentation at Wayne State, the nurse theorist Rosemarie Parse (1988) said that it is naive to believe that nursing conceptual frameworks are created from knowledge unique to nursing and that, once formulated, they do not change. Instead, all viable conceptual frameworks are constantly evolving through both inductive and deductive thinking processes, critical examination of the relationships between constructs, and assimilation of new knowledge over time. Consequently, nursing conceptual frameworks are a synthesis of the creator's personality and life experience, context, and relevant existing knowledge leading to a unique perception of the relationships between the acting components of the process of nursing. The evolution of the framework of systemic organization has been no different. Bits and pieces of the thinking and writing of scientists and practitioners in nursing such as Martha Rogers (1980) and Margaret Neuman (1979, 1983), and family specialists from related disciplines, among others David Kantor and William Lehr (1975), Salvador Minuchin (1974), Jay Haley (1976), W. Robert Beavers (1976, 1981), and Larry Constantine (1986), have been reformulated and become part of this author's universe of discourse.

The framework of systemic organization has been taught to several classes of undergraduate nursing students. In the clinical setting, undergraduate students have helped families and managers of residential facilities to better manage the chronically mentally ill and prevent further need for hospitalization. Upon follow-up after discharge, family members have made many favorable comments: for example, about improved patient compliance with the medication regime or increased willingness of patients to assume responsibilities. The framework was also used by graduate students in a family therapy course. Of 10 dysfunctional families all showed significant improvement in parenting and interpersonal relations. The therapy of four families was recorded in a case study format and improvement in family functioning was documented (Friedemann, Jozefowicz, Schrader, Collins, & Strandberg, 1988). The students involved have evaluated the framework as helpful in guiding the analysis of complex mental health problems and directing them toward logical goals for the family. Such evidence has inspired this author to share the promising theoretic base.

ENVIRONMENT

Propositions

1. All existing things are organized as open systems of energy and matter in movement.
2. The basic order of the universe encompasses the organization of all systems on Earth.
3. The order of the universe is ruled by conditions largely unknown to humans. It is timeless and limitless, and its power is awesome.
4. The organization of systems on Earth follows a secondary order; the laws of the earthly conditions of time, space, energy, and matter.

The environment is the inescapable context in which humans are living. The environment consists of all things outside a persons's physical boundary. All matter and energy is organized in systems: microsystems, such as atoms and cells, material systems as in rocks or metals, living systems of plants and animals, social systems such as schools or the work place, and macrosystems including political systems, economic systems, ecosystems, and nature as a whole, the total organization of this planet's resources ruled by nature and by man, and, finally, the universal systems. All systems are defined by rhythms and patterns. Rhythm involves the time of revolutions of matter and the flow of energy around a system's center of gravitation, whereas pattern describes the system's use of space.

The view of the universe as systems purports that all that exists is complex and organized. General systems theory is applicable here since it deals with organized complexity (Weinberg, 1975). The system view is global in that it looks at phenomena in their totality and explains process in its full complexity. It does not reduce the whole to simpler parts but instead explains the parts by the function they perform as part of the total system (Constantine, 1986).

Since all systems are open systems that exchange matter and energy with each other, they are interrelated and interdependent and form a terrestrial system. The terrestrial system is specific to Earth since it depends on the specific to Earth since it depends on the specific earthly conditions of time, space, energy, and matter. The terrestrial system is subordinated to a universal system that is timeless, limitless, and ruled by conditions largely unknown to humans. Its functions are predetermined and its power is awesome.

HUMANS

Propositions

1. Humans define their identity and the nature of their environment by the relationships they have with the human, material, and other living systems in their environment.
2. Human reality is limited to human perception.
3. Human knowledge is limited to the earthly conditions of time, space, energy, and matter.
4. The human ability to recognize the dependency on natural forces and to foresee death has the potential to evoke a human system disturbance that disrupts the organizational congruence with subsystems and primary and secondary environmental systems.
5. Humans have the need and the capacity for transcendence in their attempt to reestablish organizational congruence with their environment and the universe.
6. Humans who realize their vulnerability and dependency on natural forces have the need to create and maintain a sense of power in a manmade environment or civilization.
7. Civilization is becoming increasingly complex through the transmission of culture to new generations and the incorporation of new knowledge in the human way of life.

Since forces that move electrons around the nucleus of an atom also move planets around their suns, human system organization is universal organization and as a result humans are intrinsically one with their environment and the universe. Humans have direct relationships with primary environmental systems in that they continuously exchange energy and matter with them. Humans have indirect relationships with all other systems that are part of the terrestrial subsystem and the universe.

The terrestrial subsystem of the universe is determined by the earthly conditions of time, space, energy, and matter. As part of the terrestrial subsystem and equal to all other systems on Earth, the human system of body and mind, created and constantly evolving, is dependent on the earthly conditions. Therefore, the human system is responding to a perception of reality relative to its senses and nervous system and its movement is determined by anatomic structure, shape, and gravity. Human knowledge of the environment is restricted to the secondary organization of terrestrial energy and matter evidenced as bodies, shapes, colors, sounds, and odors.

From birth on, humans are forming their personal identity in relation to a reality perceived through their senses. Objects are not defined by their universal meaning but by the meaning relative to the objects' relationship with the human system. For example, a cup is a cup because humans drink from it and its atomic structure or its relationship to all matter that forms the Earth's crust is irrelevant to human thinking. Similarly, fellow humans are defined by their relationship to the individuals with whom they interact, or to their reference groups. For example, fellow humans who become part of a defined interpersonal relationship are parents, friends, spouses, or playmates, and people whose relationship is determined by services they offer are carpenters, teachers, or doctors. Consequently, human understanding of the functions of the total universal system is limited. Human knowledge does not encompass universal truth since knowledge of one small part of the system, the terrestrial subsystem, cannot explain the whole.

While humans, equal to other living systems, are generally absorbed by their own limited reality of things to touch, taste, see, hear, and smell, they distinguish themselves by their ability to realize their physical limitations and their dependency on conditions such as the availability of food, drink, and shelter, temperature and weather, rhythms and patterns of day and night, the seasons, or human growth and development. In addition, humans foresee their end. They experience a glimpse of the universal truth in becoming aware of the process of transformation of all matter and the law of decay of all living things on Earth. The resulting sense of helplessness and vulnerability may effect tension that has the potential to destroy the given organization of the human system and subsystems. Human systems under tension may experience a disturbance in their spatial and temporal patterns, their rhythms, and their structure and process. Since systems are interdependent, tension will affect all human subsystems ranging from those of microscopic dimension to the organic organization of the human body. Ultimately, ongoing tension may result not only in incongruence between the human body subsystems but also between the human system, other human systems, and primary and secondary environmental systems. Humans have two defenses against tension and system incongruence: spirituality and control.

Spirituality is a need and practice unique to humans. While all material objects, plants, and animals in nature have an organization that is undisturbed and inherently congruent with other earthly subsystems, humans continuously need to reestablish system congruence that is being destroyed by tension each time vulnerability becomes evident.

Humans living in primitive conditions are relatively unprotected against the forces of nature and spirituality is their major defense against helplessness and system tension. Even though the need for protection may be less pronounced in humans of modern civilizations, system incongruence leads all humans to search for meaning in life through spirituality or submission to the awesome and incomprehensive universal order. Humans have the capacity for transcendence and a mode of perception that goes beyond logical reasoning and leads to a sense of unity with the universe and a sensation of inner peace.

Control is the second measure humans use in defending themselves against their vulnerability and their dependency on such terrestrial and extraterrestrial conditions. In controlling external forces, humans have established elaborate systems such as economic systems for the supply of food, clothing, and shelter, political systems to enforce and control leadership, and subordination and social systems to assure cooperation and division of labor. As a result, modern humans have achieved considerable control over their dependency through a superimposed civil system or civilization, and a sense of power that allows them to deny the awesome power of the universe. Within their civil system humans perceive themselves as the center of world action and reduce their need for spirituality.

Civilizations or civil systems are the purposeful organization of culture, and culture can be defined as the totality of the human way of life that includes control of natural forces through the knowledge of terrestrial laws as well as the institutionalization of spiritual practices. Culture is passed on from generation to generation. Consequently, the ongoing development of civil systems depends on two processes: transmission of culture and increase of knowledge. New knowledge, as it becomes incorporated into a generation's way of life, becomes culture with each new generation. Consequently, over time the civil structure adopts characteristics of its own and becomes increasingly incongruent with the subsystem of nature and the universe. This makes it more difficult for humans to achieve spirituality or congruence with universal order.

As various civil systems around the globe have become increasingly independent of nature, they are also turning more interdependent and complex. An individual person's contribution to the total civil system has become insignificant and no longer provides personal gratification. Many individuals have lost their sense of control even over small segments of their environment such as their workplace. Ironically, with the increased ability to control natural forces, the civil systems have become so complex and intertwined that their reactions to changes are hard to predict even by experts. This has made individuals painfully aware of their powerlessness and dependency not only on the natural and universal forces, but on their own civil system now ruled by forces beyond human control. Consequently, the civil system created to relieve tension has become a new source of tension and human system disturbance.

This leads to the realization that modern humans are in ever increasing need of a system, namely the family, that allows them to experience some control over a small portion of their environment and to practice spirituality.

FAMILIES

Propositions

1. The family functions in conjunction with the human civil structure in transmitting culture, the most basic human patterns and values.
2. The family shares with the civil structure the responsibility to provide physical necessities and safety, to procreate, to teach social skills to its members, to provide for personal growth and development, to allow emotional bonding of members, and to promote a purpose for life and meaning through spirituality.
3. The family satisfies its members' needs for control over their environment and guides them in finding through system congruence comfort with each other and a meaning for life.
4. All family processes include collectively accepted and co-ordinated behaviors that aim at regulating the earthly condition or access conditions of space, time, energy, and matter in order to gain the target conditions of stability, growth, affect, and meaning for all family members.
5. The family strives to keep the four process dimensions in a dynamic equilibrium: system maintenance, system change, togetherness, and individuation.

While families early in history were the only civil system available to humans this is no longer true. As the body of knowledge and its organization has become too complex for any one person to understand, knowledge now belongs to the larger civil system incorporated in community systems and governments. Likewise, the human socialization process once unique to the family occurs to a great extent in schools and in social and recreational organizations. Even basic tasks such as reproduction, physical care for family members, or the management of finances are often carried on outside family boundaries by persons other than family members.

It follows that the family functions, the provision of physical necessities, and safety, procreation, and the socialization of the young today are complementary to those of the larger civil structure. However, the family is no less important in that it is often the only system capable of meeting directly the individuals' needs for control and spirituality, or congruence with other systems. Individuals in a functioning family experience a sense of control based on the order and predictability of family processes and they sense a glimpse of the universal order by tuning into each other's systemic organization through emotional bonding. In addition, free-flowing energy connects the family system and each individual with the environment, nature, and the universe.

The family needs to be understood first as a unit with its own organization that interacts with its environment. Second, the family is a system with interpersonal subsystems of dyads, triads, or larger units defined by emotional bonds. Third, the family is a system of individuals, personal subsystems who have their own distinct relationships with the primary environmental systems, the family system, and other family members. The purpose of the family is the transmission of family culture, namely the most basic human patterns and values that represent the backbone of culture at large.

Family-specific culture is the sum of all family processes. A representation of the pathways of family processes is pictured in Figure 1. Family processes are aimed at regulating the earthly conditions, or addressing conditions of time, space, energy (Kanto & Lehr, 1975), and matter (Constantine, 1986) in order to achieve control and congruence for each individual within the system. As is true for culture transmission at large, family culture transmission consists of two processes: transmission of patterns and values and the acquisition of new knowledge. Therefore, the target of control is achieved by meeting two target conditions: (a) stability that refers to stable patterns transmitted over generations and (b) growth made possible through the incorporation of new knowledge into the system. The target of congruence, the goal of spirituality, is aimed at each individual. It is equally divided into two target conditions: (a) affect or emotional bonding based on interactional patterns and values learned from previous generations, and (b) meaning individuals acquire through critical thinking and opening of the mind that leads to new knowledge and new realizations (Kantor & Lehr, 1975).

The regulation process consists of strategies or collective family behaviors. For example, in the attempt to regulate space with the purpose of achieving the target condition of affect and, consequently, congruence, a family may institute a weekly gathering at the grandmother's house. Another family may attempt growth necessitated by a family member who has a crippling illness. Regulating matter, the family may buy books for information or acquire equipment such as a wheelchair; regulating energy, family members may ask for help from a visiting nurse agency.

The Framework of Systematic Organization

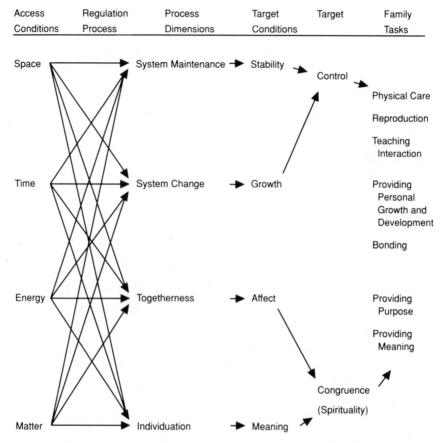

Access Conditions	Regulation Process	Process Dimensions	Target Conditions	Target	Family Tasks

Figure 1. Family processes; transmission of family culture.

The family processes are organized along process dimensions relative to each target condition. The system maintenance dimension includes family processes that organize and structure the system. A family may set up rules to share space, assign roles to family members, coordinate activities, make decisions, or schedule family time. The organizational structure is consciously controlled and preserved as family values and learned patterns are passed on to new generations. Family maintenance processes lead toward the target condition of stability that provides individuals with a sense of control and the family system with an identity.

The process dimension of system change includes processes that lead to the incorporation of new knowledge and assumption of new family behaviors. The family allows a free flow of energy and material out of the system to the environment and adjusts its time and spatial arrangements in response to environmental feedback. Thus, the family system reaches the control target by accommodating changes from within, such as new developmental needs of family members, and from the environment. Over time, the system focusing on the target condition of growth develops into a unit with new characteristics.

The process dimension of togetherness includes all processes that lead to family system-personal system congruence. It consists of a series of learned behaviors based on a set of firm values that permit energy to flow freely between family members and regulate space and time in such a way as to bring members together. The target condition is affect or emotional bonding between members that leads to a sense of commitment to the family unit and individual satisfaction with the family system.

Individuation is the second process dimension relative to the congruence target, this time environmental systems-personal systems congruence or spirituality. Individuation processes in a family encourage the acquisition of new knowledge and values leading to actions that allow individuals to establish their own relationships with external systems. Individuals use their talents and strive for spiritual growth or the target condition of meaning by connecting with systems outside the family unit and with the universe.

All four process dimensions are interrelated. There is a negative correlation between the two dimensions pertaining to each target: control and congruence. Thus, system maintenance and system change are negatively correlated. For example, a family that promotes strict control over its internal environment and limits exchange with external systems will automatically restrict its potential to assimilate new knowledge and respond to changes of the environment. Likewise orientation toward congruence between family members (togetherness) is negatively correlated with the individual's ability to establish congruence with the environment (individuation). For example, a family with extremely high unity requires commitment and sacrifice from the individuals and restricts independent thinking and acting, thereby restraining them from unfolding their full potential. Conversely, of the process dimensions relative to both, control and congruence/spirituality targets, one focuses inward toward the family system, while the other is directed outward toward the environment. Both inward-oriented dimensions (system maintenance and togetherness) and both outward-oriented dimensions (system change and individuation) are necessarily positively correlated, but each maintains enough distinction to exert individual influence on family functioning. The family is thus a unit that transmits culture and keeps in a dynamic equilibrium the four target processes that assist individuals to achieve well-being.

HEALTH

Propositions

1. Health is system congruence evidenced on all levels of an individual's system, the subsystems, and the primary environmental systems.
2. Physical disease is a condition that refers to the organizational disturbance at the organic system level.
3. Physical disease and a high level of health can occur concurrently.
4. The crucial determinant of lack of health is anxiety that results from system incongruence while well-being is the result of high level health.

Health is the maintenance of the human relationship with the universe. Health is the congruence of the universal rhythm and pattern of movement of matter and energy with the pattern and organization inherent in each person. In a person with an ideal state of health the universal rhythm and pattern are one with those of body and mind. The uninhibited movement of energy and matter within and without the person exhibits perpetual rhythms and patterns that are calming and soothing and thus promote a supreme sense of well-being. Such a state is rarely achieved except for limited periods of spiritual tranquility and through meditation.

Disturbances of the internal dynamic organization or the blockage of energy flow between the internal systems and the environment are experienced daily by all humans due to tension and the resulting feeling and sensation is anxiety. Anxiety is basic to all other emotions and is the antithesis of well-being. Both anxiety and well-being are evidenced as a sensation of the dynamic organization of body and mind and as a feeling at the interface of the human system with its environment. The relationship between the two is linear and negatively correlated.

As all parts of a system and all external systems are interrelated, anxiety experienced by the individual at one system level, if uninhibited, will spread and affect all patterns of the individual's subsystems and the primary environmental systems. Simple linear causality is not applicable in systems theory (Constantine, 1986). Instead, causality is circular in that anxiety arising at one system interface is fed back to the personal system where it is interpreted. If it is perceived as a threat to the personal system, anxiety may become the cause of new disturbance and new anxiety to be reinterpreted and reinforced.

In addition to this horizontal circular spread, the effect of anxiety moves vertically to all contact systems and subsystems down to the microscopic system level. For example, anxiety experienced by an individual at the interface between the personal system and the workplace may affect the individual's organic health or emotional connectedness with other family members. These new disturbances may then evoke new anxiety and effect further disturbance in the congruence between the individual and other persons or between the system and its organic subsystems. The search for a cause of anxiety is often in vain. Since patterns of system function that evoke anxiety are transmitted as part of culture, the actual roots of the anxiety may be dated back generations. Prolonged incongruence between system levels may lead to the loss of health and physical disease or emotional illness.

Physical disease is defined as a malfunction of one or more human organic systems or microsystems. As such physical disease is not equivalent to lack of health or the disturbance of congruence between human systems and their environment, and/or between system levels within the human body. Instead, physical disease may occur in the absence of anxiety. For example, since the process of infectious agents gaining access to a host involves a process that is intrinsic to universal order, physical disease is congruent with universal order and may represent health. Such is the case of a person with a terminal illness who is weakened through age and has accepted mortality through submission of the self to the universe. In most cases physical disease happens concurrently with lack of health in that disease is either evoked by system incongruence and anxiety, or the anxiety occurs when the person interprets the disease as a threat to the personal system, or both. Nevertheless, the concepts of health and disease are separate. Disease takes a major focus where it affects a person's well-being. The treatment of disease includes not only those measures that lead to improved congruency and less impairment of organ and microsystems but also those factors that sustain the improved flow of energy within the body and lead to congruency among the personal, family, and environmental systems.

Consequently, the concept of disease is included in the concept of health. In addition to an assessment of organic system disease, the estimation of health needs to include a measure of the person's level of control in various areas of life and the individual's congruence with the family interpersonal system, the family unit, the larger environment, and the universe. Since system congruence signifies spirituality, the concept of health also encompasses spirituality.

FAMILY HEALTH

Propositions

1. Family health encompasses three criteria: the presence of all four family process dimensions, congruence between the family system and its primary environmental systems, and congruence between all subsystems.

2. The family style is the product of weighing and emphasizing the process dimensions of (a) system maintenance, (b) system change, (c) togetherness, and (d) individuation.
3. Family functioning consists of the processes that families use in pursuing the targets of control and congruence/spirituality.
4. No single family functioning process or family style can be judged as effective or ineffective. Effectiveness of family functioning is equal to the criteria of family health.

Family health is a dynamically balanced state in which all four family process dimensions are present: (a) system maintenance, (b) system change, (c) togetherness, (d) individuation. Consequently, family health is achieved by weighing and emphasising family structural and organizational processes that lead to family stability against those that lead to growth through exchange with the environment. Family health is also a process of weighing family togetherness and commitment to the family unit against the striving of individuals to develop their own potential. The four target dimensions are emphasized, combined, and balanced in such a way that none of the family members have to compromise their personal growth and sense of well-being for the sake of the family system in their interaction with other family members and with primary environmental systems. Consequently, family health is present if (a) all four target processes are present, (b) the family system is congruent with its primary environmental systems, and (c) there is congruence between all subsystems and between the interpersonal and the personal subsystems; that is, all family members are satisfied with the family system.

Families have many options in achieving a dynamic equilibrium between these seemingly oppositional processes and none can be valued as better than the other. Therefore, the family style, defined as the sum of all family processes involved in weighing and emphasising the four family dimensions, and family health are separate concepts. Family functioning consists of the processes that families use in pursuing the targets of control and congruence. Neither singular processes of family functioning nor their collective, the family style, can be judged as effective or ineffective by themselves. Only by using all the criteria of family health, including the family's exchange with the environment, can a family's effectiveness be evaluated. Therefore, the effectiveness of family functioning is defined as family health.

NURSING

Propositions

1. Nursing occurs on the various system levels from microsystems to the larger environmental systems in the community.

2. All nursing focused on individuals includes the influence of family and environmental systems on the individual's well-being.
3. All nursing interventions at the level of family systems or the community also heeds to individuals and their subsystems.
4. The art in nursing consists of the nurse's creative ability to shift position from the role of a participant and actor in the system to that of a bystander, and to shift from one system level to another.

Nursing is the act of assisting humans in their attempt to reestablish control over their systems and congruence between their own system, their subsystems, and their primary environmental systems. In the sense that the well-being of humans is dependent on the individual's congruence with the family system and the larger environment, community nursing and family nursing are one with individual nursing. Nursing occurs at the interface of system levels. Each system level can become the main focus of nursing interventions; however, the focus is shifted to other system levels as the need arises.

Nursing is a science because its interventions depend on the understanding of system operation and processes. Energy can flow between system levels only if each level operates smoothly. Nursing is an art in that individuals are assisted in seeking congruence with their own subsystems, other humans, nature, and the universe through the nurse's use of self.

Nursing of the individual is the process in which nurses temporarily unite their own personal system with that of clients by letting energy flow between the systems so that patterns and rhythms adjust to each other. In this manner the client becomes receptive to change and interventions can be effective. Interventions include those targeted to act at the microscopic level, such as medications, and at the organic level, such as wound care or relaxation techniques. At the personal level nursing care addresses well-being, anxiety, and other emotions; at the interpersonal level the focus is on relationships with family members and other people; and at the family level nursing is concerned with the person's role and contribution to the family system as well as the family's ability to meet the person's needs for individuality. Nursing at suprasystems levels assesses and assists in changing the client's relationship with environmental systems in terms of using them more fully or reducing conflict. Environmental system interventions also include spiritual care and assisting clients in accepting the unavoidable by the nurse reaching out and sensing together with the client the order of the universe and a moment of peace.

On occasion, nurses will find that the focal system incongruency is located at the family system level and has a secondary influence on individual persons in the family. This is true in situations where family demands exceed coping resources, where family cooperation falters and individuals become hurt in interpersonal struggle. Alert nurses will recognize the need for family nursing. Nurses who practice family nursing allow themselves to become a part of the family system. As all system parts maintain their own properties while they contribute to the characteristics of the whole, nurses may fully apply their own self within such systems without losing their own identity. They can sense the energy flow within the system, the rhythms and patterns. The mere presence of nurses in an ailing system will effect change. Consequently, nurses joining family systems have powerful effects on the system unit and, as a result, on each individual.

In summary, nursing is the act of the nurse's frequent shifting from the position of a participant in a client, family, or community system to that of an objective bystander and evaluator. It also involves shifting from lower to higher system levels in balancing and meeting the client's needs for control and congruence. The act of nursing depends on the art of the nurse's use of self and the extensive knowledge of the science relative to all systems involved in the nursing process.

This leads to the conclusion that all nursing needs to include mental health and spiritual nursing. Physical care alone ends at the organic level and ignores those qualities that distinguish one person from another. A personal system is defined by the ways input and feedback are perceived, processed, and responded to. Each personal system reacts with feelings and behaviors and interprets input by ascribing meaning to it in unique ways. Each of these unique systems in turn interacts with other systems in special ways, again ascribing meaning to each relationship. Nurses need to be aware of the beauty inherent in each individual, in the processes of life, and in the interaction between themselves and others. It is such beauty that reflects the systems of nature and the order of the universe.

REFERENCES

Beavers, W. R. (1976). A theoretical basis for family evaluation. In J. M. Lewis, W. R. Beavers, J. T. Gossett, & V. A. Phillips (Eds.), *No single thread*. New York: Brunner/Mazel.

Beavers, W. R. (1981). A systems model of family for family therapists. *Journal of Marital and Family Therapy, 7,* 299–308.

Bradburn, N. M. (1969). *The structure of psychological well-being.* Chicago: Aldine.

Clements, I. W., & Roberts, F. B. (1983). *Family health: A theoretical approach to nursing care.* New York: Wiley.

Constantine, L. L. (1986). *Family paradigms: The practice of theory in family therapy.* New York: Guilford.

Fawcett, J. (1975). The family as a living open system: An emerging conceptual framework for nursing. *International Nursing Review, 22,* 113–116.

Fawcett, J. (1977). The relationship between identification and patterns of change in spouses' body images during and after pregnancy. *International Nursing Studies, 14*, 199–213.

Friedemann, M. L., Jozefowicz, F., Schrader, J. L., Collins, A. M., & Strandberg, P. (1988). *Advanced family nursing with the Control-Congruence Model.* Unpublished manuscript. Wayne State University, College of Nursing, Detroit.

Haley, J. (1976). *Problem solving therapy.* San Francisco: Jossey-Bass.

Kantor, D., & Lehr, W. (1975). *Inside the family.* San Francisco: Jossey-Bass.

King, I. M. (1981). *A theory for nursing: Systems, concepts and process.* New York: Wiley.

Miller-Ham, L., & Chamings, P. A. (1983). Family nursing: Historical perspectives. In I. W. Clements & F. B. Roberts (Eds.), *Family health: A theoretical approach to nursing care.* New York: Wiley.

Minuchin, S. (1974). *Families and family therapy.* Cambridge, MA: Harvard University.

Murphy, S. (1986). Family study and nursing research. *Image, 18*(4), 170–174.

Neuman, M.A. (1979). *Theory development in nursing.* Philadelphia: Davis.

Neuman, M. A. (1983). Newman's health theory. In I. W. Clements & F. B. Roberts (Eds.), *Family health: A theoretical approach to nursing care* (pp. 161–176). New York: Wiley.

Parse, R. R. (1988, July). *Man-Living-Health Theory of Nursing.* Paper presented at the Summer Conference of the College of Nursing, Wayne State University, Detroit.

Rogers, M. E. (1980). Nursing: A science of unitary man. In J. P. Riehl & C. Roy (Eds.), *Conceptual Models for Nursing Practice* (2nd ed.). New York: Appleton-Century-Crofts.

Weinberg, G. M. (1975). *Introduction to general systems thinking.* New York: Wiley-Interscience.

Whall, A. L. (1981). Nursing theory and the assessment of families. *Journal of Psychiatric Nursing and Mental Health Services, 19*, 30–36.

Whall, A. L. (1986). *Family therapy theory for nursing.* Newark, CT: Appleton-Century-Crofts.

Closing the Gap Between Grand Theory and Mental Health Practice With Families.
Part 2: The Control-Congruence Model for Mental Health Nursing of Families

MARIE-LUISE FRIEDEMANN

The control-congruence model is based on the framework of systemic organization and presents a mental health nursing approach to families with physical, emotional, interpersonal, social, or environmental problems. Special instruments are available to assess and evaluate family functioning. The model distinguishes itself by encouraging self-diagnosis, strengthening effective family behaviors already practiced, and introducing new behaviors in tune with the family's usual patterns. The model allows flexibility for nurses to reach families through practicing the art of nursing.
© 1989 by Grune & Stratton, Inc.

The second part of this series suggests one of many possible ways to put the framework of systemic organization described in part 1 into nursing action. Thus, as the title suggests, the practice model presents a link between grand theory and nursing practice. The proposed mental health model is applicable to a wide variety of family systems that are experiencing emotional, physical, social, or situational problems. The control-congruence model (CC-Model) as presented here represents a contextual

Reprinted from *Archives of Psychiatric Nursing, 3,* 20–28, 1989.

approach to nursing practice. However, in order to apply it to specific focal populations, the interventions built into the model must be based on an expert specialist's knowledge and judgment. As advocated by Krauss (1987), there is a need for the inclusion of context as well as specialization in psychiatric nursing, and the CC-Model allows nurses to combine the two dimensions without creating conflict.

The CC-Model operates by focusing on the processes described in the framework of systemic organization that are common to all individuals and families. Consequently, it is applicable to families of various compositions, developmental stages, and cultural backgrounds, and of differing social and economic status. Within the common context of human function, the model explains differences of human responses as adaptive and learned variations of coping. The focus on sameness permits nurses to see patients functioning at an equal level, a condition necessary for empathy and caring, and the view of individual responses as being dependent on the environment blocks crippling prejudice and value judgment.

THE STRUCTURE OF THE CC-MODEL

The following sections describe how the key concepts of control and congruence derived from the framework of systemic organization are also rooted within research and clinical practice. This is followed by a description of the actual nursing process that aims to strengthen behaviors relative to the control and congruence dimensions on the personal, interpersonal, and family system levels.

The family is considered the most important system to which an individual belongs and that exerts its influence for a long time. After members break their ties with the original system, they often recreate a family with new members that has similar characteristics (Bowen, 1976; Whitaker & Keith, 1981; Yalom, 1970). The concept of family nursing has been generally understood as giving nursing care to the total family system (Miller-Ham & Chamings, 1983). Many nurses in mental health practice have eagerly used the techniques of family therapy and excellent attempts have been made to apply to family systems nursing conceptual frameworks originally designed for individuals (Whall, 1986). Nevertheless, confusion exists in nursing theory building and practice about the interrelationship between system levels, individuals, interactional units, and the family system within its larger environment (Murphy, 1986).

Nursing with the CC-Model takes place on all system levels. As described within the framework of systemic organization, the ultimate aim of nursing is to reduce anxiety that is felt by individuals. Since individuals are interdependent with all systems of which they are part, nursing interventions directed at any of the subsystems may be effective.

At times it is best to address each member's personal needs. On other occasions the relationships between individuals may come into focus, but often the most effective nursing intervention may involve a change in family structure or process, or a manipulation of the family's immediate environment.

According to the framework of systemic organization the key to reducing anxiety pertains to the two targets of control and congruence. A close look at the literature shows that researchers and clinicians of various disciplines find most family functioning processes to fall into two dimensions relative to these targets. For example, differentiation of the self (Bowen, 1976), enmeshment and disengagement (Minuchin, 1974), closeness, self-disclosure, expressiveness, and empathy (Lewis, Beavers, Gossett, & Phillips, 1976), or family cohesion (Moos, 1986; Olsen, McCubbin, Barnes, Larsen, Muxen, & Wilson, 1984) address congruence. Family control is best expressed by power structure, negotiation of problems (Haley, 1976), mapping of family structure, boundaries (Minuchin, 1974), coalitions, rules, and roles (Haley, 1976; Lewis, Beavers, Gossett, & Phillips, 1976), control and family organization (Moos, 1986), and adaptability of family organization (Olson, McCubbin, Barnes, Larsen, Muxen, & Wilson, 1984).

In interacting with the environment, families take active control over external influences. They open or close their boundaries, screen information, and select what should be incorporated into family knowledge (Kantor & Lehr, 1975). Family congruence with the environment, on the other hand, occurs between the individuals and the systems of which they are part. Research in social ecology (Moos, 1974; Roberts & Feetham, 1982) and social learning (Bandura, 1969) suggests that individuals attempt to establish congruence with their environment, and, inversely, that the environment shapes the behaviors and characteristics, for example, of workers in organizations (Porter & Lawler, 1965), or of children in hostile families (Couch, 1970). Consequently, research in family functioning, social ecology, and social learning support the four process dimensions outlined in the framework of systemic organization:

1. System maintenance (control within the family system) — processes that serve to organize and structure the family and maintain a stable core.
2. Togetherness (congruence within the family system) — processes that lead family members to bond together, commit time and energy to each other, and feel part of the family.
3. System change (control of environmental influence) — processes that let the family system grow, adapt to changes in the environment, and incorporate new knowledge.
4. Individuation (congruence between individuals and environment) — processes that encourage individuals to use

their potential and let the family accept differences and changes in individuals.

Family processes of system maintenance and togetherness promote family stability. If exposed to stress, the family uses these processes to reestablish homeostasis, a dynamic state that has been advocated as ideal by early family therapists (Bateson, 1961; Haley, 1959; Jackson, 1957). The other two dimensions, system change and individuation, reflect the concept of morphogenesis originally discussed by Buckley in 1967, who described functional family systems as growth oriented and responsive to change from within the system and the environment. A functional family needs both homeostasis and morphogenesis. A stable family core or family identity is needed to define the system so that individuals can commit themselves to the unit, and system growth that involves changes in system structure and processes is needed to accommodate the individuals' changing needs and to adapt to external pressures.

The same targets of control and congruence, and within them the processes relative to stability, change, affect, and meaning, are equally applicable to individuals and interpersonal systems. Thus, nursing of individuals may focus on both maintaining a stable core (the personality, self-concept, identity) and controlling change (adapting to developmental and environmental change). Likewise, nurses may assist individuals in establishing emotional bonds (effect) and finding fulfillment and meaning by becoming congruent with other persons and larger systems.

Interpersonal units have stability in terms of structure and interaction rules, but there is also a need for growth as the relationship adapts to the changing needs of the individuals involved. Nursing that promotes the control and congruence targets on the interpersonal system level involves assisting the clients to balance controlling and dependent behaviors. Health of interpersonal units implies that the control balance is satisfactory for all parties or that there is congruence between them. Thus, the control and congruence targets and the processes relative to stability, growth, effect, and meaning on all three system levels are the building blocks of the CC-Model.

NURSING WITH THE CC-MODEL

The Treatment Goal

The goal of treatment based on the framework of systemic organization is family health. It consists of a family's ability to emphasize and weigh against each other the processes relative to system maintenance, system change, togetherness, and individuation in relation to the family context and larger environment. Family health is dependent on the health of all members, which is evidenced by a low level of anxiety and a free exchange of system energy with the environment. Thus, the corresponding objectives of treatment are:

1. The presence of processes relative to all four process dimensions.
2. Absence of negative responses from the environment (e.g., involvement of court and legal authorities, school reports of truancy, job dismissal based on violation of work rules).
3. Satisfaction of all family members with the family system.
4. Absence of incapacitating anxiety in all family members.

Steps of Treatment

In pursuing the above goals, the following basic steps of treatment are necessary:

1. Assess health and verify with client(s).
2. Describe the model.
3. Determine one or more focal process dimension(s) and desired change within the relative target condition.
4. Highlight existing strengths within the focal process dimension(s).
5. Enact and advance with client(s) existing functional family behaviors (strategies).
6. Advocate new functional family behaviors (strategies).
7. Lead experimentation with mutually chosen new strategies.
8. Test changes and evaluate success in reaching the targets of control and congruence and performance of family tasks.
9. Honor the client(s) effort.

The acronym **ADD HEALTH** expresses the goal of the nursing process. The sequence of the steps may be changed as the need arises. Steps 5 to 7 usually occur concurrently. There is often a need to reassess success or problems and to direct the emphasis to another dimension. In such a case, the nurse goes back to step 3. Also, step 9 needs to be practiced throughout the process.

Assessment of Health

The assessment of health is relative to the treatment goals. Its purpose consists of determining the difference between what is and what should be and the mutually agreed upon need for nursing intervention. Three assessment instruments are available that take the respondents about 30 minutes to complete. The following sections outline the model-specific assessment areas.

Assessment of Processes Relative to the Four Process Dimensions. This assessment consists of three parts: (a) the emphasis the family places on each process dimension, or its style of functioning; (b) the effectiveness of family functioning relative to each dimension; and (c) the actual strategies used and their effectiveness.

Emphasis on the Process Dimensions. This is measured by the Assessment of Strategies in Families – Family Functioning instrument (ASF-F) (Friedemann, 1986). The tool is filled out by all adult and teen family members and measures the emphasis on the four dimensions without judging success in functioning. Respondents rate strategies pertaining to each dimension according to how much they apply them in their own family on a 4-point Likert scale. The tool has 20 items, 5 relative to each dimension. Psychometric testing of this instrument is in process. Initially, 132 subjects from the community representing families of all life stages completed the instrument. A factor analysis of the responses confirmed the defined process dimensions with one factor relative to each individuation and togetherness. System maintenance and system change were represented by two factors each. Internal consistency was acceptable for three dimensions ($\alpha = .63$ to $.74$). System maintenance items were modified to improve reliability before retesting. Test results of a reapplication of the tool are not yet available. The instrument in its new format has shown clinical merit with numerous multiproblem families in that it has demonstrated change in the desired direction during the course of treatment.

Effectiveness of the Strategies. This is measured with the Assessment of Strategies in Families – Effectiveness (ASF-E) that is completed by all adult and teen family members. The ASF-E has been tested with 622 adults representing clinical and healthy families of various constellations, family life-stages, and ethnic backgrounds (Friedemann, 1988). The ASF-E has 15 items of three statements describing outcome levels of family functioning strategies. One is picked by the respondent as being most like his or her family. Reliability was found satisfactory with a Cronbach Alpha coefficient of .84. Evidence of validity is based on the involvement of expert family clinicians in item construction (content validity), confirming factor structure (construct validity), and a significant difference in family effectiveness between families from the community and clinical families (discriminant validity [$t(616) = 33.3; p < .001$]).

Actual Strategies Used. The assessment of the actual strategies used consists of recognizing strategies and appraising them with the family members in terms of their effect on individuals and the family system. The CC-Model does not prescribe an assessment format. Some clinicians may want to construct a check list of possible strategies. An effective repertoire of strategies pertaining to each process dimension needs to include behaviors that regulate all four access conditions: space, time, energy, and matter. Table 1 lists a selection of such strategies. The relative access conditions are listed in column 3. The 4th column de-

TABLE 1. Family Processes

Process Dimensions	*Strategies*	*Access Conditions*	*Family Tasks*
Control system maintenance	Screen friends, screen and withhold information, select external resources, categorize environment into "like us" and "not like us," establish rules and roles, establish decision-making and leadership, assign tasks and divide labor,	Matter/Energy	Provision of physical necessities for all members through interchange with the environment and division of labor; Safety through organization of space and matter to procure housing and material needs Reproduction
	Monitor persons' whereabouts, regulate and share space, assign space for activities,	Space	
	Schedule activities, assign curfews, schedule use of facilities, coordinate schedules, accept values of the past, structure the future	Time	
Control system change	Collect information freely; share and incorporate information; use community for recreation and education; accept help from outside; participate in community activities; exchange information,	Matter/Energy	Provision of interaction skills through teaching and modeling intra- and intersystem social exchange Provision of personal growth and development through exchange of knowledge with the environment

(*continued*)

TABLE 1. Family Processes (*continued*)

Process Dimensions	Strategies	Access Conditions	Family Tasks
	knowledge, and materials with outside systems; test old values; Experiment with new thoughts and social interaction; handle challenges with confidence; reorganize system;		
	Rearrange system space use; do not plan for the future; expect the unpredictable; act spontaneously	Space/Time	
Congruence togetherness	Share interests and belongings, express affection, do things for each other, respect each other, understand each other, enjoy each other, live by family values, conform to family standards, think like the others,	Matter/Energy	Provision of affect and bonding through love
	Share space with each other, gather together routinely,	Space	
	Arrange family times, have family rituals, give time to the family	Time	
Congruence individuation	Be enthusiastic about job, school, helping in the community;	Energy	Provision of purpose and goals in life; Provision of meaning

TABLE 1. Family Processes (*continued*)

Process Dimensions	Strategies	Access Conditions	Family Tasks
	enjoy outside stimulation; form own opinions; defend own position; use community resources to learn and grow; seek information; enjoy each other's differences; be active in community, church, politics; form personal beliefs about meaning of life or religion; seek unity with the universe;		through spirituality
	Be part of environmental systems; share space with friends;	Space	
	Adjust to rhythms and schedules of outside systems; adjust to each other's differing schedules and rhythms; spend private time outside the family.	Time	

scribes the family tasks or output of the system pertaining to each dimension. Some clinicians may share the list of sample strategies with client families while mutually exploring additional options. Others may assess strategies gradually while engaged in the working stages of the CC-Model. Family members may be helped to explore how they deal with each other or to play out interaction strategies during treatment sessions.

Congruence Between Family System and Environment. A preliminary congruence estimate is provided by ASF-E scores on the environment-focused dimensions: family change and individuation. However, the instrument is limited to the perception of the respondents. For a more complete estimate, it is necessary to obtain additional information from external systems interacting with the family and its members. The assessment includes interviews with representatives of external systems in contact with the family, such as teachers, clergymen, supervisors, case workers, doctors, friends, or extended family members.

Assessment of Satisfaction with the Family System. The Assessment of Strategies in Families — Satisfaction instrument (ASF-S) has ten items, two relative to each process dimension and two based on an additional dimension of external support. The adult and teen family respondents rate their satisfaction with strategies on a 4-point Likert scale. The tool was tested for reliability and validity in conjunction with the ASF-F (Friedemann, 1986). Upon factor analysis, a factor structure of two theoretically sound factors resulted. One was related to satisfaction with the internal family operation and the other reflected satisfaction with the family's exchange with the outside world. The internal consistency coefficient of the satisfaction scale was .82.

In addition to the ASF-S score, qualitative satisfaction data invariably emerge as a byproduct of the assessment of family strategies.

Assessment of Individual and Interpersonal Health. This area of assessment has as its goal the estimation of each individual's level of personal control and congruence with the other members in the family and with external individuals and systems. The focus on individual control and congruence is preferred over an assessment of anxiety since no available anxiety tool includes the many possible covert manifestations that are often unnoted or misinterpreted by family members.

The assessment of interpersonal health includes a qualitative estimation of controlling and dependent behaviors and each persons's satisfaction with the assigned role or power position within the relationship. This is of particular importance when family members become more dependent due to a physical or mental illness. These patients' new roles need to be negotiated relative to the remaining level of control they are able to assume over their activities of daily living and functions within the family.

ASF measures relative to the togetherness and individuation dimensions reflect individual health in terms of congruence among the individuals within the family and between individuals and external systems. Differences in perception of congruence become apparent if the scores of various family members are compared. The discussion uncovers areas of conflict, disagreement, and interpersonal friction that can be fully explored in treatment.

For example, a domineering father who sets rules and demands strict order responds positively to the ASF-S individuation section, whereas other members express unhappiness with the lack of autonomy, ability to pursue their interests, and freedom of expression. The imbalance of control and dependency becomes evident in discussing the stifling effects of the power structure in this family.

Description of the Model

Leaders of family therapy of various orientations are debating the issue of how much theoretical thinking the therapist should disclose to the family. While strategic therapists (Haley, 1976) use techniques that appear deceptive to the observer, this author has found that the majority of nurses involved with families are uncomfortable with experimentation and "fooling" the clients into action. Instead, they favor an informative approach. Work with this model has shown that a positive, honest, and open approach can be effective and lead to change.

The model functions with the assumption that if nurse and client share their basic understanding of how individuals and families function and mutually agree on the changes needed, trust is formed and client resistance is lowered. The essential ingredient needed for change to take place is acceptance. In working with systems of different structures, cultures, and values, the model helps both nurse and clients to understand that a wide variety of family processes are possible within each process dimension and puts the client in charge of choosing the ones most suitable. Consequently, the nurse gains objectivity and reduces prejudice while the client acquires autonomy.

In the example of a family in which the husband had been a heroin user for 20 years and wanted to break the habit, resolving the problem of resistance involved the wife's change of attitude from anger and blaming to understanding and support and of behavior from attempting to control her husband to helping him assume independence. The ASF-F graph that indicated a low score for individuation, particularly the husband's score, made evident the need for both to grow and develop independent personal skills. Even though goals toward independence were set mutually, the wife's resistance became strong. Against her better judgment, she fell back into a pattern of reminding and nagging, and her cooperation with home assignments was minimal. During several sessions the need for control, individually and within the family, was interpreted by the nurse and much praise was given for using strategies that led to self-development and mutual support. A cycle of alternate improvements and crises was the first indication of change. The destructive effect of falling back to old patterns became evident and predictable. Encouraged by repeated signs of success, the spouses broke resistance and provided their own solutions, namely a plan of shared household responsibilities, mutual problem solving, and involvement in activities outside the family.

The CC-Model needs to be translated into the clients' language and ways of thinking about life. The concepts of control and congruence are

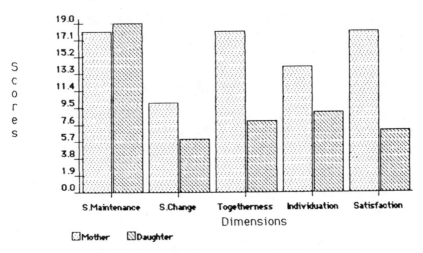

S
c
o
r
e
s

Figure 1. Mother—daughter scores on ASF-F and ASF-S.

explained in simple terms as they function on the individual and family levels and the four family process dimensions are described. It is the art of nursing, or the ability of the nurse to extend the self to the level of the client, that will determine success or failure. A bar graph depicting the ASF-F scores reflecting two family members' emphasis on the four process dimensions and the ASF satisfaction score is helpful in explaining the model in terms specific to a family (Fig 1).

Figure 1 refers to an example of a family who had a mentally ill daughter. Mother and daughter scored uniformly high on control emphasis. Mother's satisfaction score was high but the patient's was low. The bar graph was used to explain the target dimension of control. The nurse acknowledged the family's strong emphasis on control and stability. The positive aspects of families that value tradition and have firm methods of coping was stressed, in particular the ability to solve problems quickly (Kantor & Lehr, 1975). The family verified the nurse's description of their family with pride. In assessing the actual strategies used in getting daily tasks done, it became evident that the patient's mother was controlling the patient more than necessary. However, the nurse stressed and encouraged the family's effective strategies: for example, the supervision of the patient's medications that was done in an encouraging fashion. Next, the control-dependency problem of the patient was explained to the family members. Loss of control over mental and physical functions during acute outbreaks of the illness had produced severe anguish in the patient. The result was her strong urge to regain control at home. However, these attempts were frustrated since the mother was making all decisions, including the daughter's daily schedule of activities. The only way the daughter could be in control was by refusing to follow the mother's orders. Thus, by hearing about the control-dependency relationship applied to their situation, family members were learning about themselves and the functions of their family.

The Treatment Process

Treatment starts with the interpretation of the model and the assessment data and ends when the evaluation process shows significant improvement and the family is confident in continuing functional strategies independently. An ongoing assessment and evaluation of progress in small steps is interwoven in the treatment process. This is not unique to the CC-Model.

The unique components are delineated in the ADD HEALTH process. Its steps provide the necessary structure. Step 3, the determination of the focal process dimension(s), follows naturally as the family recognizes on the bar graph and from the ASF-E scores where the shortcomings are. Families familiar with family process are able to pinpoint their trouble spots easily and independently. Self-assessment helps them to stay in charge and accept the role of the nurse in guiding them toward the changes they want.

Step 4, highlighting the strengths of the strategies families use, further confirms the supportive rather than directive relationship the nurse has with the family. It is a motivating force, especially for long-suffering individuals who have never before believed that they have qualities. Trust develops at the point where the family accepts the nurse's genuine desire to help. The nurse is often able to redefine strategies family members use to show that they serve a purpose. Thus, family members start to believe that they have power to influence their future.

Step 5 strengthens the belief in the power of control. It is easiest for families to engage in strategies with which they are familiar, strategies previously used but never evaluated consciously. With encouragement to activate these processes to a greater extent, they become significant reinforcers of confidence and self-concept. Here, the art of nursing consists of guiding the family to rehearse the processes with each other through role playing, games, or media of art and expression. For example, a family working on system change needs to learn to adjust to the growing independence of their child. Father reports that his son likes to associate with another boy in school, but the family disapproves of the boy as a bad influence. The nurse stresses the value of their ability to pick up quickly what is good and what is bad in other people and their effort to protect the children from bad influences. The nurse may then suggest that children learn these qualities from their parents very early and ask the parents to test how much their son knows about finding good and bad things in people. The parents are given the assignment to invite the boy to their house after school. During that time, the mother will watch how the two children play together and will note all the good and all the bad things about the boy. Her son is given the assignment to also watch for good and bad things in his friend. In the next session, the nurse helps them to compare their impressions and is instrumental in interpreting some of the boy's behavior in light of his development stage. The decision whether the boy should come back is left to the family, but the exercise itself with the nurse's interpretation suggests that children be given more credit for sound judgment in their choice of friends and that it may be worthwhile to explore positive qualities of systems external to the family.

This example not only shows how to reinforce already existing qualities, but it illustrates how enforcing existing strategies can be used to gently guide the family into accepting and experimenting with new processes (steps 6 and 7) by realizing through practical experience that these processes are within their realm of possibilities and could be useful.

As previously mentioned, the CC-Model is broader than mere family therapy in its focus on the environment. The above example shows the introduction of an external system (the son's friend) in the effort to assist individuals to open up their minds toward their environment. To include the environmental dimension is focal to all those families whose main problems consist of environmental stress: the poor, the homeless, the unemployed, or the chronically mentally ill. Within the system change dimension, mental health nursing becomes one with community health nursing. Nurses involved with needy families will recognize that there is a basic requirement of environmental stability required before individuals and family systems are able to make changes toward growth. Through the ADD HEALTH process, nurses help families to ease stress by learning to use community resources. Connecting families with other family systems to help each other is a vital option if community resources are lacking. The challenge to the nurse consists of meeting the needs of the poor beyond mere survival. This is only achieved if families start to control their own environment, accept into their system what they need for growth, and resist those forces that are destructive to their existence. Through nursing with the CC-Model, family members gain confidence in directing functional processes toward suitable environmental systems, for example, using certain social skills in applying for a job. In addition, family members are taught new skills. Community resources such as vocational rehabilitation or a literacy class are frequently used where deficiencies are extensive.

The Evaluation Process

The evaluation of the effects of new strategies is ongoing. Generally, families who are successful in implementing new ways of coping and get much recognition of their efforts (step 9) are motivated to do even better or to continue what they have started. If a family has changed its course from self destruction to a constructive process and family members honor and recognize each other's efforts in supporting the family, there is little help needed by the nurse. Time has come to disengage from the family system. As Minuchin (1974) describes, the enthusiasm induced by the experience of a better functioning family system is ongoing and the effects of even a short period of successful therapy can be long lasting.

To decide termination, all instruments are readministered and shared with the family, as in the assessment phase. A sizable increase of emphasis and effectiveness within the focal process dimension(s), greater satisfaction, more or improved functional strategies, and favorable reports of key persons in systems with which the family has contact point to increased family health. The final decision to terminate is achieved mutually between nurse and client.

CONCLUSION

The CC-Model is suggested for those nurses who have experienced frustration with conventional approaches or those who would like to become involved with a more difficult population. It is necessary for nursing to experiment with new models in assisting the poor, the disadvantaged, the minorities, the homeless, in short all those who are denied access to traditional health care or find traditional care unacceptable. The model has the advantage of including individuals, family systems, and environmental systems. It allows nurses to be flexible in helping families to solve problems not only within their system, but in interacting with their environment. The CC-Model leads the nurse to assess priorities of needs with the clients and the family approach is instrumental in working with individuals in supporting each other. Often, individuals do not have families or have separated from their family. The CC-Model can be applied to these persons as well in that the nurse will aim at creating "families" or primary support systems. Therapy involves two or more individuals invested in each other's well-being, and the CC-Model guides the nurse in the formation of a mutual support system that is better able to cope with the environmental stress than each individual would be able to alone. While the CC-Model can only be as effective as the nurse who uses it, its value lies in the approach to thinking that is rooted in an overall theory, the framework of systemic organization, and in interventions that open up possibilities for nurses to expand their role into the community and the health care system.

REFERENCES

Bandura, A. (1969). *Principles of behavior modification*. New York: Holt, Rinehart & Winston.

Bateson, G. (1961). The biosocial integration of behavior in the schizophrenic family. In

N. W. Ackerman, F. L. Beatment, & S. N. Sherman (Eds.), *Exploring the base for family therapy*. New York: Family Service Association of America.

Bowen, M. (1976). Theory in the practice of psychotherapy. In P. J. Guerin (Ed.), *Family therapy: Theory and practice* (pp. 42–90). New York: Gardner.

Buckley, W. (1967). *Sociology and modern systems theory*. Englewood Cliffs, NJ: Prentice Hall.

Couch, A. (1970). The psychological determinants of interpersonal behavior. In K. Gergen & D. Marlow (Eds.), *Personality and social behavior* (pp. 77–89). Reading, MA: Addison-Wesley.

Friedemann, M. L. (1986). *Family functioning: Theory and measurement*. Unpublished manuscript, Wayne State University. College of Nursing, Detroit.

Friedemann, M. L. (1988). *Effectiveness of strategies in families: An instrument to evaluate family functioning*. Unpublished manuscript, Wayne State University, College of Nursing, Detroit.

Haley, J. (1959). The family of the schizophrenic: A model system. *Journal of Nervous and Mental Diseases, 129,* 357–374.

Haley, J. (1976). *Problem solving therapy*. San Francisco: Jossey-Bass.

Jackson, D. D. (1957). The question of family homeostasis. *Psychiatric Quarterly 31*(Suppl.), 79–90.

Kantor, D., & Lehr, W. (1975). *Inside the family*. San Francisco: Jossey-Bass.

Krauss, J. B. (1987). Nursing, Madness, and Mental Health. *Archives of Psychiatric Nursing, 1*(1), 3–15.

Lewis, J. M., Beavers, W. R., Gossett, J. T., & Phillips, V. A. (1976). *No single thread: Psychological health in family systems*. New York: Brunner/Mazel.

Miller-Ham, L., & Chamings, P. (1983). Family nursing: Historical perspectives. In I. W. Clements & F. B. Roberts (Eds.), *Family health: A theoretical approach to nursing care*. New York: Wiley.

Minuchin, S. (1974). *Families and family therapy*. Cambridge, MA: Harvard University.

Moos, R. H. (1974). Systems for the assessment and classification of human environments: An overview. In R. Moos & P. Insel (Eds.), *Issues in social ecology* (pp. 5–28). Palo Alto, CA: National.

Moos, R. H. (1986). *Family Environment Scale: Manual* (2nd ed.). Palo Alto, CA: Consulting Psychologists.

Murphy, S. (1986). Family study and nursing research. *Image, 18*(4), 170–174.

Olsen, D. H., McCubbin, H. I., Barnes, H. L., Larsen, A. S., Muxen, M. J., & Wilson, M. A. (1984). *Families: What makes them work*. Beverly Hills, CA: Sage.

Porter, L., & Lawler, E. (1965). Properties of organization structure in relation to job attitudes and job behavior. *Psychological Bulletin, 64,* 23–51.

Roberts, C. S., & Feetham, S. L. (1982). Assisting family functioning across three areas of relationships. *Nursing Research, 31*(4), 231–235.

Whall, A. L. (1986). *Family therapy theory for nursing*. Norwalk, CT: Appleton-Century-Crofts.

Whitaker, C. A., & Keith, D. V. (1981). Symbolic-experiential family therapy. In A. S. Gurman & D. K. Knistern (Eds.), *Handbook of family therapy* (pp. 157–225). New York: Brunner/Mazel.

Yalom, L. (1970). *The theory and practice of group therapy*. New York: Basic.

COMMENTARY

Friedemann's first paper represents a theory synthesis effort. The theory that was developed built upon earlier theoretical efforts by the editors of this book as well as other nursing perspectives. The family unit is emphasized here. The major theoretical statements address family health and family environment.

Friedemann has made a distinctive contribution to family theory development in nursing by demonstrating the utility of synthesis in the formulation of new middle-range theories. Her work is an interesting and important "second-generation" effort that used existing nursing literature as a foundation. The paper serves as a fine example of this approach to theory building.

The second paper by Friedemann is an excellent example of further explication of the theory presented in the first paper and discussion of its empirical implications. Especially noteworthy is Friedemann's presentation of steps required for empirical testing of the theory, including instrument development work.

The congruence between the conceptual, theoretical, and empirical components of the research program outlined by Friedemann is evident and represents a substantial contribution to the family nursing literature. Also of note is the discussion of family nursing practice based on the perspective advanced here.

ANN L. WHALL

CHAPTER
17

Family System Theory: Relationship to Nursing Conceptual Models

ANN L. WHALL

Kaplan (1963) stated that fields of knowledge know no boundaries, that is, no one discipline "owns" a particular area. All disciplines are therefore free to "borrow" from one another, but just as surely must reformulate that knowledge according to their own discipline. Nursing for the most part has borrowed theories of family functioning as presented within other disciplines without bothering to reformulate (Whall 1980).

This chapter presents the reformulation of one substantive knowledge area, family systems theory, according to what, in a sense, is the syntax of nursing, the nursing models. However, just as the past influences the future, the substantive knowledge base of family theory is patterned by its own past. But before the background of family systems theory is discussed, a few points need to be made.

The approach to family theory used here is to consider as a family systems theory any theory that views family in a unitary manner, and considers the members to be interacting parts of that unit. A second point is that, although family systems theories are related to general systems theories, few theorists discuss the family system using the terminology of

Reprinted from J. J. Fitzpatrick, A. L. Whall, R. L. Johnston, & J. A. Floyd, *Nursing models and their psychiatric mental health applications* (pp. 69–94). Bowie, MD: Brady, 1982.

a pure systems theorist. Rather, such terms as systems, subsystems, open systems, closed systems, and optimal system state dominate the family systems discussions. Therefore these terms and others are used in this chapter. Finally, there are many ways to classify family systems theories. Some consider group dynamics and communication theories to be forerunners of family systems theory. Although this is undoubtedly true, there are other disciplines and approaches that have had greater influence on the family systems perspective, and that nursing uses more often. These influences are from sociology, from the crisis perspective, and from the psychologically based family therapy theories. These approaches are discussed initially in relation to each other. Certain therapy theories are then analyzed according to the nursing models of Rogers (1970, 1980), Orem (1980), and Roy (1976).

BACKGROUND OF FAMILY
SYSTEMS THEORY

Family systems theory has a rather varied past. The approach to the family system found in sociology and family therapy theories, however, are quite distinct. In the early stages of family theory development, the field was dominated by the family sociologists. By perusing the early sociological journals, one can identify that theory building efforts, at least in terms of research, have focused primarily on exploratory and exploratory-descriptive studies. A good example of an early family system theory building effort from the discipline of sociology is the work of Hill (1949) in "Families Under Stress." Considered a forerunner of the crises approach to families, Hill describes the family as a living system, a group of interrelated persons, that changes over time acting, reacting, and changing in response to the challenges of wartime separation, loss, and reunion. In this early study, Hill did not emphasize the term family systems; this was to come later.

Nye and Berardos's (1966) work, *Emerging Conceptual Frameworks in Family Analysis*, identified a great deal of variability in the sociological and other approaches to the study of the family system. The 11 plus conceptual frameworks that were identified included the major frameworks discussed earlier by Hill, Katz, and Simpson (1957). In rereading the early conceptual models such as the structural functional and situational approaches, the reader is struck with the diversity that springs from different approaches when viewing data. In an approach sometimes called the home economics approach, for example, the focus is on the family-environmental interchange. The family is seen as a system bartering, conserving, and exchanging within the environmental setting. Conversely, in the structural functional approach, the focus is definitely on the internal family structure and function, e.g., role structure and concomitant functional patterns. The importance of the conceptual model used to view the data becomes most evident when the same phenomenon, the family system, is examined from the differing perspectives of the various sociological frameworks.

Family sociologists have attempted to classify the family frameworks, but in general, these theoretical positions have changed over time and some are no longer distinguishable (Broderick 1971, Hill and Hansen 1960). Hill (1974) discusses the relationship between the structural-functional and developmental approaches and the modern family systems model. Influenced by one another, the sociological conceptual frameworks have thus tended to merge, the result has many times been to approach the family from more of a systems perspective.

An additional component of family systems theory is that developed by the family therapists. Psychologically based and less interested in exploring and describing primarily "what is" than the sociologists, the therapists were concerned with what could be done to facilitate change in "dysfunctional" families. The theory developed by the therapists is therefore concerned with what is most functional to the family both in terms of the individual and the group. The first statements of this new family systems approach are found in the early writings of Jackson (1957), Ackerman (1967), Haley (1959) and others. This family systems approach does not have a very long history. Napier and Whitaker (1978) discuss that the therapy theories that viewed the family as a system were very long in developing because the first half of the nineteenth century was dominated by individual therapy approaches.

Although psychiatric mental health nursing has been influenced by both the sociological and family therapy approaches to the family system, by far the greatest influence is that of the family therapists. This influence is perhaps because of differences both in the intent and level of theory. Whereas the sociologists discussed variables to be measured when describing or exploring the family system, the therapists were more concerned with assessing specific family functioning, identifying and treating problem areas. The difference in the theory produced by the two disciplines is more readily understood by the schema developed by Donaldson and Crowley (1978). There are academic disciplines and professional disciplines; within the professional disciplines, questions regarding practice are entertained. The academic discipline seeks to describe and explore in order to understand, not treat. Thus the family systems theory developed by the sociologists is less readily applicable to treatment issues.

A third historical portion of the family systems approach is that of the crisis theorists. Stemming from the early work of Lindemann (1944) and Hill (1949), there was an explication of the crises perspective with regard to the family system. Parad and Caplan (1965) developed a model for family assessment that was related to this crises perspective.

In terms of specificity of treatment, however, the family systems theories developed by therapists are much more specific and detailed than either the sociological or crises approaches. Thus, the family systems theories discussed in the remainder of this chapter are those of the family therapists.

GENERIC FEATURES OF THE FAMILY SYSTEM APPROACHES

There are several common approaches to the family system utilized by the family therapists. Those discussed here are the unitary conceptualizations of the family system, the assumption of some optimal functional state, be it homeostasis, equilibrium, or synchrony, and the assumption that the system is an open system, a closed system, or some variation of these.

Perhaps the most important feature of the family systems approach is that of a unitary conceptualization of family. By midtwentieth century, the family system was conceptualized as a whole, a totality different from the sum of the parts but yet with interrelated parts. The family unit was discussed as having a group psyche with certain identifiable types of interaction patterns. Scapegoating, rulemaking, and other types of small group patterns were identified and discussed as occurring within families. The unitary conceptualization of the family system is exemplified by the work of Smoyak (1975). The assumption is made that the whole affects the parts and vice versa, and that a problem with a part is reflective of a problem within the whole. The insistence of family therapists that the entire family be seen at one time in therapy sessions is reflective of this unitary concept.

The degree to which this is adhered varies with the individual therapy theory. When family system theories are examined for this unitary conceptualization, the question also arises, is the approach really unitary or is it merely a sum of the parts? A unitary approach seeks to understand the system, not individuals per se.

The second feature common to family systems theory is the assumption that there is an optimal functional state. Jackson's (1957) early work indicated that mental illness may serve to maintain the family or the homeostasis. Homeostasis in this instance has a negative connotation, but whether used in a positive or negative sense, the term means that the family system maintains a balance or steady state in which one factor balances the other. In the negative sense the schizophrenia of a child may hold together a strife-torn marital union. Later theorists, especially those influenced by the crises perspective, indicated that family equilibrium is a state to be regained after a disequilibrium-producing event. In the balancing of forces implied by equilibrium, a steady state is positive and is indicative of the optimal condition of the family system. Equilibrium in this sense implies a balance of forces within the family, a balance of roles, for example, within the family so as to counteract an upset state. When a parent dies, the family is sent into disequilibrium, in the crisis view, due to the loss of a member who performed many vital roles. As the family redistributes role functions, perhaps by reaching out to a support system in the community, equilibrium again may be reached.

If homeostasis is used to connote sameness or calmness as an optimal family quality, then the question needs to be asked, what occurs so that growth is possible within individual members and family as a group? When an adolescent child begins the individuation or breaking away process, for example, most families experience an upset in sameness and calmness. Yet growth of individual family members, most would agree, is necessary and unavoidable. A theory that seeks an optimal state of calmness (stasis) may not account for growth needs.

The term equilibrium utilized as an optimal state may or may not account for growth needs. Equilibrium as a state of rest attained by a counterbalance of forces is very similar to the homeostatic concept just described and probably will not account for growth. But if equilibrium is utilized in the sense of synchrony, then the term may account for growth processes. Synchrony, from the word synchrone, means to be joined in the same period but so that changing phases are possible. In other words, family members may grow, change, and develop within the family system. For example, the person who used to prepare meals may no longer perform this function because of an individual need, but within the family system, food may be available and prepared in some other manner. Thus, individual change (or growth) was possible and yet the family system remained intact.

Barnhill (1979), in a study of the optimal family system states discussed by most of the major family therapy theorists, presents eight dimensions of family health. These states are: individuation versus enmeshment; mutuality versus isolation; flexibility versus rigidity; stability versus disorganization; clear versus distorted perception; clear versus distorted communication; role reciprocity versus role conflict; and clear versus breached generational boundaries. Although there is a loss of specificity, these categories may be summarized to mean that the healthy family system is one which allows the full development of all members and yet remains a functional whole. In this idealized family, communication is clear (synchronous), generational boundaries are not breached because this would adversely affect individuation. The terms homeostasis and equilibrium if used to mean only a balance would not account for growth states. For example, enmeshment is a homeostatic state, whereas, individuation might cause upheaval and reformulation into a new form of family system.

It is possible to extrapolate primarily an open or closed system perspective from the various family system theories. One way to describe the difference between closed and open systems is to use the discussion of meta models developed by Hultsch and Plemons (1979). The importance of this discussion to family systems theory has been identified by Fawcett (1980). There are two basic models utilized to define human beings and their relationship to the world around them — the organismic and the mechanistic models. The mechanistic model proposes cause and effect relationships. The machine is considered to be basically at rest until acted upon by some outside force. There is some time lag sequence implied as one waits for one part of the machine to affect the next. In this sense the machine is separate from the environmental field and additive in that the machine is the sum of the parts. The parts are very important in this model, for one part causes the next to function. The parts do not grow and change; patterns are repetitive. Machines (closed systems) do not take in extra stimuli, and unless the proper sequence of order is utilized to activate the machine, the machine will not function. For each machine action, there is a resultant reaction. For machines, processes are reversible, i.e., the whole procedure may be stopped and repeated in precisely the same manner and with little change in the machine. Machines in general do not regenerate, they wear down, wear out, and cease to function. Primarily linear in concept, machines close down, become entropic.

The organismic model according to Hultsch and Plemons is designed after a living organism and emphasizes wholeness; the parts are thus less important. Qualitative changes are possible within the organismic model (Hultsch and Plemons 1979, p. 5). Classical cause and effect relationships do not exist in the organismic model for with any given set of stimuli, the organism may act or not act in any given way. Living processes are not reversible in the sense that an organism progresses through time and space and is always growing older. The organismic model does not assume an at-rest state, rather this model assumes simultaneous activity, change, and growth (Hultsch and Plemons 1979). These theorists may be interpreted as positing that open systems are not repetitive and continuously patterned in the same way, that courses of action change. In systems terminology, living organisms display negentropy and equifinality. Each of the therapy theories chosen for discussion will be discussed in terms of unitary approach and conceptualization, assumption of optimal state, and a closed/open system perspective. These theories are then analyzed for reformulation utilizing specific nursing models.

SPECIFIC THERAPY APPROACHES OF HALEY, MINUCHIN, AND FRAMO

Haley, Minuchin, and Framo were chosen for this discussion because these theorists represent three distinct approaches to family therapy (Jones 1980). Haley, in his book *Problem Solving Therapy* (1978), states the basic concepts and propositions of his approach as it has evolved over time. It is important to note that, because Haley has written much and because his theoretical statements have changed over time, one of his latest theoretical works is used in this discussion. The approach of Haley in this work is unitary, not additive, for "to begin therapy by interviewing one person is to begin with a handicap" (Haley 1978, p. 10). Not only does Haley propose approaching the family as a unit, he emphasizes the need for discovering the social situation which makes the problem possible.

Some of the concepts of Haley are: the therapist, the field, family unit, family problem, directives, practice behavior, communication sequences, and communication hierarchy. Included as propositions are: the therapist becomes part of the field, or important to the family and influential in the situation before change can occur; therapy situations that are defined in terms of specific presenting problems are more amenable to change; it is the social situation, which displays a certain pattern and sequence, that makes the problem possible; assigned tasks solidify the gains of therapy as well as better illuminate the problem; change in communication sequences repatterns the behavior; and finally, secret coalitions across lines of authority produce confusion within the family system. Thus Haley is primarily concerned with the family as a unit and the interaction patterns which produce problems within the unit. The environment external to the family is considered important to the problem but not addressed at any length. An optimal family unit would be one in which there was a great diversity of response patterns, none of which deprived a member of his or her ability to grow and change (Haley 1978, p. 105).

Haley's approach indicates that he considers the family a living and somewhat open system that must accommodate growth needs. Although a few propositions, such as sequence of communication producing a problem situation, are cause/effect in nature, most propositions do not indicate classical cause/effect relationships. Haley states that in his approach the complexities of human life are simplified to reveal the structure, but that this is rather like describing a human being as a skeleton without flesh. Haley uses a few closed system terms such as control and resultant behavior. Haley's (1978) discussion of the drawback of family systems theories, i.e., steady state, equilibrium, not accounting for growth, is in essence a discussion of the drawbacks of a closed system model being applied to an open system, the family. The tasks or directives that Haley suggests are an effort to repattern the system. The tasks are expected to work directly and often call attention to an alternate pattern and at times emphasize a different aspect of the family system. The placing of emphasis on one aspect of the system in order to repattern may be understood as consistent with an open system approach. Thus, Haley's approach to the family indicates a sometimes open, sometimes closed system.

A hypothetical example of Haley's repatterning through the stages of therapy follows. This same example will be used throughout the chapter. The example is purposely made simplistic to emphasize differences in the approaches. It is important to note that any therapeutic approach would include much more than the simplistic steps identified in each · example.

Although not specifically addressed here, the first session would have drawn out all family members as to their opinion of the problem. No interpretations would be made. A mother and father with a ten-year-old boy with cerebral palsy also have an eight-year-old boy who has developed night fears to such an extent he is afraid to fall asleep at night. The mother has been sleeping with this child to reassure him. The mother is intensely involved, however, with the care of the disabled child and the father works two jobs to raise more funds for the treatment of this child. Entering the family system through the parents, the therapist might approach disengagement of the mother from the over-involvement with the disabled child by assigning the father to assume the responsibility for reorganizing the care of the disabled child to include outside assistance. As the father has management skills, he might be directed to be the authority in an area in which he had been closed out. The therapist would be careful not to imply the mother as been incompetent, but rather acts in this manner to free her for other duties. The mother who has spent little time with the eight-year-old might be assigned to take this child out on several nights now that she is relieved of care, and spend the time talking with, enjoying, and getting to know the eight-year-old with enjoyable activities. The mother might also be directed to stop sleeping with this child and to have the father handle any problems or questions that arise in this matter. All of this initial process should be designed to involve the peripheral person, the father, in order to repattern the over-involvement of mother with the disabled child. Also, by entering the family system via parental concerns for the children, the therapist becomes central to the parents and thus engages them more fully in the therapy. By assigning tasks also, the therapist becomes part of the field for the period of time between sessions.

In the next phase of therapy, the parents might be encouraged to engage in adult activities by arranging time away from the children. At this step Haley might expect some resistance. The assumption would be that somehow the over-involvement of both parents is a means of keeping the parents separate. Any resistance to change might be dealt with perhaps by getting at anger between the two adults by discussing disparities. Perhaps the troubled marital relationship is related to feelings of despair and/or guilt over the disabled child. The child's night fears are assumed to be somehow connected to both stress in the marriage and the evening's sequence of events when the mother stays with the disabled child. This sequence has the effect of eliminating both the husband and also the eight-year-old child from involvement with the mother. The night fears might be thought to serve as some means of uniting the parents in the fearful child's room. Haley uses the identification of the sequence of events surrounding the behavior to illuminate the social situation that surrounds the problem. Unless the problem behavior ceases, however, Haley believes the therapy to be a failure.

It is important to note several things about Haley's approach. The family is assessed as a unit, not as a sum of parts, and there is no attempt to assess the individual's physical, social, and psychic needs. This individual assessment approach would contribute to continuance of the problem from the stages of therapy point of view. The family is approached as a dynamic unit, capable of change. An indirect manipulation via "directives" might be expected to result in a cause/effect result unless the therapist understands that several outcomes are possible from any directive. It is assumed in Haley's approach that optimal family functioning, i.e., more diverse patterns, would result from blocking the cross-generational coalitions. The intense involvement with the child on the part of the mother would be replaced with a joint new parental approach. The change and diversity that are sought eschew an equilibrium approach on the part of Haley.

Minuchin's approach in *Families and Family Therapy* (1974) indicates more of an open systems approach. Some of Minuchin's concepts are: family system, family structure, therapeutic system, and subsystems, or hierarchical groups of family members. Some of the propositions of Minuchin are: the individual is influenced by and influences constantly recurring sequences of interaction; an individual is reflective of the family system of which he is a part; stress in one part of the system affects other parts of the system; and changes in family structure contribute to changes in behavior of individuals within a given system.

Minuchin is primarily concerned with the family as a unit, not as a sum of individuals. Minuchin focuses more fully upon the contextual patterns operating within the unit. The optimal family functioning that Minuchin seeks to facilitate is flexible adaptation and the ability to restructure over time according to the demands of each new situation, keeping subsystem boundaries clear. This open system allows the members to grow and develop as needed. As with Haley, the emphasis is on present-day processes, not influences of the past. Although specificity is lost in a summary, the optimal family state for Minuchin is one which stresses flexibility, clear system boundaries, and growth needs of all members. Minuchin's model indicates an emphasis upon an open growing family system. Use of such phrases as "the therapist contributes to change" rather than "the therapist directs," indicates little cause/effect orientation. Although the assumption is made that changing the context will change the individual behavior, this change usually is not implied to be the one-to-one relationship of a closed system. Minuchin does state that when deviation goes beyond the systems tolerance, mechanisms are used by the family to re-establish equilibrium (Minuchin 1974, p. 52). His position is that the family must learn to adapt to change. Use of the term adaptation is not in the sense of an outside force acting upon the family, but rather a mutual change. A steady state or equilibrium is definitely not the goal, rather it is an evolving system with clear intra-system relationships that values the worth of the individual subsystems. The environment external to the family is not discussed in detail.

In the hypothetical situation that is simplified to emphasize differences, a Minuchin therapist would first attempt to join the family system for the purpose of engagement. By joining the system, the therapist experiences the context of the system and develops a "working diagnosis" (Minuchin 1974, p. 129). The therapist might join the system, through giving support, while the family discusses the problem. There is no attempt on the part of the therapist to assess individual physical, social, and psychic needs and no interpretations are made. The therapist tracks or asks clarifying questions about, for example, the sleeping arrangements and boundaries this family displays. The therapist might explore the parental systems functioning and functioning of the sibling subsystem. During a first session the therapist evolves a "working diagnosis" similar to this: A non-functioning sibling subsystem is having difficulty operating effectively, and this is related to practically non-existent boundaries between the parental system and the child subsystem. The parental system is having difficulty functioning with several cross boundary problems.

The therapist in the initial session directs the participants to discuss the situation with each other; the children also are encouraged to discuss the issue that brought in the family. The therapist might thus illuminate the idiosyncratic system as well as recreate communication channels. Space might be changed and boundaries identified by sitting the children together. The children, with the help of the therapist, might agree to share a room at night. This arrangement would recognize that the youngest child is able to call for help if needed for the older child, and that the older child is thus able to assist with family functioning by serving as a companion to the younger child. The therapist thus might join the weak sibling subsystem supporting the boundaries. The therapist might also escalate stress by blocking the mother from verbally controlling the therapy session and also by emphasizing differences of opinion between the parents and children. Homework is sometimes assigned to be carried out, e.g., the parents might be asked to allow the children to handle the identified problem. This approach is to strengthen the sibling subsystem before working with the troubled parental system. Gradually, the therapist could move to a new area, e.g., the parents' troubled marital union.

Although the system is in a sense manipulated, Minuchin points out that any task given may elicit any number of responses. The responses, however, tend to expand the family's repertoire and hence tend to be change enhancing. Although identification of boundaries seems inflexible in a change model, Minuchin perceives boundaries as harmonious with functioning systems.

Framo's approach in *Rationale and Techniques of Intensive Family Therapy* (1965) also demonstrates a unitary approach to the family system. However, terms indicative more of a closed system perspective seem clearer. Some of Framo's concepts are: family system, past unresolved problems, family rules, resistance, and transference. Some derived propositions of Framo are: the therapist must stop old patterns before change can occur; rules hold the family in a repetitious cycle; past unresolved problems tend to be acted out in the present family; the attachment of past feelings to present family members tends to hold the family in a repetitive cycle; and accumulated experiences with present family members and the mutual accommodations made to these experiences tend to account for present behaviors.

Framo is primarily concerned with the family as an operating system or unit. The focus is on the psychodynamics and resultant behavior. The goal of therapy or the optimal system state is a clear perception by members of one another, as free as possible from past influences and misperceptions. The emphasis is more upon the past affecting the present. Framo's approach is primarily a closed system perspective for the family therapy addresses past problems. It can be interpreted that the family will remain enmeshed unless acted upon by some outside force. Since the family rules hold the family in a state of equilibrium, the goal of therapy is to establish a new equilibrium based upon accurate perceptions of the here and now. The environment external to the family is not addressed to any great extent.

In the hypothetical situation, a Framo approach would take place over time. The family would need to agree to work over time with the therapist. The family also must be willing to bring into the therapy sessions any extended family members identified as essential to the primary family unit (Framo 1965, p. 147). Several evaluation sessions are held to determine underlying situations. The initial presented problem is rarely thought to be indicative of the underlying situation. The family is asked to identify the changes they would like to occur. In the simplifeid example, family members, including the child with cerebral palsy, would be asked to discuss their version of the problem and this would assist with identifying transactional patterns. The parents would be encouraged to discuss their feelings regarding their families of origin, as well as events in their early and present marriage. The therapist thus works to clarify feelings regarding the past, thereby assisting the parents to gain some insight. The therapist might confront the mother with her absenting behavior in terms of the marital relationship and make some interpretation in this regard. Perhaps anger is related to some past event or perhaps some anger at their families of origin.

The therapist at the end of several evaluation sessions develops his or her diagnosis: there are coalition patterns, e.g., between the mother and the disabled child; there are family myths, e.g., that the relationship problems occur because of the disabled child; and that the fearful child's acting out is somehow related to holding the family together. During the middle phase of therapy, the therapist would most likely focus on working through feelings and working out new relationship patterns. The therapist would be careful not to perpetuate the family system status quo. According to Framo, resistance to change is expected and must be identified and challenged. In the final or termination phase of therapy, the attempt is to solidify gains. In the optimal case, the parents would be better able to discuss feelings openly and decrease the overinvolvement with the children. The children are thus free to pursue their own interests. Resistance to termination might be encountered, e.g., the "well" sibling (the disabled child) and later the index child (the fearful child) might act out their separation and dissolution fears. Termination issues are handled directly and the family should be freer to relate on the basis of present reality to one another.

The family system in this view is seen as repetitive, and entropic in its initial state. Changing the family by breaking the old rules or equilibrium and establishing a new relational system is the goal. The internal environment of the family is of prime importance and the family is approached without much utilization of the external environment. Physic processes are important and related to the system problems.

CORRELATES OF PERSON, HEALTH, ENVIRONMENT, AND NURSING WITHIN THE THERAPY MODELS AND THE NURSING MODELS

In Haley's model, the person is seen as part of the total family system, a subsystem, as it were, whose behavior is understandable in terms of the whole family system. Health in Haley's schema is the ability to change, grow, and develop a repertoire of diverse ways of handling life situations (1978, p. 105). The environment external to the family is now addressed although Haley identifies that external events should be considered. The therapist (or nurse) in Haley's model is a participant in the system but is also a director, in control of the therapy.

In Minuchin's model the person is understood in terms of the total family system. Behavior, although not totally predictable, is understandable primarily in terms of family system functioning. Extrapolated, health is the ability to grow, change, develop, and function as a member of the family system. The environment external to the family affects the family, such as economic depression. The nature of the relationship to environment is not, however, addressed at any length. The nurse (or therapist) in Minuchin's model would be much less the director, but more of a facilitator of repatterning within the context of the system.

In Framo's model, the person is more influenced by past situations that affect the present family system. Health is interpreted as the freedom from past experience so as to live more fully in the present with clearer perceptions. Environment external to the primary and extended family is not generally considered. In all of the above family therapy theories, person, health, and environment are viewed in light of psychosocial considerations. Physical or biological considerations are not usually addressed.

The therapist-nurse in Haley's model would be more of an active director who assigns tasks. At times, to influence change in the family system, paradoxical injunctions might be given. The therapist-nurse in Minuchin's model is also an active participant within the system. Not in control but rather participating and influencing, the therapist joins this system and might attempt to escalate stress in the system so as to facilitate change. A therapist-nurse in Framo's model is more of an evaluator, analyzer, and a reflector. The therapist-nurse might at various times clarify, confront, and support as new patterns are worked out.

In Rogers' (1980) conceptual model, the study of the environmental field is considered integral with the study of person (man in her terminology). In contrast, all three family therapists discuss that the individual can only be understood in his or her context—the family system. Man according to Rogers is conceived of as a four-dimensional energy field embedded in a four-dimensional environmental field. Rogers conceives of man as an indivisible unit—by studying only an individual's biology, for example, one cannot know the whole person. Man as a four-dimensional energy field manifests openness, or negentropy and pattern and organization. The environment is also a four-dimensional negentropic energy field characterized by pattern and organization; environment encompasses all that is outside the human field (Rogers 1980, p. 332). Thus it seems that Rogers would consider the family, although not specifically addressed, a negentropic energy field embedded in the larger environmental field. Nursing as a verb is seen as working with the energy field, not for or on the client (Falco and Lobo 1980, p. 173). The nurse is part of the co-extensive energy field, not separate. Health, although not addressed specifically, may be extrapolated as symphonic interactions between persons and their environment, a coherence and integrity of the human field (Falco and Lobo 1980). Rogers' conceptual model requires consideration of development, or unidirectional change in her words. That is, since each person is progressing (or developing) in one direction only, this progression must be accounted for in the interaction pattern of the energy field.

Roy's conceptual framework views person as a biopsychosocial being (Roy 1980). Roy states persons are also related to others in the group (Roy 1980, p. 3). The person as a whole should be viewed therefore from biologic/psychologic and social science perspectives. It is unclear if the biopsychosocial parts are assessed separately and from this, knowledge is applied to the adaptive modes, or if the sum of the parts can never equal the whole. It seems that environment is all that is external to the person. Health is considered an inevitable dimension of life and extrapolated health is optimal adaptation or high level wellness on the health-illness continuum (Roy 1976). The goal is to maintain the integrity of the whole. Roy discusses developmental processes, developmental stages, and crises. The nurse as a person external to the client evaluates and determines whether the individual is experiencing an adaptation problem or is in need of additional assistance. The nurse might then assist the family to adapt more fully or to change the nature of the focal stimulus so that it falls within the adaptive range. The person, although in constant interaction with his environment, seems to be the prime focus; family is not addressed in great length.

Orem's model views person (man in her terminology) as a psychophysiologic organism with rational powers (Calley, et al. 1980, p. 303). Nursing gives direct assistance to those unable to meet their own self-care needs. Health is a state of wholeness or integrity of the individual human being, his parts, and his modes of functioning (Orem 1980, Foster and Janssens 1980). Orem states that man's functioning is linked to his environment (Orem 1971). It would seem that environment is all that is external to the person. Orem, in an interesting discussion of the way family is to be approached, suggests that within the concept of wholeness, families are important. However, the parts (individual members) have existence and operations apart from the whole and, it would seem, must be assessed separately. Orem suggests that the nursing of families requires a special knowledge base different from, yet complementary to, that of individuals alone. It would seem that congruence between Orem's model and a family systems theory might be approached from her nursing systems perspective. That is, nursing systems are formed when nurses use their abilities to provide for groups by performing systems of action.

Congruence and Reformulation Issues

It is important that nursing as a discipline reformulate, according to its purposes and needs, the theories derived from other fields (Fawcett 1978, Kaplan 1963). The issue is that a discipline changes, adapts, and reformulates for its purposes, extant concepts, and groups of concepts. In this section the nursing models are utilized to reformulate selected aspects of the above family system theories. The family systems theory of Haley is compared to Orem's model and needed reformulations are addressed. Both Haley and Orem are considered to utilize both mechanistic and organismic concepts. The assumption is made in terms of both theorists of sometimes open, sometimes closed systems. Orem identifies that an important first step in nursing care is the diagnosis or identification of the problem. This is quite similar to Haley's insistence upon definition of the family problem in terms of a specific behavior. Orem's way of arriving at the problem statement is to assess: (1) what is the self-care demand (what is the problem); (2) does the patient have a deficit for engaging in self-care (what are the abilities of family members to handle the problem); (3) what is the reason for the problem's existence (what is the relationship of subsystems, the hierarchical sequence that makes the problem possible); (4) should the patient be helped to refrain from self-care (is the family system capable of participating in the therapy, or must the nurse therapist temporarily direct and control); and (5) what is the patient's potential for engaging in self-care (what is the optimal functioning that can be expected of this family system in relation to the problem) (Orem 1980, p. 203)?

The most evident areas of congruence between Haley and Orem deal with the therapist (nurse) as the director of therapy. Orem states that step one in the nursing process is determining why the patient is under care (see above diagnostic steps). Step two is to design a system of nursing that will contribute to the goals. If the goal is to change a problematic family behavior, the nurse identifies changes that are needed in roles and resources, for example, and identifies the approach so that the changes might be most effective. This is similar to Haley's concept of giving specific directives to the family that involve details in terms of time and specific frequencies. Whereas Orem seems to indicate that the nurse is separate during assessment, this could be interpreted as using much the same approach as Haley, i.e., the care giver experiences the context and then, as it were, steps back and directs. In the final step of the nursing process, the caregiver, according to Orem, compensates for self-care deficits, overcomes self-care limitations, and fosters and protects self-care abilities and limitations. This might be interpreted as an area of difference between Haley and Orem. In this last step Orem could be interpreted to indicate that environmental resources might be utilized to overcome any inherent deficits. Haley does not deal with the environment to any great extent.

In the hypothetical situation presented, these differences between Haley and Orem are apparent. That is, community agency, such as Crippled Children's Commisssion, might be employed to take over some of the financial burden felt by the father. Self-care limitations might be overcome by utilizing some ongoing community resource such as home-making service to free the mother from some of her duties. The father and mother thus would be freer to function as marriage partners. In the areas of fostering and protecting development, an Orem therapist would recognize that the fearful child's development might be limited or thwarted in terms of allowing him to learn to care for himself by the overprotection of his mother. The Orem therapist might identify the disabled child as a self-care resource within the family and thus suggest, after discussions, that both children sleep in the same room, thus assisting one another. In terms of fostering self-care and protecting the self-care abilities, it seems that an Orem therapist would not insist on termination within a specified number of sessions as Haley does. Recognizing that the newly established family self-care system needs support, some sort of continuing assistance would be offered for continuity of care.

Two other points of disparity between Orem and Haley are that Orem indicates that family collaboration and physical needs should be considered. Orem states that the family's interest or ability to collaborate in care must be assessed (Orem 1980, p. 204). In other words, an Orem therapist would consider reviewing the plan for therapy with the family, rather than using a non-informed manipulation approach. Orem states that meeting the immediate self-care need is a first step towards collaboration and/or participation in family self-care. Once the family is functioning so that a state of wellness of the family system is near, then collaboration and participation in self-care would definitely be addressed. It thus might be reviewed with the family that the child's fears were related to the family's pattern of coping, that the closeness of the mother with the children, although designed to help them, was not allowing for the growth and assumption of responsibility of which the children were capable. It would also be reviewed with the parents that friction between them is always felt in the system and the direct discussion of differences between the parents is necessary. An Orem therapist might temporarily give directives and control, but at some later point the family would be enlisted as collaborators.

In terms of the physical needs, Orem sees man as a psychophysiologic organism, as a biologic organism in an environment with physical and biologic components (Calley et al. 1980). As such, an Orem therapist would recognize that physiologic responses, such as gastrointestinal problems of the fearful child, have a psychological aspect. Therefore, the therapist would consider these GI problems as secondary to the family system problem. The nurse therapist, however, would assess the physical state of all the members, realizing that just as the mind may affect the body, the opposite is also true.

The family systems theory of Framo (1965) is compared to Roy's (1976) model and reformulations are addressed. Both Roy and Framo utilize more mechanistic than organismic concepts. Assumptions appear to be made that the family is sometimes a closed and sometimes an open system. Although Roy does not discuss the family as a system to any great extent, her consideration of the whole person with his or her total environment, as well as insistence upon considering the developmental state of the person, leads one to conclude that, within her model, the family system should be considered.

Galbreath (1980 p. 206) discusses Roy's model and the family system. She refers to Boszormenyi-Nagy, an associate of Framo. The reference is to the way in which an enmeshed (or closed) family system, keeps a child from individuation. The parent adapts to a focal stimulus, a need for companionship, by disallowing the child to separate. This is considered a case of maladaptation in terms of the system because the child's developmental needs are stifled and hence his or her integrity is threatened. A central concept in Roy's model (1976, p. 3), adaptation, is discussed as being carried out in the physiological, self concept, role function, and interdependence modes. Adaptation is thought to occur within an acceptable range; a response outside of this range is considered maladaptive.

If one considered the family system to incorporate the above modes, the concept of adaptation as utilized by Roy might be applied quite readily. For example, family systems have physiologic needs such as food, clothing, and shelter. As part of this need, it is necessary that the family provide adequate amounts and types of these supplies. An overcrowded family, for example, might lead to problems in one of the adaptation modes. Family systems have self-concept needs, both of the family subsystems, or individuals, and the family as a whole. An inadequate self-concept on the part of the parent might lead the parent to adapt by utilizing his or her children, over whom he or she has more control, as life companions. A deficit in the parent's self-concept would be hypothesized in terms that the parent views himself or herself as inadequate in terms of relating to adults. This child companionship thus would eliminate the need to seek other adult companions who might find the adult wanting. This turning inward would lead to an enmeshed or closed down family. Such families are described by both Framo (1965) and Boszormenyi-Nagy (1965).

Role function needs and interdependence needs might be seen as leading to maladaption within the hypothetical family system. Every family has a number of roles that must be fulfilled such as child caregiver, fund raiser, companion, etc. When these roles are not fulfilled, role conflict occurs and maladaptation may result, i.e., the integrity of the system is threatened. In the hypothetical situation, the role of caregiver to the disabled child was superceding all other roles. The roles such as mother of the fearful child, marital partner, and adult were not being handled and interdependence maladaption existed in the sense that the children were not allowed to separate from the parents.

Intervention in Roy's model is the key to nursing activity; the nurse changes the perceived parental inadequacy by manipulating the environment by increasing, decreasing, removing, or altering stimuli (Galbreath 1980). The person is seen basically in an "at rest" state, and the nurse is seen as the operator, altering the input stimuli. These relationships suggest a mechanistic view.

In Framo's approach to the hypothetical family, the parents may be seen as living out past problems in terms of the present family. In other words, there are definite problems with self-concept. By manipulating the environment, the stimuli is altered; that is, by allowing the parents to ventilate, and work through their past feelings in the present therapy sessions, the self-concept changes and the perceptions are brought into normal range. These relationships also suggest a closed system conceptualization.

A Roy approach to the family system would include assessment of the various adaptive modes. A deficit would be found in the role function, self-concept, and interdependence modes. It is doubtful that the intervention would include only a catharsis. A nurse therapist approaching the family from the Roy model likely would utilize the environment. The parents would be separated from the children. The space in the home probably would also be assessed in terms of the children's sleeping arrangements and be changed to facilitate the care. Because of Roy's emphasis upon developmental stages, the children and parents would be encouraged to individuate with support and find companions in their own age group. Other developmental tasks would be assessed and addressed.

Because of Roy's emphasis on physiologic adaptation, the physiologic needs of the members would be addressed. Roy's approach to the family system would therefore be more comprehensive with more attention to other environmental factors than that of Framo. In the interventions identified by Roy (1980), there is emphasis on teaching and educating the patient; most likely the family would be taught what were the bases of their problem. Roy suggests with dysfunctional interdependence modes that cognitive and affective structuring may be changed through insight therapy (1976, p. 392). Insight therapy is of course related to Framo's approach. Outlets for the parents would be identified to decrease temporary spillover of tension onto the children. The manipulation of the environment is encouraged to provide for independence as congruent as possible with developmental level.

Because of similarities, the structural family theory of Minuchin is compared with Rogers' conceptual framework. Both are considered primarily open systems approaches. Reformulations are addressed and the reformulated model is used to analyze the hypothetical situation. The areas of similarity between Minuchin and Rogers have to do with Minuchin's field approach. Energy fields extend to infinity (Rogers 1980) and in Minuchin's model, the contextual field of the family, as well as the extended field, is the unit of analysis. Rogers is interpreted to extend this to mean that the family may be conceived of as an energy field. The family field is considered in Minuchin's structural theory to be greater and different from the sum of the parts or the individuals. Otherwise, Minuchin would assess the parts or individuals separately rather than in interaction; this is not the case. The approach to the whole rather than parts is an area of congruence with Rogers. In Rogers's conceptualization, energy fields are always open. Minuchin's view that the family is a system that must change and grow according to internal and external forces would seem compatible with Rogers. Openness in Minuchin's terms is related to the constantly evolving patterns that are never entirely predictable.

Pattern and organization identify energy fields (Rogers 1980); patterns and organization also are continuously changing. In part, Minuchin's position that the family system must account for changing requirements is a recognition of this continuous change. As children grow, the family system is repatterned. Adults in Minuchin's view also grow and change and these simultaneous events account for the dynamic nature of the family system. Just as the family system continuously grows, changes, and repatterns, Minuchin indicates and Rogers stresses that so also does the environment. The environment is, in Rogers' conceptual model, an energy field, a system that grows, changes, evolves, and repatterns. The fluctuations in weather patterns are examples of this change as well as fluctuating patterns manifested in the development of towns and cities. Rogers's concepts seem compatible with Minuchin for he specifically addresses the repatterning of the economic system — economic depression — as one pattern that affects the family. The point made by Rogers is that she considers the effect of the environmental field upon the family to be, not one of cause and effect, but rather one of mutual interaction. This position would seem fairly compatible with Minuchin. The therapist in influencing the family system never directly controls the situation. Rogers's principle of helicy postulates that change is continual, innovative, probabilistic, and characterized by increasing diversity (Rogers 1970, 1980). Minuchin's approach can be interpreted as identifying the need to handle change although this is less true than with Rogers. When Minuchin states one "works with" the system, this might be interpreted to mean that change is innovative and probabilistic rather than cause and effect. In other words, although all adolescents come to individuation, the general pattern is there, no two adolescents separate from the family in quite the same way. The situation probably has certain features, the fearful parent, the rejecting adolescent — but none of this is certain.

Rogers further postulates that the human and environmental fields are characterized by resonancy. That is, wave patterns manifest change from longer waves, lower frequency to higher frequency shorter waves. One might postulate that each family member manifests different field patterns and that the entire family thus manifests some diverse yet unified pattern. The environmental field also manifests a diverse yet whole pattern. Perhaps Minuchin's approach to synchronous subsystem boundaries is an attempt to effect a synchrony between and among the various system patterns. But just as there is no cause/effect in Rogers's approach; Minuchin's approach can be interpreted to indicate the therapist attempts repatterning, not that repatterning is caused to happen. Minuchin emphasizes that only by working with the family system will individual patterns change.

Minuchin's concept of working within the context of the family can be interpreted in a Rogerian sense, i.e., that the total field context or family system is an influential force in terms of the individual field. With both Rogers and Minuchin, the whole is most important and approaches are nonadditive, change models.

Rogers's third principle is complementarity or that interaction between human and environmental fields is continuous, simultaneous, and mutual. A corollary of the principle is that there is no separation between man and environment. Minuchin's concept of boundaries seems incongruent with both resonancy and complementarity. That is, if fields extend to infinity and are in mutual simultaneous interaction, then there are no boundaries. Rogers does state, however, that use of the term boundaries is acceptable to aid perception. The human ability to perceive fields is very limited and what seems to be a boundary may in essence be a different field pattern. What Minuchin refers to as marking boundaries may be effecting a decrease in the invasive repatterning of one field by another.

Other terms of Minuchin, such as adaptation, stress, and equilibrium, also need to be changed or deleted in light of Rogers's model. If adaptation means the process of accommodating to some outside force from a state of rest, then this concept would be incongruent with Rogers's position. Minuchin, however, states that by facilitating the use of alternative modes, the therapist makes use of the family matrix (field) in the process of healing (facilitating synchrony). This interpretation would be acceptable in Rogers's terms. However, Minuchin goes on to say that the family structure must be able to adapt. As previously discussed, this implies a closed system perspective and needs to be changed. The continued existence of the family as a system depends on a sufficient range of patterns, availability of alternative patterns, and flexibility to mobilize as necessary. This is an area of congruence for both theorists. Minuchin's approach could be reformulated to mean that, in a particular family system, the greater the range of complex patterns available for the subsystem, the more likely the total field is to exhibit synchrony.

Rogers's definition of health, as extrapolated from Newman (1979), is symphonic interaction between persons and their environment, a coherence. An invasive field that, in effect, attempts to repattern another according to its own needs, is not a coherent force within the family unit. Thus cross-generational coalitions inhibit the development and change of the less developed unit. Perhaps the more established field of the adult is one of more intensity, and if a coalition develops, the newer evolving field may not develop its own pattern. Minuchin's extrapolated definition of health is flexible adaptation and the ability to restructure over time according to the demands of each new situation. Flexible adaptation might be reformulated to non-invasive synchrony between field forces within the family system.

In the hypothetical situation, a reformulated structural approach might be relabeled to indicate less of a mechanistic nature. In the reformulated theory, the nurse using Rogers's model might approach the hypothetical situation differently. Because in the example the family unit is composed of several members, the nurse would seek to identify the points of disharmony within the field. The fearful child is symptomatic of family disharmony. The nurse, as part of the environmental field, seeks to promote synchrony and development of emergent field patterns by influencing the family field towards a more synchronous patterning. Recognizing the dysynchrony related to invasive closeness of one field (the mother) with another field (that of the child with cerebral palsy), the nurse seeks to influence the repatterning of this relationship. The fears of the other child are considered to be a manifestation of a field which is in distress. Part of the disharmony of the family field is related to the absence of the father, or at least disparity of approach between the mother and the father. The nurse, in assessing the situation, might attempt to experience the family system or field using all of her senses and skills.

Any attempt at repatterning would be developed with the family and addressed as attempts at reformulating or trying out a new pattern. Although the Rogers approach might parallel Minuchin's in the hypothetical situation in many ways, the differences would revolve around working with the family, not manipulating, not by identifying boundaries, but by identifying the different growth patterns and needs. Placing the children in the same bedroom is an example of an attempt to synchronize fields of similar frequency.

The physical needs of the family members are considered as manifestations of the total field. Consequently these are addressed if disharmony is evident. But, rather than addressed as a separate entity, the needs are looked upon as manifestations of the whole. The child with cerebral palsy may be quite healthy and display little physical disharmony, whereas the fearful child may display some type of physical disharmony, such as dietary and gastrointestinal problems. Thus, parts of individual subsystems may be addressed but always considered in terms of the whole. In a particulate approach, gastrointestinal problems of the fearful child would be treated alone, and probably with little success as separate from the total family field.

RESEARCH AND PRACTICE ISSUES

Although all three reformulated models are quite different, there are common elements. These commonalities have to do with approaching assessment from a holistic stance. That is, the psychic state of health of a family or individual is not the total focus in the reformulated nursing approach, whereas many of the family therapy theories utilize a psychic assessment approach only. The nursing therapies focus more broadly; a recognition is made that, for example, a mother with severe iron deficiency anemia may very well handle her fatigue by interacting with a parental child. A second area of commonality is that the nursing therapy approaches deal with family/individual participation. Most of the nursing models eschew a silent manipulation as the nurse assesses and treats; all the models suggest an openness with clients. That is, the silent, never revealed manipulation of the system is not the approach indicated by the nursing models. Roy, for example, states that environmental manipulation must be approached, and attempts to solidify gains through teaching and other explanatory attempts. The family or client is seen as active, more as a partner in therapy rather than in the passive sick role posture. Even Minuchin, who is relatively open with families, does not share with them what he believes to be the underlying situation. Finally, the nursing therapies, when compared to some other therapy theories, seem an optimistic approach. The family is not seen as totally foretold by past family systems, living out past echoes as it were. The family is conceived of as primarily healthy or tending toward health and capable of learning, growing, and changing as completely as needed. The nursing approach therefore includes discussing with the family the patterns that are seen as dysfunctional, and working with the family utilizing strengths to change these patterns and interrelationships. Because the deep-seated, intractable, and pathology-laden interpretations of the family dysfunction are not made, the traditional loathing to share the diagnosis of the underlying problems with the family is less.

The research and practice issues in a sense revolve around the reformulations. Not many of the therapy theories have been systematically explored in terms of outcomes (Wells et al. 1978). Rather than address outcome evaluation, which all therapy theories need to do, some of the research issues that revolve around the reformulated nursing therapy approaches will be addressed. With the Rogers approach, there are several basic and applied questions:

Is family dysfunction an invasiveness of one field force with another?
If family health is synchrony, how is repatterning best accomplished?
Is there a family energy field that may be considered in relation to other energy fields?

There are many more research issues that may be readily identified.

In a reformulation with Orem's model, some research issues might be:

What is the nature of a total family assessment that also includes individual data?

How does one maintain a family perspective using individual assessment data?

How does one assess a family self-care deficit?

What is the nature of family self-care agency, etc.?

Orem discusses that the nursing of groups requires a specialized knowledge base. The nature of the knowledge base most complimentary with an Orem approach should be explored.

In a reformulation with Roy's model, there are several research issues that might be addressed:

Do the adaptation modes transfer readily to the family system?

Is family health an additive concept comprised of individual assessments?

Does one assess family adaptation modes and then only intervene in the stimuli?

The practice issues flow from the theoretical reformulations.

The effect of educating the family to the underlying problem also needs to be assessed. The traditional individual psychoanalytic approach held that teaching and education were of little value. The troubling situation had to be relived and experienced before insight and resolution could result. If a Roy approach incorporates both education and insight goals, then the relationship of education to insight needs to be addressed. The traditional view is that after insight, little education is needed. Another important issue in the Roy approach has to do with manipulation of the external environment, and whether this is effective when dealing with the family unit.

The above reformulated nursing therapy approaches are a first attempt to accomplish what Kaplan (1963) and Fawcett (1978) indicate lies before us. That is, rather than borrowing in total extant family theories, nursing must reformulate to its own purposes. Some might question the effect of nurse therapists practicing from a variety of approaches, but, after all this is currently the case, for nurses are practicing using a multiplicity of unchanged theories.

REFERENCES

Ackerman N: Prejudice and scapegoating in the family. *In* Zuk G, Boszormenyi-Nagy I (Eds.): Family Therapy and Disturbed Families, Palo Alto, Science & Behavior Books, 1967

Barnhill L: Healthy family systems. Fam Coordinator, (January), 94–100, 1979

Boszormenyi-Nagy I: A theory of relationships: experience and transaction. *In* Boszormenyi-Nagy I, Framo J (Eds.): Intensive Family Therapy: Theoretical and Practical Aspects, New York, Harper & Row, 1965

Broderick C: Beyond the five conceptual frameworks: a decade of development in family theory. J Marriage and the Family, 33:139–159, 1971

Calley J, Dirksen M, Engalla M, Hennrich M: The Orem self-care nursing model. *In* Riehl J, Roy C: Conceptual Models for Nursing Practice (2nd Ed.), New York, Appleton-Century-Crofts, 1980

Donaldson S, Crowley D: The discipline of nursing. Nurs Outlook, 26:113–120, 1978

Falco S, Lobo M: Martha E. Rogers. In the Nursing Theories Conference Group. Nursing Theories: The Base for Professional Nursing Practice, Englewood Cliffs, Prentice-Hall, 1980

Fawcett J: The "what" of theory development. *In* Theory Development: What, Why, How? New York, National League for Nursing, 1978

Fawcett J: Address to a nursing doctoral seminar on family health, May 14, 1980. Jacqueline Fawcett, PhD, RN, is an Associate Professor, School of Nursing, University of Pennsylvania

Foster P, Janssens N: Dorothy E. Orem. In the Nursing Theories Conference Group. Nursing Theories: The Base for Professional Nursing Practice, Englewood Cliffs, Prentice-Hall, 1980

Framo J: Rationale and techniques of intensive family therapy. *In* Boszormenyi-Nagy I, Framo J (Eds.): Intensive Family Therapy: Theoretical & Practical Aspects, New York. Harper & Row, 1965

Galbreath J: Sister Callista Roy. In the Nursing Theories Conference Group. Nursing Theories: The Base for Professional Nursing Practice, Englewood Cliffs, Prentice-Hall, 1980

Haley J: The family of the schizophrenic: a model system. J Nervous and Mental Disorders, 129:357–374, 1959

Haley J: Problem Solving Therapy, San Francisco, Jossey Bass, 1978

Hill R: Families Under Stress, New York, Harper & Row 1949

Hill R: Modern systems theory and the family: a confrontation. *In* Sussman M: Sourcebook in Marriage and the Family, Boston, Houghton-Mifflin Company, 1974

Hill R, Hansen D: The identification of conceptual frameworks utilized in family study. Marriage and Family Living, 22:299–301, 1960

Hill R, Katz A, Simpson R: An inventory of research in marriage and family behavior: a statement of objectives and progress. Marriage & Family Living, 19:89–92, 1957

Hultsch D, Plemons J: Life events and life-span development. *In* Baltes P, Brim O (Eds.): Life Span Development and Behavior, Vol. 2, New York, Academic Press, 1979

Jackson D: The question of family homeostasis. Psychiatric Quarterly Supplement, 31:79–90, 1957

Jones S: Family Therapy: A Comparison of Approaches, Bowie, Maryland, Robert J. Brady Co., 1980

Kaplan A: The Conduct of Inquiry, New York, Harper & Row, 1963

Lindemann E: Symptomatology and management of acute grief. Am J Psych, 101:141–148, 1944

Minuchin S: Families and Family Therapy, Cambridge, Harvard University Press, 1974

Napier A, Whitaker C: The Family Crucible, New York, Harper & Row, 1978

Newman M: Theory Development in Nursing, Philadelphia, F. A. Davis, 1979

Nye F, Berardo F: Emerging Conceptual Frameworks in Family Analysis, New York, The Macmillan Company, 1966

Orem D: Nursing: Concepts of Practice (2nd ed.), New York, McGraw-Hill, 1980

Parad H, Caplan G: A framework for studying families in crises. Social Work, 5:3–15, 1960

Rogers M: An Introduction to the Theoretical Basis of Nursing, Philadelphia, F. A. Davis, 1970

Rogers M: Nursing: a science of unitary man. *In* Riehl J, Roy C (Eds.): Conceptual Models for Nursing Practice, New York, Appleton-Century-Crofts, 1980

Roy C: The Roy adaptation model. *In* Riehl J, Roy C (Eds.): Conceptual Models for Nursing Practice, New York, Appleton-Century-Crofts, 1980

Smoyak S: Introducing families to family therapy. *In* Smoyak S (Ed.): The Psychiatric Nurse as a Family Therapist, New York, J. Wiley, 1975

Wells R, Dilkes T, Trivelli N: The results of family therapy: a critical review of the literature. Family Process, 7:189–207, 1972

Whall A: Congruence between family theory and nursing models. Adv Nurs Sci, 3:59–67, 1980

COMMENTARY

From Fitzpatrick, Whall, Johnston, and Floyd's book focuses on the theory development strategy of reformulation. This three-step strategy involves

1. identification of the underlying assumptions and major propositions of an existing conceptual model and a middle-range theory
2. comparison of these assumptions and propositions to determine their logical congruence
3. modification of the theory, if needed, to yield a logically consistent conceptual-theoretical structure that can be used for empirical research and clinical practice.

This chapter explains linkages of conceptual models of nursing with a middle-range theory developed within the context of other family sciences, including family sociology, family therapy, and the crisis perspective. Three conceptual models of nursing are used as starting points: Orem's Self-Care Framework, Rogers's Science of Unitary Human Beings, and Roy's Adaptation Model. Family systems theory is the middle-range theory that is modified for logical linkage with each of the conceptual models. Given the emphasis on the family as a system, this theory can be classified as family nursing theory. Examination of future research based on the proposed conceptual-theoretical structures to determine the extent to which methodology is in keeping with the whole family perspective is warranted.

JACQUELINE FAWCETT

Family Adjustment To Heart Transplantation: Redesigning the Dream

MERLE H. MISHEL
CAROLYN L. MURDAUGH

The processes family members of heart transplant recipients use to manage the unpredictability evoked by the need for and receipt of heart transplantation were explored. Twenty family members were theoretically sampled using the grounded theory approach. Three separate family support groups, each of 12 weeks duration, provided data for constant comparative analysis. Redesigning the dream was identified as the integrative theme in the substantive theory that described how family members gradually modify their beliefs about organ transplantation and develop attitudes and beliefs to meet the challenge of living with continual unpredictability. The theory consists of three concepts — immersion, passage, and negotiation — which parallel the stages of waiting for a donor, hospitalization, and recovery.

Heart transplantation has become an acceptable therapeutic intervention for patients with end-state heart disease, but little attention has been focused on the needs of the patients' families as the patients proceed from diagnosis through surgery into recovery phases.

Reprinted from *Nursing Research, 36*, 332–338, 1987.

Effects on the family of patients' having other cardiovascular conditions, such as myocardial infarction and coronary artery bypass surgery, have been studied. Conclusions of these investigations supported the position that both the surgery and the recovery process are tremendous sources of stress, as the integrity of the family is threatened. Changes in roles of family members add further stress to the already overburdened family system. Personality changes in the patient increase tension and stress in the family (Mayou, Foster, & Williamson, 1978).

Spouses of patients undergoing coronary artery bypass surgery also have reported numerous sources of stress during hospitalization and recovery (Sexton & Munro, 1985). These include a lack of control of hospital events, lack of privacy, and fear of responsibility for caring for patients after discharge. The most commonly identified stressor for spouses was waiting for the surgery.

The adaptation of patients with cardiac conditions who undergo heart transplantation has been considered in only four studies (Evans et al., 1984; Lough, Lindsey, Shinn, & Stotts, 1985; McAleer, Copeland, Fuller, & Copeland, 1985; Wallwork & Caine, 1985). Only Evans et al. considered the interpersonal nature of the patient's life. Nor has the literature recognized the unpredictabilities that require adaptation by the partner and the patient.

Unpredictability refers to the unknowns involved in heart transplantation. The initial unknown is whether the precarious condition of the patient can be maintained until a heart is available and whether the patient will survive the surgery. The instability of the postoperative period follows and culminates in the unpredictable occurrences of infections, rejections, and secondary illnesses. Life span with a heart transplant is known to be limited; therefore, the events remain uncertain with the patient's status being subject to sudden and catastrophic change.

The purpose of the present study was to identify processes used by family members to manage the unpredictability elicited by the need for and receipt of heart transplantation.

METHOD

Design: The method used was grounded theory (Glaser & Strauss, 1967) which involves concurrent collection, coding, and analysis of data. Data that are similarly coded are grouped into categories. Core or central categories emerge, explaining the major action in the area under study.

Sample: The sample consisted of family members of patients who underwent heart transplantation. The subjects were labeled as partners, to designate the particular family member considered the significant other by the patient. The total sample consisted of 20 subjects who were participants in three separate support groups. There were seven partners in Group 1, eight in Group 2, and five in Group 3. The groups consisted of 14 wives, 5 mothers, and 1 sister. Age of the family members ranged from 24 to 72 years; almost half ($n = 9$) were in their thirties.

All husband–wife pairs had children, with the number ranging from 1 to 12. The children's ages ranged from 3 months to 52 years. Most subjects had at least a high school education. One-third had been employed prior to the patients' illness and had quit their jobs; only one had continued to be employed. Jobs included retail clerk, hair dresser, secretary, and sales representative. The subjects came from 13 states, and all had permanent homes in a city other than the one where the transplant surgery was performed. Eighteen families had relocated temporarily and two permanently to the medical center city.

Data Collection: Data were collected from family members who attended a support group conducted by the investigators. Subjects were referred to the group by the nurse transplant coordinators and social workers with approval of the surgeon who headed the transplant team. Informed consent was obtained from each subject after an individual explanation of the study. All data were kept confidential. Group meetings were structured to focus on any topic expressed as a concern. At the beginning of the group, the subjects were asked: "What has been happening with you?" Initially, the conversation centered on what was happening with the patient, but as the group progressed the subjects were better able to talk about their own experiences.

Data collection took place over 2½ years and included data from the three separate groups. For 12 weeks the groups met weekly for 1½ hours in a comfortable meeting room in a building attached to the medical center. At the conclusion of each weekly meeting the investigators recorded the data on audiotapes. The investigators attempted to record all content discussed, the subjects' reactions, group dynamics, and the investigators' thoughts about what occurred in the meeting. Thirty-six transcripts provided the data for constant comparative analysis.

Data Analysis: Open coding was used for the analysis of transcribed data. The data were partitioned into relevant sentences, phrases, or anecdotes. This coding continued until properties and categories emerged. Selective coding was then used to sort data bits into the emerging categories. Concurrent coding and analysis continued until unique categories no longer appeared in the data. The category structure was refined by merging categories and their properties into a smaller set of higher-level concepts to refine and expand the emerging theory.

The emerging themes directed additional data collection. The groups contained participants who were in all three stages in the heart transplant program. Thus, themes relevant to certain stages and to variables within a stage were explored with current group members, facilitating the use of theoretical sampling methods. Data collection and analysis continued until theoretical saturation was achieved.

Trustworthiness of the Data: Guba (1981) and Lincoln and Guba (1985) suggested that four factors can be used to assess the rigor of a qualitative investigation: credibility, transferability, dependability, and confirmability.

Credibility refers to having confidence in the truth of the findings. Six methods were used to check credibility. Prolonged engagement at the site and persistent observation were made possible by the long data-collection period. Peer debriefing, exposure of the investigators' thinking to a jury of peers, was done through scheduled discussions with transplant team members who worked closely with the patients and their families. Triangulation was accomplished by comparing the emerging perspective with lay articles by transplant recipients, professional articles on life following transplantation, literature on spouses' experiences living with a chronically ill partner, and television documentaries on transplantation.

The investigators' findings were compared with recorded information from consultations provided to the patient and/or family member to achieve referential adequacy. Member checks, the last credibility method used, allowed the conceptualizations that emerged to be verified and modified for accuracy in group meetings.

Transferability is concerned with verification that the results are not context-bound (Sandelowski, 1986). The sample covered all adult age groups, education levels, and adult role activities. Therefore, the subjects, content, and range of data were sufficient to provide the basis for assessing relevancy to related contexts and care providers. Data on patients were provided by partners, thus the results of the analysis are limited to the perspective of the partner.

Dependability refers to both the stability and the trackability of the variance over time. An audit trail was established by a research assistant who reexamined a portion of the transcribed notes of the group sessions. The research assistant arrived at comparable conclusions, given the data, perspective, and situation.

To support *confirmability*, the interpretational objectivity of the data (Lincoln & Guba, 1985), the investigators gathered information from the heart transplant team members in addition to the subjects. Alternative explanations were explored with these individuals. Confirmability was further addressed by reflecting on notes depicting initial directions in organizing the data, enabling changes in the early formulations.

FINDINGS

Redesigning the Dream: The basic social psychological process emerging from the data that explains family adjustment to heart transplantation is the process of redesigning the dream. This process refers to cognitive and behavioral changes that occur in the partner from the time the patient enters the heart transplantation program to an unknown period posttransplantation. When the families are accepted into the program, they have a dream that life will return to normal after the patient receives a new heart. Yet as they wait for a donor and experience hospitalization for transplantation and recuperation after discharge, their attitudes, beliefs, and behavior undergo an evolution. The initial dream is reformulated and reshaped to fit the reality of the medical–technological treatment environment. Data are unavailable to determine when the redesign is completed or whether it is ever completed.

During the pretransplantation stage and up to 3 months posttransplantation, the process of redesigning the dream is comprised of three inter- and intrapersonal concepts, immersion, passage, and negotiation. Immersion occurs during the waiting for a donor stage, passage is experienced during hospitalization, and negotiation characterizes the recovery after discharge. The three phases illustrate the experience of the partners in interaction with the patients and are limited to the significant dyad.

IMMERSION. During the wait for a donor heart, unknowns center on whether a heart will become available before the patient dies. A major characteristic of the uncertainty is that the patient and the family can do nothing to influence organ availability. The only avenue open is to attempt to maintain the patient's condition so that deterioration or death can be averted.

Immersion is a series of behaviors in which one family member, usually the partner, pledges self to the welfare of the patient. Partners direct all effort toward keeping the patient alive and relatively comfortable. Any conflicts that exist within the family or marital relationship, or in general life, are blocked or submerged. All the partner's cognitive activity is directed toward planning for the patient's welfare; all affective activity is a reflection of the patient's emotional state. Information about

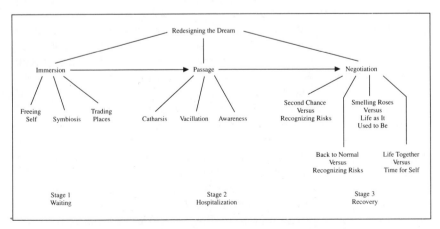

Figure 1. Substantive Theory-Redesigning the Dream

the posttransplant phase is irrelevant. The perspective on the posttransplant period is that "life will return to normal." Three categories of immersion occur concurrently: freeing self, symbiosis, and trading places.

The partner *frees the self* from home tasks, childrearing, work, and social commitments and transfers all attention to the patient. Families relocate, terminate jobs, and establish a temporary shelter near the hospital. Priorities are reassigned and former responsibilities transferred, if possible, to other persons. Some examples include sending the children to live with relatives, weaning a baby who was breast-fed so the grandparents could take over the care. Partners are able to free themselves because they believe the situation is temporary.

The term *symbiosis* is used in its broadest sense to include parasitism or antagonistic symbiosis in which the association with the patient is destructive to the partner. Patients benefit from the close union because they are taken care of by partners. Partners suffer from the relationship because they lose their sense of self. Partners who free themselves from other commitments reassign the freed energy into a bond with the patient. The strength of the bond is reflected in the partners' inability to discuss their own feelings. Instead they respond to questions in terms of the patient's emotional state. Use of "I" as the personal pronoun is absent and replaced by "we," "she," or "he." All emotions, thoughts, and feelings expressed as how the patient feels; personal experience is absent. All interests and activities are those of the patient or those jointly shared by patient and partner. A personal illness or a child's illness are only attended to as a threat to the well-being of the patient.

Partners find the close union stressful, but feel guilty if they attempt to change the relationship. The committed partner conveys the attitude that a personal life is not justifiable at this time. Life is on hold, with no roots, commitment, or involvement with anything other than the patient. The partner is unable to show any disappointment, and, instead, must work to maintain the transplant patient's spirits. Partners complain that there is no time to be alone and thus devise activities to provide a modicum of privacy and time for themselves. One partner said she was interviewed by a newspaper reporter who asked, "Why don't you break down?" She said: "Because I can't. There is no time to break down now. Maybe in 6 months I may break my favorite dish or stub my toe and I will just cry and break down and fall into pieces, and then I will express how I am feeling, but during the waiting period, I can't."

Filtering information and monitoring are two properties of symbiosis that serve a protective function. Filtering information is designed to protect the patient from encountering information that could be upsetting or distressful. Partners decide what information they will convey to the patient about their medical condition, family events, or future plans. Partners withhold news about family illnesses or deaths from the patient until after surgery. Some partners censor the literature on heart transplantation so the patient is not exposed to media that has a tragic or problematic outcome. Visits with recovering transplant recipients are selected according to the recipients' health and recovery course; transplant recipients who are not doing well are not visited or discussed.

Monitoring involves checking the patient's physiological state to determine if the patient is maintaining enough strength to survive until a heart is available. The patient's behavior, sleep–wakefulness pattern, food and fluid intake and output, activity level, respiration, and skin turgor are constantly observed. Partners describe waking up suddenly in the middle of the night and listening for their husband's breathing. If they did not see the chest move, they checked to see if the patient was alive.

In the third category of immersion, accentuated in the waiting for a donor phase, the partner *trades places*, that is, takes on many of the traditional roles and behaviors the patient performed prior to the illness. A major statement of partners was, "Never say never," implying (a) they were doing things they never thought they would do and (b) they might take on other responsibilities in the future that they could not comprehend in the current situation. One partner flew home to manage the family business every weekend. Prior to the patient's illness, no business activities were shared and the partner had no preparation for her responsibilities. Other partners spoke of shoveling snow, carrying big suitcases, becoming major wage earners, and managing finances, activities they had never been involved in before the patient became ill.

PASSAGE. Beginning with transplantation surgery, the patient moves from imminent death toward another chance at life, and the partner moves from immersion toward independence. Although passage is initiated by surgery, the stage continues into the postdischarge period and culminates when both the patient and the partner move from a belief in the return to normal to recognition of permanent vulnerability. Passage consists of three categories: catharsis, vacillation, and awareness.

While the patient regains strength and receives attention from the heart transplant team, partners have an opportunity to recognize their exhaustion and fatigue, and begin to nurture themselves. The partner believes the worst is over and the patient will steadily recuperate. Belief in the return to normal life is reinforced by seeing the patient continually gain strength.

Although the ties to the patient continue after surgery, they do not retain the character of absoluteness that existed during immersion. When the partner is away from the patient, the symbiotic relationship begins to disintegrate. During immersion, the close symbiotic attachment was necessary for the partner to support the terminally ill family member. Disintegration of the symbiosis is reasonable as the patient progresses and is pushed toward independence. Partners begin to solidify their perceptions about their personal growth and start to differentiate from the patient. Part of this differentiation process, labeled *catharsis*, begins in the passage stage.

Catharsis refers to the expression and reliving of stressful events. It consists of emotional ventilation by the partners to discharge the tension accumulated during immersion. The partners begin to relive the stressful events by sharing them repeatedly and by experiencing the emotions repressed during immersion. The reliving enables them to integrate the trauma of continual unpredictability that characterized the waiting for a donor period. One partner recounted how she had allowed her husband, who was physically unstable, to drive her young son to nursery school, knowing that he could collapse at the wheel, killing himself and the child. Yet the partner reasoned the risk was necessary for her husband to maintain his self-esteem. Retelling allowed her to release the emotions that accompanied the event but could not be expressed at the time. Other partners related nightmares of car wrecks or feelings of vulnerability. Vulnerability was expressed as headaches, nightmares, shaking, inability to concentrate, anxiety, and the need to find a safe place. One partner stated, "I break out into tears suddenly now when our situation is better than it's been in years." Others stated that when their husbands were beginning to do well, they felt emotionally vacant, blunted, or consumed with anger that was difficult to repress. In other partners, the emotional expression occurred as tremendous anxiety or fears of leaving the house. Purging the trauma begins in the passage phase and continues to reappear in the negotiation phase as partners start to structure their future.

A second category of the passage phase refers to the ebb and flow in the belief of a return to normal. *Vacillation* is caused by unpredictable complications that occur the first 6 weeks postoperatively. This phase often strikes the partners by surprise. Even though the partners were informed about the unstable posttransplant period, all hoped the potential complications would not happen to their loved one. Initial complications function to crack the dream that all will be normal.

The partner begins to develop and use a cadre of unpredictability management and hope maintenance methods to buffer the growing realization that a new heart does not mean a return to normal. Unpredictability management is defined as the use of selected techniques to enhance the relationship between cues and outcome (Seligman, 1975). The techniques are designed to reinforce the belief that cues indicating complications can be anticipated, prevented, or reversed. Hope maintenance is defined as the positive evaluation of transplant-related events. Hope maintenance and unpredictability management methods are directed at managing the slowly growing realization that the patient's life span is unpredictable and can end suddenly with little warning. Thus, only selected amounts of this realization are integrated into the belief system at a time. The buffering methods prevent partners from being overwhelmed by the unpredictability and enable them to gradually integrate this realization as they begin to accept a new view of the patient's life.

The belief in a normal life is gradually eroded and the partner becomes *aware* of the necessity to redefine the term *normal*. As the partner learns the entourage of medications, diet restrictions, and the dangers of immunosuppression, the possibility that life will not return to normal gradually emerges. When patients approach discharge and the protection of the transplant team is lessened, partners express fear that they will be unable to help the patient maintain stability.

In the immersion phase, the partner is uninterested in hearing about the posttransplant phase. In passage, as the patient's discharge approaches, the partner absorbs as much information as possible about what life will be like when the patient returns home. The partner listens to accounts of infections, secondary illnesses, and interpersonal family problems. The partner tends to believe these accounts are due to some characteristic of the other transplant recipient and are not applicable to one's own loved one. However, these accounts cannot be totally dismissed, and awareness grows that surgery has provided not only a new heart, but new threats that will not disappear after discharge from the hospital.

When the patient is discharged, the patient and partner gain pleasure from sharing everyday events. Joy is experienced from the simple task of watching the patient cut an onion or eat in a restaurant. Along with this joy is the awareness that the patient is different from the person one knew prior to surgery. Sometimes it is the recipient's slowness, "It took him 40 minutes to put on a pair of pants." At other times the change is the patient's reluctance to do normal activities of daily living. Statements included, "Why do I have to wait on him hand and foot? He's capable of getting his own glass of water." Other partners note that the patient is not affectionate, "He ignores me, he's not interested in me anymore." Others complain because their spouse has lost interest in sexual activity. Mood changes such as deep depression, irritableness, unreasonable anger at children, listlessness, agitation, or shaking are noted. Changes in appetite and irregular and inconsistent food urges also are observed.

As the partners begin to notice differences in the patient, they reinitiate the checking and monitoring behavior performed in immersion. When the patient is at home, partners have to rely on their own judgment for answers. Whenever complications occur in a patient, checking and monitoring behavior increases. Partners acknowledge the fragility of any sense of stability, and grief is expressed for loss of what was viewed as normal. Recognition of the patient's vulnerability necessitates constructing a new dream and a new definition of normal.

The partner and patient begin to use more elaborate methods of unpredictability management and hope maintenance to create a more certain immediate environment and future. These techniques are considered successful when rejection or infection are preceded by recognizable cues and averted, or when the harm to self-esteem from secondary effects of medications is diminished by techniques fostering optimism. To the degree that success is achieved, the future can be viewed in a positive light. Notice of death or complications in another transplant recipient or unpredictable events involving the patient upsets the balance achieved.

NEGOTIATION. The negotiation stage differs from the stages of immersion and passage in that the prior stages in the redesigning process emphasized the partners' cognitive, psychological, and social evolution, but negotiation refers to the dynamic interaction between the patient and the partner. Although data were elicited only from partners, the focus is now on the partners' experience in interaction with the patient. A dialogue begins between the patient and partner about their future life. Negotiation begins when the partner speaks of living with continual unpredictability. When the partner and the patient complete the passage phase, their perspective on their future life has radically changed. The partner, and often the patient, realize that a new life-style must be structured that considers the patient's vulnerability and unpredictable future. Negotiation results from the differing views of a new life held by the partner and patient. Each view involves a realignment of power in the significant dyad relationship. Four negotiation patterns were identified in the data.

One form of negotiation, *recognizing the risks versus second chance*, involves a partner who recognizes the risks to a stable life and begins to focus on obtaining some security for self and children. The partner is able to describe two life images: one with her husband and children, and the other as a widow with her children. Children become extremely important, cherished and protected because the partner views them as healthy and secure. Children are thought to be permanent for a set number of years but the transplant recipient can die suddenly, without warning. The partner seeks employment to prepare for an uncertain future. Security is also sought by retaining some control over family finances. Partners are unwilling to relinquish all of the roles gained when they traded places in the immersion phase. Partners of heart transplant recipients state they will never let themselves be powerless again. They find themselves in conflict between their commitment to a patient with an uncertain future and the drive for survival for themselves and their children.

Meanwhile, patients are not interested in seeking security. Instead, they are motivated to enjoy a second chance at life which takes the form of a hedonistic pursuit of desires. The opportunity for a second chance can require moving to a new location such as a mountain town or interrupting life's goals to pursue a personal dream in their remaining time. The discrepancy between the partner's and the patient's goals for the future creates interpersonal conflict. This was exemplified by a patient who went out for an early morning walk and returned 3 hours later than planned. When he arrived home, his wife was very angry and he responded, "Why should you be so angry, I have the right to go any place I want." The wife responded, "No, you don't. I'm concerned about you when you are not back in a set time. Things are different now, they'll never be the same."

A second negotiation pattern, *back to normal versus recognizing the risk*, involves a partner who recognizes the risks to a stable life and a patient who refuses to recognize any vulnerability. In this pattern, the patient views the new heart as a cure and maintains the same career goals and life objectives that existed prior to the illness. Often partners report patients refuse to tell business contacts or new relationships they are a heart transplant recipient. Great effort is directed toward viewing and presenting the self as a totally healthy person. Mood changes and decrements in functioning such as memory loss, or changes in perceptual relations are denied or attributed to the partner's behavior. For example, the spouse may be blamed for misplacing objects or distracting the patient.

Meanwhile, the partner feels unable to make the patient aware of potential dangers and to take precautions to avoid exposure to infection, overwork, dietary indiscretions, and so on. Partners respond by planning for their security by refusing to return all the roles assumed in the immersion phase. One woman refused to relinquish all of her ties to the family business. Another demanded that the family relocate near the transplant center so that medical care would be accessible. Partners continue to monitor the patient because the patient often ignores signs of vulnerability. Interpersonal conflict is not overtly expressed. Instead, partners try to indirectly influence the patient's behavior while they insure a means for their own future security.

A third negotiation pattern, *smelling the roses versus life as it used to be*, involves retiring. Smelling the roses differs from second chance in that patients have no desire to pursue unfulfilled dreams in their lives. These patients do not exhibit the same egotistical behavior toward their partners. Instead, they have a desire to prepare the partner for life without them. The patient reevaluates life goals and pursues the pleasure of constant contact with and care from the partner during the remaining years. The partner, though wanting to retain some power and control over family affairs, prefers returning the primary provider role to the patient. Patients may retire to a recreational life, entrusting the partners with more role responsibilities by teaching them how to repair the car, or making plans for rearing the children. Often partners object to learning more of the patient's traditional roles and feel they are being prepared for widowhood. Some patients attempt to reinforce their dependency by requiring the partner to care for them as they did during immersion (i.e., pouring medicines or bringing them food). Immersion behaviors from an earlier stage are perpetuated by minimizing any illness the partner experiences. One partner who shared information about her arthritis pain said her husband responded, "What do you mean, you're sick? I'm the one who had the surgery!"

In a fourth form of negotiation, *life together versus time for self,* both the partner and patient desire to relinquish former goals and enjoy their remaining time together. Although the pattern does not appear conflictual, the absolute availability required by the patient generates feelings of being trapped. Partners complain that there is no time for self. Development of the individual is supported, as the patient desires that the partner share only the patient's interests. Complaints of boredom are heard by partners who expected life to offer more excitement or variety than the future portends. One partner complained that her husband did not want her to return to school; he only wanted her to be interested in his hobbies. Many partners desperately sought ways to have some time alone such as a nightly bath for a half hour, sitting in an empty chair in the garage, or driving across the city to find tofu yogurt.

These four patterns of interpersonal conflict comprise the negotiation process which assists in redesigning the dream. The success of negotiation is reflected in the degree of interpersonal conflict and level of cohesion and stability in the family. Negotiation for role realignment may persist for an indefinite period of time posttransplant. The stability of the patient and success of the unpredictability management and hope maintenance methods influence the amount of negotiation, thus the amount of dream redesigning. In an unstable situation, negotiation is more extensive and heightens following each unpredictable complication. The result of the negotiation process is the resolution of interpersonal conflict culminating in negotiated roles that address both the patient's vulnerability and the partner's needs.

DISCUSSION

Redesigning the dream applies to families who experience heart transplantation. Qualifiers of this process include age, prior experience with illness, childrearing responsibilities, and relocation. The process was experienced with more intensity and distress in partners who were in their thirties, had young children, and had relocated to the transplant center. Older partners often had chronically ill spouses with ongoing cardiovascular disease, thus they were either better prepared or more amenable to future treatment options, including transplantation. The younger partners were catapulted from life with a healthy spouse into a catastrophic illness experience. The rapidity with which the younger partners faced the transplant surgery caused them to view themselves as victims in the sense the word applies to anyone who suffers a physical and/or psychological loss incidentally or accidentally (Janoff–Bulman & Frieze, 1983). This sense of victimization was not seen in partners who were led gradually to transplantation.

Although partners of patients with a long-term illness had less sense of victimization, their sense of coherence in the world was also shaken by the unpredictability of the waiting period. Their history of near-miss experiences when the patient almost died undermined any illusions of safety and enhanced their feelings of vulnerability. The vulnerability was managed by immersing themselves in their situation to enhance predictability and decrease the uncertainty of events. All partners exhibited a heightened state of vigilance in order to anticipate any signs of danger that could destroy their precarious stability.

The nature of the sense of vulnerability changes throughout the process of redesigning the dream; however, the experience of vulnerability continues and is slowly integrated into a new model of reality. Coming to terms with living with continual unpredictability requires establishing a view of the world in which stability is not assumed as normal, and the partner and patient never again view themselves as invulnerable.

Consistent with adaptation to threatening events, this evolution is characterized by a period of total involvement, followed by a slow integration of the meaning of the situation. As described by Horowitz (1980) and found in this study, integration of the meaning of stressful events occurs through an ebb-and-flow process. Clues that life will be different are gradually acknowledged at the same time the patient and the partner are buffered by strategies denying the reality. As the family member accepts the reality of a different life, the buffering strategies gradually diminish. The ebb and flow of awareness and buffering strategies is a major activity in progressing through the process of redesigning the dream.

As the view of life is gradually modified, the partner and patient engage in actions to adapt to the changes wrought by the reality of a different life. Family members' perceptions of the situation and the management strategies they choose influence the process of coming to terms with the new definition of reality (Fife, 1985). The patterns of behavior may represent efforts to protect themselves from the continual unpredictability, yet these behaviors may require drastic and long-lasting modifications in roles and expectations. In the process of negotiation to structure a new view of life, role diffusion and discontinuity increase the potential for conflict. These kinds of disruptions in the family are likely to increase the level of stress and vulnerability to secondary psychosocial problems (Fife). Resolution of the negotiation process appears to be gradual. When partners and patients return to the transplant center a year after the surgery, they report that role changes are continuing and have not returned to their previously defined status.

Contribution to Nursing Theory and Practice: Modern medicine has been termed a *halfway technology* because no matter how wonderful, the sophisticated technology with its accompanying procedures does not completely cure illnesses. Instead, the major advances allow persons to live longer with their illness and perhaps enjoy a better quality of life.

However, the medical perspective is not adequate for dealing with psychosocial issues emerging from transplantation or assisting nurses to meet the psychosocial needs of patients and their families waiting for or following transplant surgery. Substantive nursing theories that address these major nursing practice problems must be developed. The substantive theory, redesigning the dream, is a step in this direction.

REFERENCES

Evans, R. W., Manninen, D. L., Overcast, T. D., Garrison, L. P., Jr., Yagi, J., Merrikin, K., & Jonsen, A. R. (1984). *The national heart transplantation study: Final report*. Seattle: Battelle Human Affairs Research Centers.

Fife, B. L. (1985). A model for predicting the adaptation of families to medical crisis: An analysis of role integration. *Image: The Journal of Nursing Scholarship, 17*(4), 108–112.

Glaser, B. G., & Strauss, A. L. (1967). *The discovery of grounded theory*. New York: Aldine Publishing Company.

Guba, E. G. (1981). Criteria for assessing the trustworthiness of naturalistic inquiries. *Educational Communication and Technology Journal, 29*, 75–92.

Horowitz, M. J. (1980). Psychological response to serious life events. In V. Hamilton & D. Breznitz (Eds.), *Handbook of stress* (pp. 711–732). New York: John Wiley & Sons.

Janoff–Bulman, R., & Frieze, I. H. (1983). A theoretical perspective for understanding reactions to victimization. *Journal of Social Issues, 30*(2), 1–17.

Lincoln, Y. S. & Guba, E. G. (1985). *Naturalistic inquiry*. Beverly Hills, CA: Sage Publications.

Lough, M., Lindsey, A., Shinn, J., & Stotts, N. (1985). Life satisfaction following heart transplantation. *Heart Transplantation, 4*, 446–449.

Mayou, R., Foster, A., & Williamson, B. (1978). The psychological and social effects of myocardial infarction in wives. *British Medical Journal, 1*, 699–701.

McAleer, M., Copeland, J., Fuller, J., & Copeland, J. (1985). Psychological aspects of heart transplantation. *Heart Transplantation, 4*, 232–233.

Sandelowski, M. (1986). The problem of rigor in qualitative research. *Advances in Nursing Science, 8*(3), 27–37.

Seligman, M. E. P. (1975). *Helplessness*. San Francisco: W. H. Freeman & Co.

Sexton, D., & Munro, B. (1985). Impact of a husband's chronic illness (COPD) on the spouse's life. *Research in Nursing and Health, 8*, 83–90.

Wallwork, J., & Caine, N. (1985). A comparison of the quality of life of cardiac transplant patients and coronary artery bypass graft patients before and after surgery. *Quality of Life and Cardiovascular Care, 1*, 317–322.

COMMENTARY

Mishel and Murdaugh's paper is a report of a family-related theory development effort. Wives, mothers, and a sister of men who received heart transplants provided the data from which a theory, called redesigning the dream, was induced.

The methodology for this qualitative study follows the tenets of Grounded Theory, with concurrent coding and analysis as well as theoretical sampling. A special feature of the paper is the explicit attention given to factors or criteria that assess the rigor of qualitative research, including credibility, transferability, dependability, and confirmability.

The influence of Grounded Theory also is seen in the labeling of the major study findings as a basic social psychological process. Thus, Grounded Theory provided a conceptual perspective as well as the methodological direction for theory generation. Readers familiar with Mishel's writings will also recognize a theoretical overlay from her work on uncertainty, which is evident in the stated purpose of this study: "to identify processes used by family members to manage the *unpredictability* elicited by the need for and receipt of heart transplantation" [italics added].*

The concepts of the theory of redesigning the dream are clearly identified and defined, as are the dimensions of each major concept. The explicitly described and diagrammed connections between the major concepts exemplify the temporal processes that are a typical feature of the Grounded Theory approach.

*Readers interested in the uncertainty perspective are referred to Mishel, M. H. (1988). Uncertainty in illness. *Image: Journal of Nursing Scholarship, 20,* 225–232.

JACQUELINE FAWCETT

CHAPTER

19

Effect of Role Clarity and Empathy on Support Role Performance and Anxiety

LILLIAN BRAMWELL
ANN L. WHALL

The purpose of this study was to examine wives' anxiety in response to their husbands' first myocardial infarction from the perspective of perceptions and interpretations of their support roles, their husbands' experience, their abilities to act supportively, and how these and other factors contributed to their degree of anxiety. Major study variables were: role clarity (measured by an instrument developed for the study), empathy (measured by the Barrett–Lennard [1978] Relationship Inventory), support role performance (measured by an instru-

This study was funded by the Canadian National Health Research and Development Program through a National Health Fellowship.
The assistance of Mary Denyes, Thomas Duggan, and Effie Hanchett is acknowledged.
Reprinted from *Nursing Research, 35,* 282–287, 1986.

ment developed for the study), and anxiety (measured by the State–Trait Anxiety Inventory Form A [Spielberger, Gorsuch, & Lushene, 1970]). Four exogenous variables, husband's condition, previous experience in the support role, self-esteem, and trait anxiety, were used to test alternate hypotheses. Subjects were 82 wives of men admitted to three cardiac care units. Data were collected prior to the husband's hospital discharge and at 3 weeks postdischarge. Data were analyzed with path analysis procedures. Study findings supported two hypotheses, that support role performance has a direct negative effect on anxiety and trait anxiety has a direct positive effect on anxiety. Descriptive data obtained during the postdischarge interview provided documentation of uncertainty as another source of anxiety.

This study focused on wives' perceptions as they attempted to develop a support role during the rehabilitation phase following a first myocardial infarction (MI) of their husbands. An illness crisis, such as an MI, has long-term consequences for life-style change. Wives, who are able to support their husbands during rehabilitation, can assist with development of behaviors that are health-promoting rather than self-defeating.

Work by Meleis (1975, 1981) and Meleis and Swendsen (1978) on role insufficiency and role supplementation as well as other literature sources were used to develop the theoretical perspective of this study. Meleis used the symbolic interactionist concept of role developed by Mead (1934, 1968) and elaborated upon by Blumer (1969), Sarbin and Allen (1968), and Turner (1962, 1968). From this perspective, social roles evolve within the context of complementary or counterroles. For example, a wife's support role develops as her husband requires assistance with his recuperative role.

According to Meleis (1975), nurses assist individuals with health-related life transitions and attendant role transitions. This assistance includes the wife in support role transition as well as the husband in transition from illness to wellness. Nurses intervene to prevent or remedy role insufficiency through a process of role supplementation. Anxiety is one response to perceived role insufficiency, which, in turn, can interfere with adaptive role transition (Meleis, 1975, 1981).

As two major components of the role supplementation process are role clarification and role taking (adopting the perspective of the individual in the counterrole), it is assumed within Meleis's (1975) framework that understanding of role requirements and the perspective of the individual in the counterrole influence role performance.

The purpose of this study was to examine wives' perceptions and interpretations of support role requirements, the ill partner's experience, the ability to act supportively, and how these and other factors contributed to the degree of anxiety experienced by wives as they assisted their husbands with recovery from a first myocardial infarction.

REVIEW OF THE LITERATURE

Bedsworth and Molen (1982) reported on wives' psychological stress following husbands' admission to the cardiac care unit. The most frequently adopted coping strategy was obtaining more information by discussing the situation with others. The most frequently reported response was anxiety (51%), followed by helplessness (16%). Hentinen's (1983) subjects reported insomnia (89%) and fatigue (69%) which were interpreted as signs of stress. Patients' wives who attended group sessions reported feelings of anxiety over anticipated problems with care of their husbands after discharge (Harding & Moorefield, 1976).

Problems of providing support to husbands following an MI were examined in a series of studies. Wives interviewed 30 to 60 days following their husbands' hospital discharge reported feeling tension due to unanticipated problems, such as husbands' mood changes and uncertainty about husbands' physical limitations (Rudy, 1980). In interviews with wives 2 months and then 1 year after husbands' MI, anxiety was identified as a response to problems with care of husbands, partly attributable to lack of knowledge (Mayou, Foster, & Williamson, 1978). The theme of anxiety in response to lack of knowledge was supported by the work of Royle (1973), Skelton and Dominian (1973), and Wishnie, Hackett, and Cassem (1977).

Almost all reported studies, however, were of an exploratory, descriptive nature. None tested relationships among such variables as information and provision of support and anxiety. Nursing studies that seek explanation of phenomena need to go beyond description of response patterns to inclusion of subjects' perceptions and interpretations of the situation.

THEORETICAL FRAMEWORK

It was postulated that anxiety is influenced by degree of role clarity, ability to empathize with the individual in the counterrole who requires support, and self-assessed adequacy of support role performance.

Role Clarity: The understanding of behavioral requirements for role performance is known as role clarity (Cottrell, 1942; Meleis, 1975). It includes knowledge of (a) the goals of role performance, (b) behaviors and attitudes necessary for goal achievement, and (c) role boundaries, all in relation to occupants of counterroles (Meleis, 1975; Sarbin & Allen, 1968).

The degree of role clarity influences adequacy of role performance (Burr, 1972; Hardy, 1978; Sarbin & Allen, 1968). A time of crisis will result in diminished role clarity if cues for adequate role performance are not perceived (Stryker, 1964). One consequence of failure to perceive role performance cues is personal disorganization (Stryker, 1964), which may be manifested as anxiety. The literature reviewed indicates a link between lack of knowledge of how to help husbands and anxiety (Royle, 1973; Skelton & Dominian, 1973; Wishnie et al., 1977). Thus, an illness crisis, such as MI, would adversely affect support role performance and increase anxiety for wives who lack understanding of role behaviors.

Empathy: The meanings and expectations associated with roles are established within a shared context (Turner, 1962). Shared context implies the ability to assume the perspective of the individual in the counterrole, which is defined as role taking (Lindesmith, Strauss, & Denzin, 1975). Role-taking ability promotes role transition (Meleis, 1975) and, it is assumed, enhances role performance; therefore, an ability to view the recovery period through the eyes of her husband would help the wife to provide adequate support. On the other hand, an inability to comprehend the experiences of the individual in the counterrole results in anxiety (Rudy, 1980; Wishnie et al., 1977).

According to Meleis (1975), "role taking involves the empathic abilities of ego both cognitively and affectively" (p. 268). She recommended that, for research purposes, role taking could be defined as a component of empathy and measured with an empathy scale, such as that contained in the Relationship Inventory (Barrett–Lennard, 1978).

Support Role Performance and Anxiety: Support role performance incorporates Meleis's (1975) concepts of role insufficiency and role mastery. An extrapolation from Meleis's definitions of these two concepts provides the following definition of support role performance: perception of the adequacy with which role behaviors are carried out, the effectiveness of role behaviors in attainment of related goals, and the congruence of role sentiments with role behaviors.

Meleis (1975) identified one response to role insufficiency (inadequate role performance) as anxiety. Hardy (1978) and Nye (1976) postulated a relationship between perception of inadequate role performance and anxiety. The review of related literature for this study also contained references to anxiety experienced by wives regarding anticipated (Harding & Moorefield, 1976) or actual (Mayou et al., 1978; Rudy, 1980) difficulties with care of husbands following hospital discharge.

HYPOTHESES

Major Hypotheses: The path model (Marasculio & Levin, 1983) portrayed in the theoretical framework served as the basis for generation of the following major hypotheses:

I. Role clarity has a direct negative effect on anxiety and an indirect negative effect on anxiety via empathy and support role performance.

II. Empathy has a direct negative effect on anxiety and an indirect negative effect on anxiety via support role performance.

III. Support role performance has a direct, negative effect on anxiety.

Alternative Hypotheses: Four exogenous variables, the husband's condition, previous support roles, self-esteem, and trait anxiety, were considered as alternate explanations for wives' anxiety. It is possible for wives to have low role clarity, empathy, and support role performance, yet experience low anxiety because they interpret their husbands' condition to be good. Alternately, previous experiences with support roles may have equipped wives to function adequately in the support role and thus reduce anxiety. It was also necessary to identify the contribution of self-esteem to self-assessed adequacy of support role performance and thus to anxiety. Finally, trait anxiety was included to identify variance in anxiety explained by a general tendency (trait) to respond with anxiety. The following hypotheses were generated in relation to exogenous variables:

IV. Husband's condition has a direct negative effect on anxiety.

V. Previous experience with support roles has a direct negative effect on anxiety and an indirect negative effect on anxiety via role clarity, empathy, and support role performance.

VI. Self-esteem has a direct negative effect on anxiety and an indirect negative effect on anxiety via support role performance.

VII. Trait anxiety has a direct positive effect on anxiety.

The theoretical framework with exogenous variables is portrayed in Figure 1.

METHOD

Subjects: The sample consisted of 82 wives of patients admitted to three university-affiliated teaching hospitals in Ontario, Canada. Their husbands had been admitted for treatment of a first MI. Over a 10-month period all wives who met inclusion criteria were asked to participate in the study. Procedures for protection of subjects' rights received the approval of hospital and university review committees.

Twenty-four women refused to participate. Their refusals may be categorized as those who (a) reported an inability to cope with additional demands of study participation or (b) felt their contribution was not advisable for other reasons. Attrition of 7 subjects occurred for such reasons as husbands' readmission ($n = 3$), death ($n = 1$), not returning

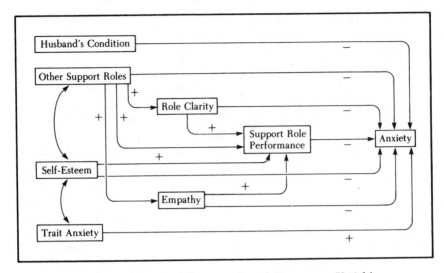

Figure 1. Theoretical Framework with Exogenous Variables

home ($n = 1$), and wives' refusal ($n = 2$). The final sample consisted of 82 women between the ages of 32 and 79.

Instruments: ROLE CLARITY QUESTIONNAIRE. The role clarity questionnaire, developed for this study, was modeled after Rizzo, House, & Lirtzman's (1970) role ambiguity scale. Items were reworded to fit perceived clarity of support role requirements and were expanded to include emotional, social, and physical support requirements. Eight items were rated on a 6-point scale from completely disagree to completely agree.

The questionnaire was screened for face and content validity by a panel of eight nurse researchers and practitioners. It was then pretested with 17 wives of MI patients before use in this study. The coefficient alpha for this study sample was .82 with item-total correlations ranging from .45 to .72.

SUPPORT ROLE PERFORMANCE QUESTIONNAIRE. The support role performance questionnaire was designed for this study to measure wives' self-assessed adequacy of their support provision. It paralleled the role clarity questionnaire and was developed, pretested, and revised in a similar fashion with 10 wives. A coefficient alpha of .88 was obtained for the study sample. Item-total correlations for the 7 items included in analysis ranged from .59 to .79.

Confidence in the reliability of the instruments as represented by coefficient alphas for the role clarity and support role performance questionnaires is tentative because both instruments were examined only in this study and the sample size was small. Further testing of these instruments is indicated.

RELATIONSHIP INVENTORY (RI). Barrett–Lennard's (1978) empathy subscale of the "myself-to-the-other" (MO) form of the RI was used to measure wives' self-assessed abilities to empathize with their husbands. The MO scale addresses empathic perception (Barrett–Lennard, 1981). Coefficient alphas ranged from .70 to .88 in the context of therapeutic relationships (Abramowitz & Jackson, 1974; Gurman, 1977; Lopez & Wambach, 1982) and .64 in a study of college student relationships (Gurman, 1977). The coefficient alpha obtained with this study sample was .56 with item-total correlations ranging from −.03 to .41 across the 16 items.

STATE-TRAIT ANXIETY INVENTORY (STAI). The STAI (Spielberger et al., 1970) form X–1 (A-State) is a measure of the dependent variable, anxiety. The STAI form X–2 (A-Trait) measures the exogenous variable, trait anxiety. Substantial information is available on concurrent validity (Spielberger et al., 1970; Zuckerman, 1960) and on discriminant validity (Auerbauch, 1973; Stoudenmire, 1972; Zuckerman, 1976) of the STAI. Internal consistency coefficients available for both state and trait scales ranged from .84 to .94 (Holtzman, 1976; Lazarus & Opton, 1966; Spielberger, Vagg, Barker, Donham, & Westberry, 1980). In this study, a coefficient alpha of .90 was obtained for the A-Trait scale and a coefficient alpha of .94 for the A-State scale, during the second interview.

HUSBAND'S CONDITION. A Cantril (1965) ladder with rungs numbered from zero to 10 was used to represent subjects' perceptions of their husbands' conditions. Subjects were first asked to imagine the worst possible outcome in terms of husbands' condition, anchored as zero, and then the best possible outcome, anchored as 10. Wives then indicated where on the ladder they would locate their husbands' present condition.

PREVIOUS SUPPORT ROLES. Information on experience with giving support to others was measured as a dichotomous variable, with previous experience or no previous experience in the support role recorded.

SELF-ESTEEM. The Rosenberg (1965) Self-Esteem Scale was used to measure wives' assessment of self-worth and thus the intrinsic ability to provide adequate support. This scale is unidimensional and has construct and predictive validity (George & Bearon, 1980; McIver and Carmines, 1981). The coefficient alpha of the self-esteem scale for this study sample was .77 with item-total correlations ranging from .22 to .61.

STRUCTURED INTERVIEW SCHEDULE. The structured interview schedule, designed for the study, was first presented to the same panel of experts that assessed the role clarity and support role performance questionnaires. Following revision, it was pretested during the same interviews in which the support role performance questionnaire was tested. It was designed to obtain descriptive information on subjects' experiences following husbands' hospital discharge and to identify other sources of anxiety.

Procedure: Data were collected at two different times, within 72 hours prior to hospital discharge and between 2 and 3 weeks postdischarge. During the first interview, demographic information was collected after which the role clarity questionnaire, the MO empathy scale, and the STAI were administered in that order. The second interview took place in a private setting, mainly in subjects' homes. The support role performance questionnaire and then the A-State anxiety scale were administered, followed by a structured interview. All data were collected by the same investigator.

Data Analysis: Path analyses were done to examine the patterns of influence on anxiety that were proposed by the theoretical model for the study. Significance level for all hypotheses testing was .05. Statistical Package for the Social Sciences (SPSS) data analysis routines (Hull & Nie, 1981; Nie, Hull, Jenkins, Steinbrenner, & Bent, 1975) were used.

RESULTS

The path coefficients in the path analysis model (Figure 2) are standardized partial regression coefficients, which represent the direct effect of each independent variable on the dependent variable, anxiety, while holding the effects of all other variables in the model constant. Path coefficients indicate the relative contribution of each variable to explained variance.

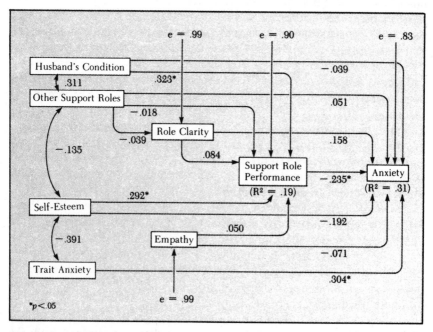

Figure 2. Path Analysis Diagram: Theoretical Framework with Exogenous Variables

Major Study Variables: Hypotheses I and II were not supported. Hypothesis III, that support role performance has a direct negative effect on anxiety, was upheld. Support role performance (maximal possible score = 42, $M = 34.66$, $SD = 5.21$) had a direct significant effect of $-.235$ on anxiety (maximal possible score = 80, $M = 41.09$, $SD = 11.75$.) The relatively high mean score for support role performance was consistent with the general contention of wives during the second interview that they gave adequate support to their husbands.

Exogenous Variables: Variance in anxiety explained by the three major study variables was .14. Addition of the four exogenous variables to the path model increased explained variance to .31. This increase was due in part to the direct positive effect (.304) of trait anxiety (maximal possible score = 80, $M = 30.93$, $SD = 3.86$) on anxiety. Most of the remaining contribution to explained variance was made by (a) the positive effect (.323) of husband's condition (maximal possible score = 10, $M = 5.78$, $SD = 1.92$) on support role performance and (b) the positive effect (.292) of self-esteem (maximal possible score = 40, $M = 30.93$, $SD = 3.86$) on support role performance.

Other Sources of Anxiety: The 68 (83%) wives who reported some degree of anxiety at the second interview were asked to identify the sources of their anxiety. For those whose anxiety related to their husbands ($n = 66$), the most frequent source was fear of recurrence ($n = 21$, 26%). These wives were not sure they could respond appropriately to another MI. The 12 (15%) wives who attributed anxiety to their husbands' stage of recovery expected that if and when recovery was complete, they would no longer feel anxious. Husbands' behavior, for example, trying to do too much too soon, created anxiety for 12 (15%) wives. Present uncertainties, such as recommended degree of physical activity and lack of information about their husbands' physical condition, were sources of anxiety for 13 (16%) wives, and 8 (10%) were anxious about an unknown future. Considered together, these sources of anxiety reflected a theme of uncertainty.

The theme of uncertainty was also evident in wives' inability to predict husbands' health status in 3 months ($n = 28$, 34%) and in 1 year ($n = 53$, 65%). They reported the existence of too many unknown factors, such as extent of full recovery possible, the possibility of recurrence, whether the husband would return to work, whether he would resume previous destructive behaviors if he did return to work, and whether current positive behavior changes were permanent.

DISCUSSION

Uncertainty: Sixty-six of 68 wives who experienced anxiety at the time of the second interview attributed their anxiety to uncertainty about the present and/or the future. It is possible that uncertainty accounted for a substantial portion of unexplained variance in the path model. Results from the present and previous studies (Bedsworth & Molen, 1982; Hentinen, 1983; Wishnie et al., 1977) indicate a need for further investigation of the relationship between uncertainty and anxiety in the context of recovery from a serious illness.

The study findings in relation to uncertainty are reminiscent of Mishel's (1981, 1983, 1984) work on measurement of uncertainty in illness. Mishel's (1983) Parent Perception of Uncertainty Scale (PPUS) contains three characteristics of uncertainty (ambiguity, lack of information, and unpredictability) that were also contained in wives' descriptions of the sources of their uncertainty. They experienced ambiguity about the possibility of recurrence and their ability to cope. Lack of information about their husbands' physical condition resulted in uncertainty about allowable physical activity. Unpredictability of husbands' future behaviors produced uncertainty about husbands' prognosis. A modified form of the PPUS would provide a measure of uncertainty experienced by those in support roles.

Major Study Variables: The findings regarding direct and indirect relationships between role clarity and anxiety may be due to adequacy of the role clarity instrument. Because this is a newly developed instrument, further assessment of validity and reliability with larger and more diverse samples are necessary before this study instrument can be accepted as a measure of role clarity within the context of a support role.

Another possibility is that the relationship between role clarity and anxiety is not linear, as multiple regression procedures assume, but curvilinear. Some indication of a curvilinear relationship was apparent in descriptive study findings that suggested subjects who lacked role clarity experienced anxiety. Seven (9%) subjects reported high role clarity due to prior attempts to control such known risk factors as: diabetes ($n = 3$), hypertension ($n = 2$), angina ($n = 1$), or heredity ($n = 1$). Despite their best efforts at prevention, an MI had occurred. Not knowing what more they could do to prevent recurrence became a major source of anxiety.

The findings for direct and indirect relationships between empathy and anxiety may also be due to limitations in the variable measure. The MO scale was tested for validity and reliability on a population that differed from the study sample. In addition, items in the empathy scale were based on a psychotherapeutic definition of empathy (Rogers, 1959). This definition may not correspond to the empathic process that occurs between husband and wife, particularly when both are involved in a crisis situation. Questions, therefore, arise regarding reliability and construct validity of the MO scale when used in other than therapeutic contexts.

Exogenous Variables: Trait anxiety provided the greatest explanation of variance in anxiety. This finding is not surprising, given the link between definitions of anxiety as "a transitory emotional state or condition . . . of tension and apprehension" and trait anxiety as "relatively stable differences in anxiety proneness" (Spielberger et al., 1970, p. 3). Although nurses can do little to modify trait anxiety, it is a factor to consider in crises situations. A usually anxious wife may be very anxious and thus might need additional assistance.

The relationship between the husband's condition and support role performance merits additional study. If wives perceived that their husbands were in good condition, they may have inferred that their support role performance was adequate. An alternate explanation might attribute the wife's perception of her husband's condition to the mediating influence of the husband's behavior. For example, husbands who actively pursued rehabilitation goals may be perceived as being in good condition. Future investigations need to include measures of behavior in the counterrole to separate out these effects.

The direction of the relationship between self-esteem and support role performance is questionable. Limited descriptive findings suggested the possibility that perceived adequacy of support role performance influenced self-esteem rather than vice versa. Comments were made by wives on several occasions that if one good thing had come from the illness crisis experience, it was an awareness of being stronger and more capable than they had previously thought. A similar pride in new-found abilities was expressed by subjects in Dracup's (1982) study.

Suggestions for Further Study: The significant relationship identified between perceived adequacy of support role performance and anxi-

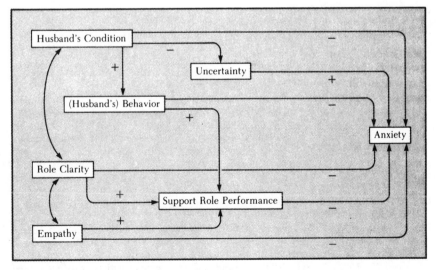

Figure 3. Direct and Indirect Effects on Anxiety Experienced by Person in Support Role

ety supported Meleis's (1975) contention that one outcome of role insufficiency (inadequate role performance) is anxiety. The tentative nature of other results limit interpretation of the remaining relationships among major study variables. In view of support in the literature, however, for the importance of role clarity and empathy to occupants of the support role and the incidence of anxiety reported by subjects in this and many other studies, relationships among these variables merit further inquiry. The mediating influence of the husband's behavior on support role performance and the contribution of uncertainty to anxiety should also be investigated. The model portrayed in Figure 3 is proposed for further investigation of the influence of selected variables on the anxiety experienced by individuals in support roles.

REFERENCES

Abramowitz, S. I., & Jackson, C. (1974). Comparative effectiveness of the there-and-then versus the here-and-now therapist interpretations in group psychotherapy. *Journal of Counselling Psychology*, 21, 288–293.

Auerbauch, S. M. (1973). Trait–state anxiety and adjustment to surgery. *Journal of Consulting and Clinical Psychology*, 40, 264–272.

Barrett–Lennard, G. T. (1978). The relationship inventory: Later development and adaptations. *Catalog of Selected Documents in Psychology*, 8(3), 57. (Ms. No. 1732)

Barrett–Lennard, G. T. (1981). The empathy cycle: Refinement of a nuclear concept. *Journal of Counselling Psychology*, 28, 91–100.

Bedsworth, J. A., and Molen, M. T. (1982). Psychological stress in spouses of patients with myocardial infarction. *Heart & Lung*, 11, 450–456.

Blumer, H. (1969). *Symbolic interactionism: Perspective and method.* Englewood Cliffs, NJ: Prentice–Hall.

Burr, W. R. (1972). Role transitions: A reformulation of theory. *Journal of Marriage and the Family*, 34, 407–416.

Cantril, H. (1965). *The pattern of human concerns.* New Brunswick, NJ: Rutgers University Press.

Cottrell, L. (1942). The adjustment of the individual to his age and sex roles. *American Sociological Review*, 7, 617–620.

Dracup, K. A. (1982). The effect of a role supplementation program for cardiac patients and spouses on mastery of the at-risk role (Doctoral dissertation, University of California, San Francisco, 1982). *Dissertation Abstracts International*, 43, 3534B–3535B.

George, L. R., & Bearon, L. B. (1980). *Quality of life in older persons: Meaning and measurement.* New York: Human Sciences Press.

Gurman, A. S. (1977). The patient's perception of the therapeutic relationship. In A. S. Gurman & A. M. Razin (Eds.), *Effective psychotherapy: A handbook of research* (pp. 503–543). New York: Pergamon Press.

Harding, L. A., & Moorefield, M. A. (1976). Group intervention for wives of myocardial infarction patients. *Nursing Clinics of North America*, 11, 339–347.

Hardy, M. E. (1978). Role stress and role strain. In M. E. Hardy, & M. E. Conway (Eds.), *Role theory: Perspectives for health professionals* (pp. 73–109). New York: Appleton–Century–Crofts.

Hentinen, M. (1983). Need for instruction and support of wives of patients with myocardial infarction. *Journal of Advanced Nursing*, 8, 519–524.

Holtzman, W. H. (1976). Critique of research on anxiety across cultures. In C. D. Spielberger & R. Diaz-Guerrero (Eds.), *Crosscultural anxiety* (pp. 175–187). New York: John Wiley and Sons.

Hull, C. H., & Nie, N. H. (1981). *SPSS update 7–9.* New York: McGraw–Hill.

Lazarus, R. S., & Opton, E. M. (1966). The study of psychological stress: A summary of theoretical formulations and experimental findings. In C. D. Spielberger (Ed.), *Anxiety and behavior* (pp 225–262). New York: Academic Press.

Lindesmith, A. R., Strauss, A. L., & Denzin, N. K. (1975). *Social psychology* (4th ed.). Hinsdale, IL: Dryden Press.

Lopez, F. G., & Wambach, C. A. (1982). Effects of paradoxical and self-control directive in counselling. *Journal of Counselling Psychology, 29,* 115–124.

Marasculio, L. A., & Levin, J. A. (1983). *Multivariate statistics in the social sciences: A researcher's guide.* Monterey, CA: Brooks/Cole.

Mayou, R., Foster, A., & Williamson, B. (1978). The psychological and social effects of myocardial infarcts on wives. *British Medical Journal, 1,* 699–701.

McIver, J. P., & Carmines, E. G. (1981). *Unidimensional scaling* (University paper series: Quantitative applications in the social sciences No. 24). Beverly Hills: Sage Publications.

Mead, G. H. (1934). *Mind, self and society.* Chicago: University of Chicago Press.

Mead, G. H. (1968). The genesis of the self and social control. In C. Gordon & K. J. Gergen (Eds.), *The self in social interaction* (pp. 51–59). New York: John Wiley & Sons. (Original work published in 1925.)

Meleis, A. I. (1975). Role insufficiency and role supplementation: A conceptual framework. *Nursing Research, 24,* 264–271.

Meleis, A. I. (1981, June). *The age of nursing scholarliness: Now is the time.* First annual Helen Nahm Research Lecture at School of Nursing, University of California, San Francisco.

Meleis, A. I., & Swendsen, L. A. (1978). Role supplementation: An empirical test of a nursing intervention. *Nursing Research, 27,* 11–18.

Mishel, M. H. (1981). The measurement of uncertainty in illness. *Nursing Research, 30,* 258–263.

Mishel, M. H. (1983). Parents' perception of uncertainty concerning their hospitalized child. *Nursing Research, 32,* 324–330.

Mishel, M. M. (1984). Perceived stress and uncertainty in illness. *Research in Nursing and Health, 7,* 163–171.

Nie, N. H., Hull, C. H., Jenkins, J. G., Steinbrenner, K., & Bent, E. H. (1975). *Statistical package for the social sciences* (2nd ed.). New York: McGraw–Hill.

Nye, F. I. (1976). The therapeutic role. In F. I. Nye (Ed.), *Role structure and analysis of the family* (pp. 111–130). Beverly Hills: Sage Publications.

Rizzo, J., House, R., & Lirtzman, S. (1970). Role conflict and ambiguity in complex organizations. *Administrative Science Quarterly, 15,* 150–163.

Rogers, C. R. (1959). A theory of therapy, personality, and interpersonal relationships, as developed in the client-centered framework. In S. Koch (Ed.), *Psychology: A study of a science: Vol. 3. Formulations of the person in the social context* (pp. 184–256). New York: McGraw–Hill.

Rosenberg, M. (1965). *Society and the adolescent self-image.* Princeton, NJ: Princeton University Press.

Royle, J. (1973). Coronary patients and their families receive incomplete care. *Canadian Nurse, 69*(2), 21–25.

Rudy, E. B. (1980). Patients' and spouses' causal explanations of a myocardial infarction. *Nursing Research, 29,* 352–356.

Sarbin, T., & Allen, V. (1968). Role theory. In G. Lindzey & E. Aronson (Eds.), *The handbook of social psychology* (Vol. 1, pp. 488–567, 2nd ed.). Reading, MA: Addison–Wesley.

Skelton, M., & Dominian, J. (1973). Psychological stress in wives of patients with myocardial infarction. *British Medical Journal, 2,* 101–103.

Spielberger, C. D., Gorsuch, R. L., & Lushene, R. E. (1970). *STAI manual.* Palo Alto, CA: Consulting Psychologists Press.

Spielberger, C. D., Vagg, P. R., Barker, L. R., Donham, G. W., & Westberry, L. G. (1980). The factor structure of the state–trait anxiety inventory. In I. G. Sarason & C. D. Spielberger (Eds.), *Stress and anxiety* (Vol. 7, pp. 95–109). Washington: Hemisphere.

Stoudenmire, J. (1972). Effects of muscle relaxation training on state and trait anxiety in introverts and extraverts. *Journal of Personality and Social Psychology, 24,* 273–275.

Stryker, S. (1964). The interactional and situational aapproaches. In H. T. Christensen (Ed.), *The handbook of marriage and the family* (pp. 125–170). Chicago: Rand McNally.

Turner, R. H. (1962). Role-taking: Process versus conformity. In A. M. Rose (Ed.), *Human behavior and social processes* (pp. 20–40). Boston: Houghton–Mifflin.

Turner, R. H. (1968). The self-conception in social interaction. In C. Gordon & K. J. Gergen (Eds.), *The self in social interaction* (pp. 93–106). New York: John Wiley and Sons.

Wishnie, H. A., Hackett, T. P., & Cassem, N. H. (1977). Psychological hazards of convalescence following myocardial infarction. In R. H. Moos (Ed.), *Coping with physical illness* (pp. 103–112). New York: Plenum.

Zuckerman, M. (1960). The development of an Affect Adjective Check List for the measurement of anxiety. *Journal of Consulting Psychology, 24,* 457–462.

Zuckerman, M. (1976). General and situation-specific states and traits: New approaches to assessment of anxiety and other constructs. In M. Zuckerman & C. D. Spielberger (Eds.), *Emotions and anxiety: New concepts, methods, and applictions* (pp. 133–174). New York: John Wiley and Sons.

COMMENTARY

This study reported by Bramwell and Whall focuses on variables associated with wives' ability to provide support during their husbands' rehabilitation following a myocardial infarction. A family-related middle-range theory was formulated from a review of the literature and theoretical assertions about role performance and empathy. The concepts of the theory and their complex relationships are clearly summarized in seven hypotheses and depicted in Figure 1.

The statistical technique of path analysis was appropriately used to determine the validity of the direct and indirect, or contingent, relationships between theory concepts. The study findings are summarized in Figure 2, which includes the path coefficients.

A special feature of this paper is the inclusion of a diagram (Fig. 3) that illustrates a new middle-range theory formulated on the basis of the study findings and further review of the literature. Note the *exclusion* of concepts not found to be associated with wives' support role performance in the reported study, as well as the *inclusion* of the new concept of uncertainty.

The conceptual perspective guiding the study and proposed future research is not identified explicitly. Symbolic interactionism is, however, mentioned in the introductory section of the report. Given the emphasis of the research on role behavior, it seems likely that the symbolic interactionist conceptualization was the implicit conceptual model.

JACQUELINE FAWCETT

CHAPTER
20

The Needs, Concerns and Coping of Parents of Children with Cystic Fibrosis*

DEBRA P. HYMOVICH
CINDY DILLON BAKER

The authors of this explanatory study examined the perceptions parents of children with cystic fibrosis (CF) have of the impact of CF on family functioning. A sample of 161 mothers and fathers completed the Chronicity Impact and Coping Instrument: Parent Questionnaire (CICI:PQ), an instrument to measure parent perceptions of their concerns, needs, and coping strategies. No significant differences were noted between responses of mothers and fathers. Parents were most concerned about their child's future and making their child comfortable or happy. Over one-half of the parents wanted information about their child's condition and growth and develop-

*The authors wish to acknowledge the assistance of Lisa Pennisi, Research Assistant, for her major contribution toward the smooth functioning of this study, and to Gloria Hagopian for her critique of the manuscript. This research was partially supported by a grant from the Nursing Research Branch, Division of Nursing, DHHS, Public Health Service grant 1-R21 NU 00827-03
Reprinted from *Family Relations*, 34, 91–97, 1985.

ment. Coping strategies used most often were talking with the nurse and physician, and praying.

The purpose of this exploratory study is to determine perceptions that parents of children with cystic fibrosis have of the impact of their child's condition on family functioning. The overall aims of the study are to sensitize health professionals to parental perceptions of needs, concerns, and coping strategies, and to provide guidelines for intervention that are specific to the expressed needs of parents. Specific questions addressed in this study are: (a) What are the parents' perceptions of their concerns and needs? and (b) What are the parents' perceptions of their coping strategies when faced with problems?

BACKGROUND

Cystic fibrosis (CF) is a genetically transmitted disorder, characterized by widespread dysfunction of the exocrine glands. It is the most common lethal genetic disease in children, with an estimated incidence of about 1 in 1800 live births in the United States. It is most prevalent among Caucasians, and has an incidence of about 1 in 17,000 in the black population. There are considerable differences in the manifestations of the disorder with wide variations in growth and the severity of symptoms. The nature of the treatment, including daily therapy, the potential for repeated hospitalizations, and an uncertain course of the disease can produce considerable stress in families. Although these families are considered to be at increased risk for psychosocial sequelae and/or management problems, relatively little research has dealt with the topic. For example, when Denning, Gluckson, and Mohr (1976) reviewed the *Cystic Fibrosis Club Abstracts* from 1962 to 1975, they found that only 2.7% ($n = 17$) of the 260 papers considered psychosocial aspects of the disease. A similar incidence was found in a search of the world's literature on the subject.

Previous studies, primarily descriptive, have contributed to our understanding of the impact of a variety of chronic illnesses on children and their families. Most studies have focused on family weaknesses and problems, while few have considered strengths of individuals or family units. The majority of these studies have based their findings on interviews with only one member of the family, usually the mother. One notable exception is Burton's (1975) study of children with cystic fibrosis, in which she interviewed both parents, all children over nine years of age, and observed all family members regardless of age.

While the majority of studies have stressed the hardships and difficulties encountered by these families, a few (i.e., Burton, 1975; Lewis &

Khaw, 1982; McCubbin, McCubbin, Patterson, Cauble, Wilson & Warwick, 1983) are beginning to note the strengths and adaptability of families. Children with CF are living into adulthood, and parents are facing many of the same childrearing issues encountered by all parents. Yet, there have been few attempts to look at parental needs that are developmentally oriented rather than disease oriented. This study is an initial step in assessing family impact from this broader developmental perspective.

Although there are a number of researchers (i.e., McCubbin, McCubbin, Cauble & Nevin, 1979; Stein & Reissman, 1980) developing instruments to assess families of chronically ill children, these measures are still in the formative stages and are usually related to either the impact of the condition on the family or the coping strategies used by family members. The Chronicity Impact and Coping Instrument: Parent Questionnaire (CICI:PQ) used in this study (Hymovich, 1983) was designed to cover both the impact and coping of family members.

The conceptual framework (Hymovich, 1979) on which this study is based has four major components. The first component consists of the developmental tasks of individuals and families. The second component contains variables that influence the impact of a child's chronic condition on the family. These variables include parental perceptions of the problems and satisfactions in their daily lives and resources available or needed by the family. The third component contains the coping strategies used by family members to manage the stresses imposed by the child's illness. The fourth component of the framework is the intervention needed by families of chronically ill children. The CICI:PQ provides information regarding the second and third components of the framework: parental perceptions of the impact of their child's chronic condition, how parents cope with the impact, and parent intervention needs.

METHODS

Procedure

Following approval of the University and Hospital Human Subjects Review Committees, each parent was introduced to the research assistant (RA) by the nurse coordinator in the CF Center. The RA explained the purpose of the study and answered questions posed by the parents. If the parents were willing to participate in the study, the RA went over the consent form with them and gave them a copy of the CICI:PQ. Those parents unable to complete the instrument at the clinic were given a stamped, self-addressed envelope and asked to return it by mail. If only one parent was present at clinic, a second copy of the CICI:PQ was sent home to the spouse. To assure anonymity, the questionnaires were coded and returned to the researcher. Of the 161 participants in the study, one-third completed the instrument in the clinic; the remainder completed it at home and returned it by mail. Most of the parents (85%) completed the questionnaire in under 25 minutes. Parents were asked to complete the questionnaire separately to determine similarities and differences in mothers' and fathers' perceptions of their concerns, needs, and coping strategies rather than a consensus. While it is possible that these individual reports may mask some of the compromise and negotiation that occurs between parents, it is equally likely that consensus may suppress some of the individual perceptions that are affecting family functioning.

Sample

The convenience sample for this study was composed of families of children with cystic fibrosis who were seen at St. Christopher's Hospital for Children Pediatric Pulmonary and Cystic Fibrosis Center in Philadelphia, Pennsylvania and its satellite clinic in Wilkes-Barre. Data were collected between November 1982 and February 1983. All parents who brought their children to the Center during those months were asked to participate in the study. Of the 175 families who came to the Center, 116 (66%) were willing to participate. Eleven percent ($n = 19$) of the families refused at the time they were asked, and 23% ($n = 40$) failed to return the questionnaire.

Twenty-six percent of the sample indicated that they had two or more children with cystic fibrosis. All of the parents were Caucasian, with the exception of one mother who was black. The sample provided a range of family structures and developmental stages in the life cycle. The majority of families (85%) had children whose CF was diagnosed over one year prior to testing. Only 15% of the sample had children diagnosed less than one year prior to testing. Parents ranged in age from under 18 to over 50 years, with the majority falling in the 30 – 39 year age bracket. Of the 116 families in the study, 82% were married, 14% were separated or divorced, 3% were single parents, and 1% were widowed. The sex of the children with CF was equally distributed between male and female. Four percent of these children were under 1 year of age, 29% were between 1 and 5.11 years, and 44% were of school age (6 – 11.11 years), and the remaining 23% were adolescents under 20 years. Most of the parents perceived the severity of their child's condition as either mild (44%) or moderately severe (49%). Only 8% thought their child's condition was very severe. Eighteen percent of the children with CF had no siblings, 40% had one sibling, and the remainder (42%) had between 2 and 7 siblings. Other demographic data are reported in Table 1.

TABLE 1.   Characteristics of Parents in the Sample[a]

Variables	Mothers (n = 103)	Fathers (n = 58)
Age in years		
Under 18	1.0%	0.0%
19–29	25.0%	38.0%
30–39	38.0%	38.0%
40–49	25.0%	29.0%
Over 50	11.0%	16.0%
Religion		
No religion	7.0%	11.0%
Catholic	30.0%	27.0%
Protestant	54.0%	59.0%
Other	9.0%	4.0%
Employment status		
Not employed	50.0%	14.0%
Employed, full-time	25.0%	84.0%
Employed, part-time	25.0%	2.0%
Occupation		
Professional	4.0%	14.0%
Managerial	22.0%	22.0%
Clerical and sales	22.0%	18.0%
Skilled trades	10.0%	18.0%
Machine operators	20.0%	18.0%
Unskilled	20.0%	8.0%
Family income		
Over $30,000	21.0%	30.0%
$21,000–$30,000	20.0%	32.0%
$11,000–$20,000	37.0%	28.0%
$5,000–$10,000	14.0%	8.0%
Under $5,000	8.0%	2.0%

Note. Some percentages do not add up to 100 because of rounding.
[a] $N = 161$.

Chronicity Impact and Coping Instrument: Parent Questionnaire

The CICI:PQ (Hymovich, 1981, 1983) was designed to measure the impact of chronic childhood illness on parents, how parents cope with the impact, and parental perceptions of their needs. The CICI:PQ is a 167-item questionnaire that measures (a) demographic data, (b) parent relationships, (c) hospitalization experiences, (d) concerns of oneself (SELF CONCERN) and of one's spouse (SPOUSE CONCERN), (e) help wanted regarding the child with CF and the siblings (HELP), (f) coping strategies of oneself (SELF COPE) and one's spouse (SPOUSE COPE), (g) communication with siblings (SIBTALK), and (h) beliefs (BELIEF). A Likert format was used for responses to items on the majority of the scales. Internal consistency reliability of the subscales was determined

TABLE 2.   Number of Items and Reliability Coefficients of the
CICI : PQ Scales

Scale	Items	r
HELP	23	.95
SELF CONCERN	16	.89
SPOUSE CONCERN	15	.91
SELF COPE	40	.80
SPOUSE COPE	15	.80
SIBTALK	9	.84
BELIEFS	9	.43
STRESSOR	54	.72

using Chronbach's alpha. The HELP, SELF CONCERN, and SPOUSE CON-
CERN scales were combined to form a STRESSOR scale. The number of
items and reliabilities for these subscales are listed in Table 2.

The HELP scale is composed of three subscales, CHCARE (physical
care of child with CF), DEVELOP (growth and development needs), and
SIBHELP (growth and development of siblings and sibling relationships).
The SELF CONCERN scale contains three subscales: SELF (concerns about
the individual), SPOUSE (concerns related to relationships with spouse
and family), and CHILD (concerns related to care of the child with CF).
The SELF COPE scale does not contain subscales. Intercorrelations were
obtained for the three scales and their subscales.

Descriptive statistics were used to determine parental perceptions of
their needs, concerns, and coping strategies as measured by the CICI : PQ.
To compare responses of mothers and fathers on the HELP, SELF CON-
CERN, and SELF COPE subscales, t tests were used.

RESULTS

The intercorrelations among the HELP, SELF CONCERN, and SELF COPE
scales and their subscales are presented in Table 3. The HELP and SELF
CONCERN scales are significantly associated with one another ($r = .39$,
$p = .006$), however their correlations are low enough to suggest they are
measuring different aspects of parent stressors. The low correlations
beween the SELF COPE scale and the HELP ($r = .07$) and SELF CONCERN
($r = .20$) scales indicate that the SELF COPE scale is a relatively independent measure.

All items on the HELP scale were positively correlated and significant
at the .001 level. Item correlations ranged from .22 to .83. The HELP
subscales were positively associated with the total HELP scale ($r = .66$ to
.71), indicating that the subscales are measuring different aspects of the
HELP dimension. Intercorrelations for the SELF CONCERN items ranged
from .02 to .75. All but two of these items were statistically significant at

TABLE 3.   Intercorrelations of the CICI : PQ Scales[a]

Scale	1	2	3	4	5	6	7	8	9
1. HELP	—	.71****	.66****	.69****	.39**	.39****	.34*	.37****	.07
2. CHCARE		—	.71****	.51****	.30****	.47****	.21*	.32****	.06
3. DEVELOP			—	.16	.09	.30*	.11	.01	.26
4. SIBHELP				—	.52****	.41****	.37****	.53****	.25
5. SELF CONCERN					—	.76****	.84****	.86****	.20
6. SELF						—	.60****	.47****	.31*
7. SPOUSE							—	.49****	.10
8. CHILD								—	.19
9. SELF COPE									—

[a]Numbers vary due to missing data on one or more variables.
*$p = .01$. **$p = .006$. ***$p = .005$. ****$p = .001$.

or below the .04 level. The correlations between the SELF CONCERN scale and its subscales ($r = .76$ to .86) indicate they are measuring different aspects of the SELF CONCERN construct.

The intercorrelations between the 42 variables comprising the SELF COPE scale ranged from .01 to .49. The majority of these correlations were low indicating that the strategies represent relatively independent ways of coping. The variables did not tend to cluster with one another, suggesting that the use of one strategy does not mean the use of another will necessarily occur.

Findings are reported for parent responses on the HELP, SELF CONCERN, and SELF COPE scales of the CICI : PQ. Since there were no significant differences between the responses of mothers and fathers on the three scales or on responses to individual items within the scales, data for the entire sample are reported. However, where there were differences of more than 15% between the two parents, these data are reported separately.

Self Concerns

A moderate amount or a great deal of concern about their child's future was expressed by the greatest number of parents (64%). Forty-two percent of the parents were concerned about making their child comfortable or happy. Others were worried about the responsibility of caring for their child (38%), the weather influencing what their child could do (39%), having enough insurance (33%), and whether they were taking proper care of their child (35%). Other concerns related to the relationship with their spouse. These concerns included having enough time together (12%), talking with one another (22%), getting out of the house together (18%), and their sexual relationship (14%). The areas of concern to the fewest parents were related to their individual needs, such as having enough fun and relaxation (10%) and getting out of the house alone (10%). More mothers (30%) than fathers (15%) indicated they felt worn out. While more fathers (38%) were concerned about making their child comfortable or happy (mothers, 18%).

Parent Needs

Over one-half of both parents wanted help with the following areas: information about their child's condition (73%), physical (66%) and emotional (62%) development, diet and nutrition (57%), physical care (56%), social (55%) and intellectual (52%) development, and expected child development (53%). Other areas in which parents wanted help were dental needs of the child (38%), managing behavior (32%), play and recreation activities (31%), play and learning experiences (29%), sleep habits (24%), and genetic counseling (23%). In regard to managing minor childhood illnesses, 42% of the parents wanted assistance with this.

About one-third of the parents also wanted help with childrearing issues related to the siblings of the child with CF. The areas mentioned most often were helping the sibling understand CF (44%) and helping the children get along (40%). Close to 33% of the parents wanted help regarding the siblings' emotional, social, and physical needs. Other areas in which assistance regarding siblings was wanted were meeting intellectual needs (29%) and expected child development (25%). Of the parents who wanted help, a higher percentage of fathers (FA) than mothers (MO) wanted guidance in helping their children understand CF (FA, 68%; MO, 48%) and get along with one another (FA, 60%; MO, 43%), and in meeting the children's intellectual needs (FA, 50%; MO, 28%).

Parent Relationships

Of the 124 parents who responded to the question regarding the relationship with their spouse, 60% were very satisfied, 26% were somewhat satisfied, 13% were somewhat dissatisfied, and 2% were not sure of their satisfaction. Regarding changes in their relationship since the diagnosis of CF was made, 34% of the parents felt there had been no change, 41% thought they were closer to one another, while 6% felt they were further apart, and another 19% were unsure of the change that may have occurred.

Parent Coping Strategies

Parents were asked what they had done in the past when they needed information or help regarding their child's development, care, and condition. The coping strategies mentioned most often were asking a physician (92%) or nurse (88%) for information. Sixty-three percent said they questioned other parents of children with cystic fibrosis, while 16% spoke to clergy, and 48% sought information from others. In addition, 55% of the mothers and 30% of the fathers queried friends or relatives.

Parents were also asked to indicate the ways in which they coped differently when they had more concerns than usual or when they were upset with their spouse. The coping strategies used more often in these circumstances were praying (47%), talking with someone (38%), busying oneself with other things (27%), crying (26%), asking for help (21%), hiding feelings (21%), smoking (14%), blaming oneself (13%), and yelling, screaming, slamming doors, etc. (12%). The following strategies were used less often: getting away (24%), exercising (15%), and ignoring (12%). The parents indicated that they took alcohol (16%) or medicine (13%) and blamed others (12%) about the same amount as they did when less stressed. Parents who smoked more when stressed tended to use more alcohol and medications, ignore the situation, and get away from it. It was not possible to identify any other consistent pattern in number or types of coping strategies used by parents.

Only 19% of the parents belonged to an association related to CF. Of those who did belong, 17% never went to meetings, 48% went occasionally, and 35% frequently attended. One-third of the parents who attended meetings thought they were very helpful, one-half thought they were somewhat helpful, and the remaining 17% did not find the meetings helpful to them.

When parents were asked if they had someone who could care for their child in case of an emergency, the majority indicated they had someone to care for their child for a day (87%) or a week (62%). Another 6% were not sure someone was available for a day and 22% were uncertain about child care for a week.

DISCUSSION AND IMPLICATIONS

Several of the limitations of this study should be recognized prior to discussing the findings. The study sample was not a random sample of all families of children with CF, but the majority of the complete population who visited the CF Center during the study period. Therefore, generalization of the findings cannot extend beyond this population. However, the findings may be suggestive of significant influences on other families of children with cystic fibrosis or other chronic illnesses. A basic assumption of this study was that one's reaction to the environment is in terms of how he or she perceives it. Consequently, the impact of cystic fibrosis on families can best be determined by asking family members to describe the impact from their perspective.

It is interesting to note that 82% of the sample in this CICI:PQ study represented intact families, and that 74% of the parents had been married only once. Furthermore, we found no differences in the number of intact families in those who participated in the study and those who did not participate, indicating that the sample did reflect the entire composition of the Center.

Although they did not compare families with the general population, Myerowitz and Kaplan (1973) have reported that families of children with CF were significantly less likely to divorce than parents of children with PKU and other forms of mental retardation. Several recent studies of families of children with a variety of chronic conditions have not found the divorce rate to be higher than the national average (Longo & Bond, 1984). Perhaps these data reflect a trend toward more families of chronically ill children remaining intact and a lowering of the divorce rate in the general population.

Venters (1981) recently noted that by the end of the first year after diagnosis, family life became less stressful, strained family relationships eased, new routines minimized initial disruption, and some agreement among family members about future goals and aspirations occurred. Since the majority of parents in the study reported here have known of the diagnosis for over a year, it is possible that the initial support they received enabled them to manage the stresses of the illness so that they had sufficient energy to cope with family relationships as well. Most of the parents expressed satisfaction with their marriage and many felt the diagnosis had either not changed their relationship or it brought them closer together. Friedrich (1979) found marital satisfaction to be the most accurate predictor of successful coping. Scores on the HELP and SELF CONCERN subscales suggest that many parents have been able to meet their own needs sufficiently so that they are able to concentrate on the developmental needs of their children.

The findings related to parent needs are particularly noteworthy in that they clearly point out the importance of providing information and guidance related to child development, in addition to that related to the child's condition. Over one-half of the parents who completed the HELP subscale of the CICI:PQ wanted guidance regarding all aspects of their child's development. At least one quarter of parents wanted help with each of the 15 items on the subscale.

About three-quarters of the parents wanted help in understanding their child's condition and its management. This is consistent with a recent finding that 74% of parents of children with over 100 chronic conditions said they had difficulty understanding their child's disease or wanted more information about it (Stein, Jessop & Reissman, 1983). The implications for intervention are clear. Health professionals from a variety of disciplines need to be available to provide education and anticipatory guidance to these families.

It is anticipated that by knowing the specific coping strategies used by clients, health professionals will be able to support those that are effective and recommend alternatives for those strategies that are ineffective. Further analysis of the data from this study may provide clues as to which strategies are most effective.

This study is significant in that it lends empirical support for the use of the CICI : PQ as a tool to systematically assess the concerns, needs, and coping strategies of parents of children with cystic fibrosis. The tool provides a practical means of helping parents express their concerns to health professionals. It has the additional benefit of helping parents realize that they are not the only ones facing these problems and, equally important, that their concerns are important to health professionals.

The results of the questionnaire can be used to develop educational programs for individual families or for groups of families within a clinic setting. It is evident from the findings that parents need information regarding the nature of their child's condition and its daily management as well as the growth and development of their children. Pamphlets, slide tapes, and videotapes could be developed to cover topics of importance to the parents.

Use of the tool may also result in more efficient use of interdisciplinary team members because it will enable the assessor to determine specific needs to be met and which team members are appropriate for meeting them.

The investigators of this study looked at impact and coping from the perspective of both mothers and fathers. McCubbin et al. (1983) point out the important role fathers have in families coping with chronic illness. The CICI : PQ can serve as a basis for parent discussions of similarities and differences in viewpoints, thus improving communication among the parents. Intervention programs can be developed for specific family members (e.g., fathers, siblings) or for the total family depending on the needs and concerns that are identified.

Awareness of the types of stressors faced by parents is necessary for health professionals who are going to work with these families. This knowledge is needed to prevent potential problems in adaptation that may impair therapeutic effectiveness and family well being. In order to provide quality care for children with cystic fibrosis and their families, it is necessary to identify those areas that are important to the families.

Health professionals have the potential to play a major role in assessing and helping these families to minimize their potential problems and enhance their coping abilities. Comprehensive care of these families includes assessing their strengths as well as their weaknesses, and assessing their developmental needs in addition to those needs related to their child's illness. Intervention strategies can then be identified and instituted to support the integrity of the family as well as the individual members. The CICI : PQ can be used to provide such an assessment.

AUTHOR NOTE

Single copies of the CICI:PQ and scoring guidelines are available for $5.00 from Debra P. Hymovich, PhD., FAAN, 929 Longview Road, Gulph Mills, PA 19406.

REFERENCES

Burton, L. (1975). *The family life of sick children: A study of families coping with chronic childhood disease*. London: Routledge & Kegan Paul.

Denning, C. R., Gluckson, M. A., & Mohr, I. (1976). Psychological and social aspects of cystic fibrosis. In J. A. Mangos & R. C. Talmo (Eds.), *Cystic fibrosis projections and the future* (pp. 127–151). New York: Intercontinental Medical Book.

Friedrich, W. N. (1979). Predictors of the coping behaviors of mothers of handicapped children. *Journal of Consulting and Clinical Psychology, 47*, 1140–1141.

Hymovich, D. P. (1979). Assessment of the chronically ill child and his family. In D. P. Hymovich & M. U. Barnard (Eds.), *Family Health Care, General Perspectives* (Vol. 1) (pp. 280–293). New York McGraw-Hill.

Hymovich, D. P. (1981). Assessing the impact of chronic childhood illness on the family and parent coping. *Image, 13*(3), 71–74.

Hymovich, D. P. (1983). The chronicity impact and coping instrument: Parent questionnaire. *Nursing Research, 32*, 275–281

Lewis, B. L., & Khaw, K. T. (1982). Family functioning as a mediating variable affecting psychosocial adjustment of children with cystic fibrosis. *Journal of Pediatrics, 101*, 636–640.

Longo, D. C., & Bond, L. (1984). Families of the handicapped child: Research and practice. *Family Relations, 33*, 57–65.

McCubbin, H., McCubbin, M., Cauble, A., & Nevin, R. (1979). *CHIP — Coping health inventory for parents*. Forb: University of Minnesota.

McCubbin, H., McCubbin, M., Patterson, J. M., Cauble, A. E., Wilson, L. R., & Warwick, W. (1983). CHIP — Coping health inventory for parents: As assessment of parental coping patterns in the care of the chronically ill child. *Journal of Marriage and the Family, 45*, 359–370.

Myerowitz, J. H., & Kaplan, H. B. (1973). Cystic fibrosis and family functioning. In P. R. Patterson, C. R. Denning, & A. H. Kutscher (Eds.), *Psychological aspects of cystic fibrosis* (pp.34–56). New York: Columbia University.

Stein, R. E., & Riessman, C. K. (1980). The development of an impact-on-family scale. Preliminary findings. *Medical Care, 18*, 465–472.

Stein, R. E., Jessop, D. J., & Riessman, C. K. (1983). Health care services received by children with chronic illness. *American Journal of Diseases of Children, 137*, 225–230.

Ventes, M. (1981). Familial coping with chronic and severe childhood illness. The case of cystic fibrosis. *Social Science Medicine. 15A*, 289–297.

APPENDIX   Sample Items on the CICI:PQ

HELP scale

Please indicate if you would like to have help with or discuss any of the following:

	Would like (1)	Not sure (2)	Would not like (3)
Physical care of child			
Diet/nutrition			
Care of minor illnesses			
Information about my child's physical development			
Helping children get along			

SELF CONCERN scale

During the past 3 months, how much of a concern have the following areas been for you?

	None/Does not apply (1)	Not sure (2)	A little bit (3)	Quite a bit (4)	A great deal (5)
Extra demands on my time					
Feeling worn out					
Making my child comfortable or happy					
Talking with or understanding my spouse/partner					
Having enough insurance to meet expenses of child care					

SELF COPE scale

In what ways do you do things differently when these problems come up?

	Does not apply (1)	Do less (2)	Do about the same (3)	Do more (4)
Cry				
Talk with someone				
Get away				
Exercise				
Pray				
Blame self				

COMMENTARY

This paper presents one of the several studies in a program of research designed to describe and to measure the needs of parents and other family members when a child has a chronic illness. This report focuses on the development and psychometric testing of one instrument used in the research program: the CICI:PQ.

The work reflects a family-related approach, with parents of chronically ill children serving as the family members of interest. The study serves as a good example of theory induction inasmuch as instrument items were generated through use of a grounded, inductive technique. The instrument represents the empirical indicator for a middle-range theory of parental needs in the particular situation of a chronically ill child. The techniques used here could easily be adopted for instrument development in other areas, such as needs of caregivers of the chronically ill elderly.

Hymovich and Baker have made a substantial contribution to family theory development in nursing. Their work is representative of nursing research programs that seek to generate middle-range theory about families and family members through instrument development efforts. Continued development and use of the CICI:PQ and similar instruments should advance nursing knowledge of family coping during stressful events.

ANN L. WHALL

I N D E X

A page # followed by an F indicates a figure; A "T" following a page # indicates a table.

Parent Perception of Uncertainty Scale
(PPUS), 369
Path analysis, 65
Pediatrics nursing, 13, 15
Personal Resource Questionnaire (PRQ),
247, 248, 249t, 251
Philosophy of science
central concerns, 43
developmental stages of, 44–47
family nursing theory, research
guidelines and, 51
historical realism, 46–47
logical positivism, 44, 48
Weltanschauungen, 46
world outlook analysis, 46
PPUS. See Parent Perception of
Uncertainty Scale
Pregnancy. See Family functioning
PRQ. See Personal Resource Questionnaire
Psychiatric-mental health nursing
family therapy models, use of, 300
nursing education, historical, 13
sociology and family therapy, influence
of, 319
standards of practice, 16
Public health nursing, 141
burn out, problem of, 172
creation of, 97–98
diminishing presence of, 172
focus for research, as a, 103–104
issue of midwifery, and, 101
peer teaching technique, 170
principles of, 10
role in sociopolitical agendas, 102–103
role of, 12, 13
school nurses, 13, 169
Push Button Test, 203

Related cases, definition of, 37–38
Relational data. See Family phenomena,
measurement of
Relationship Inventory (RI), 365
Research traditions, evaluation of, 49–50
RI. See Relationship Inventory
Rogers, M.E. See Conceptual models of
nursing and the family; Family
system theory
Role Clarity Questionnaire, 364
Roy, C. See Conceptual model of nursing
and the family; Family system
theory

Sampling, 64–65
Sarason's Life Experience Survey, 170
Science of Unitary Human Beings. See
Conceptual models of nursing
Scientific progress
goals of, 47–48

measurement, criteria of, 48–49
models of, 49
nursing knowledge, criteria for, 48–49
philosophical views
pragmatism, 48
problem-centered, 48
realism, 47–48
relative to research traditions, 49–50
Self-Care Framework. See Conceptual
models of nursing and the family
Self-Esteem Scale, 365
Sense of Mastery Scale, 127
SIMFAM. See Simulated Family Activity
Measure
Simulated Family Activity Measure
(SIMFAM), 79, 203
Single parent families (Hanson S. study),
243–257
abstract, 243
commentary on paper, 257
discussion and conclusions, 254–255
Family Environment Scale (FES), 247,
248, 249t, 251
Family Interaction Schedule (FIS), 247,
248, 249t, 251
findings, 248–254
communication and health, 251
correlations
additional results, 254
between children's major variables,
252t, 253t
problem solving and health, 251
religiousness and health, 251, 254
social support and health, 251
socio economic status and health,
249–251
Hollingshead Four Factor Index, 247
increase in number of, 244
instrumentation
Family Health Inventory (FHI), 247,
248, 249t
Personal Resource Questionnaire
(PRQ), 247, 248, 249t, 251
literature review, 244–246
healthy two parent families,
descriptors of, 245
methodology, sampling, 246–247
sampling, summary description of, 247
study of, historic overview, 244
STAI. See State-Trait Anxiety Inventory
Standards of nursing practice
family, and the, 15–16
history of, 97–98
State-Trait Anxiety Inventory (STAI), 127,
360, 365
Stern, P. See Affiliation of stepfather with
family
Structured Family Interview, 80, 203
Stuart, M. E., 31
Sullivan, J., 69